Nursing Diagnosis Index

Handbook of
Nursing
Diagnosis

THIRTEENTH EDITION

Lynda Juall Carpenito-Moyet, RN, MSN, CRNP

Family Nurse Practitioner
ChesPenn Health Services
Chester, Pennsylvania

Nursing Consultant
Mullica Hill, New Jersey

Wolters Kluwer | Lippincott Williams & Wilkins
Health

Philadelphia • Baltimore • New York • London
Buenos Aires • Hong Kong • Sydney • Tokyo

Acquisitions Editor: Jean Rodenberger
Product Manager: Michelle Clarke
Director of Nursing Production: Helen Ewan
Art Director, Design: Joan Wendt
Art Director, Illustration: Brett MacNaughton
Senior Manufacturing Manager: William Alberti
Compositor: Cadmus

13th Edition

9 8 7 6

Printed in China
ISBN-13: 978-0-7817-7793-3

Care has been taken to confirm the accuracy of the information presented and to describe generally accepted practices. However, the authors, editors, and publisher are not responsible for errors or omissions or for any consequences from application of the information in this book and make no warranty, expressed or implied, with respect to the currency, completeness, or accuracy of the contents of the publication. Application of this information in a particular situation remains the professional responsibility of the practitioner; the clinical treatments described and recommended may not be considered absolute and universal recommendations.

The authors, editors, and publisher have exerted every effort to ensure that drug selection and dosage set forth in this text are in accordance with the current recommendations and practice at the time of publication. However, in view of ongoing research, changes in government regulations, and the constant flow of information relating to drug therapy and drug reactions, the reader is urged to check the package insert for each drug for any change in indications and dosage and for added warnings and precautions. This is particularly important when the recommended agent is a new or infrequently employed drug.

Some drugs and medical devices presented in this publication have Food and Drug Administration (FDA) clearance for limited use in restricted research settings. It is the responsibility of the health care provider to ascertain the FDA status of each drug or device planned for use in his or her clinical practice.

TO OLEN, MY SON

for your wisdom and commitment to justice
for our quiet moments and embraces
for Olen Jr. and Aiden
for your presence in my life
. . . I am grateful
for you are my daily reminder of what is
really important . . .
love, health, and human trust

CONTENTS

SECTION 2

Health Promotion/Wellness Nursing Diagnoses   527

SECTION 3

SECTION 4

Diagnostic Clusters 633
**(Medical Conditions with Associated Nursing Diagnoses
and Collaborative Problems)**

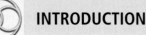
Creating a Care Plan for Your Client

Step 1: Complete the assessment from your course or the agency

Step 2: Refer to Section 4 Diagnostic Clusters in this book for the primary medical diagnosis of your client such as:

- Diabetes Mellitus
- Pneumonia
- Heart Failure

OR

the surgical procedure the client has had such as:

- Abdominal Surgery
- Hysterectomy
- Total Joint Replacement

Step 3: For a generic care plan with goals, interventions and rationale for all hospitalized persons or a generic care plan for all persons having surgery. Refer to http://thepoint.lww.com/Carpenito13e for a sample generic care plan.

Save the care plan in a word file so you can do the following:

- Add risk factors to the generic care plan from your assessment data of your client.
- Delete or revise goals/interventions not useful for your client.
- Add additional priority diagnoses not on the generic care plan as Risk for Complications of Unstable Blood Glucose if the person has diabetes mellitus and had had abdominal surgery.
- You can start your care plan with one of these plans. Now you will review the assessment data on your assigned client in Step 4.

◄◄ Carp's Cues

In addition to generic medical and surgical care plans on the web site, you can review a care plan that has been individualized based on assessment data. Consult you instructor on how you can use these generic care plans.

Step 4: Identify the Client's Risk

Factors

Risk factors are situations, personal characteristics, disabilities, or medical conditions that can hinder the person's ability to heal, cope with stressors, and progress to his or her original health prior to hospitalization, illness, or surgery.

Before hospitalization:

- Did the client have an effective support system?
- Could the client perform self-care? bathing? feeding self?
- Did the client need assistance?
- Could the client walk unassisted?
- Did the client have memory problems?
- Did the client have hearing problems?
- Did the client smoke cigarettes?
- Did the client abuse alcohol or drugs?

What conditions or diseases does the client have that make him or her more vulnerable to:

- Falling
- Infection
- Nutrition/fluid imbalance
- Pressure ulcers
- High anxiety
- Physiological instability (e.g., electrolytes, blood glucose, blood pressure, respiratory function, healing problems)

When you meet the assigned client, determine if any of the risk factors are present:

- Obesity
- Communication problems
- Movement difficulties
- Inadequate nutritional status

Write significant data on index card:

- Hearing problems
- No or ineffective support system
- Unhealthy lifestyle (little regular exercise, smokes, poor nutritional habits)
- Learning difficulties
- Ineffective coping skills (angry, depressed, unmotivated, denial)
- Obesity
- Fatigue
- Financial problems
- Negative self-efficacy
- Self-care difficulties

◄◄ Carp's Cues

Risk factors can be used as additional related factors for a nursing diagnosis on the generic plan such as:

- *Anxiety* related to loss of job and hospital costs
- *Risk for Infection* related to compromised healing secondary to excess adipose tissue (obesity)

OR

an additional nursing diagnosis not on the generic plan as:

- *Ineffective Self Health Management* related to insufficient knowledge of risks and strategies to quit smoking
- *Impaired Communication* related to unavailable interpreter and compromised hearing
- *Ineffective Denial* related to continued smoking despite recent deep vein thrombosis
- *Fatigue* (refer to list of related factors under *Fatigue*)
- *Impaired Memory* (refer to related factors under *Impaired Memory*)

Step 5: Identify Strengths

Strengths are qualities or factors that will help the person to recover, cope with stressors, and progress to his or her original health (or as close as possible) prior to hospitalization, illness, or surgery. Examples of strengths are:

- Positive spiritual framework
- Positive support system
- Ability to perform self-care
- No eating difficulties
- Effective sleep habits
- Alertness and good memory
- Financial stability
- Ability to relax most of the time
- Motivation, resiliency
- Positive self-esteem
- Internal locus of control
- Self responsibility
- Positive belief that they will improve (self-efficacy)

Write a list on a card of the strengths of your assigned client and of their support systems.

The strengths of the client and their support systems strengths can be used to motivate them to cope with some difficult activities. Strengths are not nursing diagnoses, risk or related factors. They are to be considered in planning care. For example, a person, with a strong religious affiliation and a new cancer diagnosis may benefit from a dialogue session with their religious leader.

Step 6: Create Your Initial Care Plan

Print the generic care plan (medical, surgical) for your assigned client. These generic care plans reflect the usual predicted care a client needs. Ask your instructor how you can use them to prevent excessive writing.

◀◀ Carp's Cues

In the remaining steps, collaborative problems are discussed. If you do not know about them, please refer to the section that follows care planning, The Bifocal Clinical Practice Model.

Step 7: Review the Collaborative Problems on the Generic Plan

Review the collaborative problems listed. These are the physiological complications that you need to monitor. Do not delete any because they all relate to the condition or procedure that your client has had. You will need to add how often you should take vital signs, record intake and output, change dressings, etc. Ask the nurse to whom you are assigned for the frequency of monitoring.

Review each intervention for collaborative problems. Are any interventions unsafe or contraindicated for your client? For example, if your client has edema and renal problems, the fluid requirements may be too high for him or her. Ask a nurse or instructor for help here.

Review the collaborative problems on the generic plan. Also review all additional collaborative problems that you found that are related to any medical or treatment problems. For example, if your client has diabetes mellitus, you need to add Risk for Complications of Unstable Blood Glucose.

Step 8: Review the Nursing Diagnoses on the Generic Plan

Review each nursing diagnosis on the plan.

- Does it apply to your assigned client?
- Does your client have any risk factors (see your index card) that could make this diagnosis worse?

An example on the Generic Medical Care Plan is *Risk for Injury related to unfamiliar environment and physical or mental limitations secondary to condition, medication, therapies, or diagnostic tests.*

Now look at your list of risk factors for your assigned client. Can any factors listed contribute to the client's sustaining an in-

jury? For example, is he or she having problems walking or seeing? Is he or she experiencing dizziness?

If your client has an unstable gait related to peripheral vascular
disease (PVD), you would add the following diagnosis: *Risk for
Injury related to unfamiliar environment and unstable gait secondary to
peripheral vascular disease.*

Review each intervention for each nursing diagnosis:

- Are they relevant for your client?
- Will you have time to provide them?
- Are any interventions not appropriate or contraindicated for
  your assigned client?
- Can you add any specific interventions?
- Do you need to modify any interventions because of risk factors
  (see index card)?

Review the goals listed for the nursing diagnosis:

- Are they pertinent to your client?
- Can the client demonstrate achievement of the goal on the day
  you provide care?
- Do you need more time?
- Do you need to make the goal more specific for your client?

Delete goals that are inappropriate for your client. If your client will need more time to meet the goal, add "by discharge."
If the client can accomplish the goal this day, write, "by (insert
date)" after the goal.

Using the same diagnosis *Risk for injury related to unfamiliar
environment and physical and mental limitations secondary to the condition, therapies, and diagnostic tests*, consider this goal:

The client will request assistance with ADLs.

Indicators

- Identify factors that increase risk of injury.
- Describe appropriate safety measures.

If it is realistic for your client to achieve all the goals on the day
of your care, you should add the date to all of them. If your client
is confused, you can add the date to the main goal, but you would
delete all the indicators because the person is confused. Or you
could modify the goal by writing:

Family member will identify factors that increase the client's
risk of injury.

Remember that you cannot individualize a care plan for a client
until you spend time with him or her, but you can add or delete
interventions based on your preclinical knowledge of this client
(e.g., medical diagnosis, coexisting medical conditions).

Step 9: Prepare the Care Plan (Written or Printed)

You can prepare the care plan by:

- Saving the online generic care plan into your word processor, then deleting or adding specifics for your client (use another color for additions/deletions or a different type font) then print it.
- Writing the care plan

Ask your faculty person what options are acceptable. Using different colors or fonts allows your instructor to clearly see your analysis. Be prepared to provide rationales for why you added or deleted items.

Step 10: Initial Care Plan Completed

Now that you have a care plan of the collaborative problems and nursing diagnoses, which are associated with the primary condition for which your client was admitted? If your assigned client is a healthy adult undergoing surgery or was admitted for an acute medical problem and you have not assessed any significant factors in Step 1, you have completed the initial care plan. Go to Step 12.

Step 11: Additional Risk Factors

If your client has risk factors (on the index card) that you identified in Steps 1 and 2, evaluate if these risk factors make your assigned client more vulnerable to develop a problem. The following questions can help to determine if the client or family has additional diagnoses that need nursing interventions:

- Are additional collaborative problems associated with coexisting medical conditions that require monitoring? For example, if the client has diabetes mellitus add *Risk for Complications of Unstable Blood Glucose*
- Are there additional nursing diagnoses that, if not managed or prevented now, will deter recovery or affect the client's functional status? For example, a client who has recently experienced a death of a significant person needs *Grieving* added to the plan

You can address nursing diagnoses not on the priority list by referring the client for assistance after discharge (e.g., counseling, weight loss program).

Step 12: Evaluate the Status of Your Client (After You Provide Care)

Collaborative Problems

Review the nursing goals for the collaborative problems:

- Assess the client's status.
- Compare the data to established norms (indicators).

- Judge if the data fall within acceptable ranges.
- Conclude if the client is stable, improved, unimproved, or worse.

Is your client stable or improved?

- If yes, continue to monitor the client and to provide interventions indicated.
- If not, has there been a dramatic change (e.g., elevated blood pressure and decreased urinary output)? Have you notified the physician or advanced practice nurse? Have you increased your monitoring of the client? Communicate your evaluations of the status of collaborative problems to your clinical faculty and to the nurse assigned to your client.

Nursing Diagnosis

Review the goals or outcome criteria for each nursing diagnosis. Did the client demonstrate or state the activity defined in the goal? If yes, then document the achievement on your plan. If not and the client needs more time, change the target date. If time is not the issue, evaluate why the client did not achieve the goal. Was the goal:

- Not realistic because of other priorities?
- Not acceptable to the client?

Step 13: Document the Care you provided and the client's responses on the Agency's Forms, Flow Records, and Progress Notes

Nursing Diagnoses Versus Collaborative Problems*

In 1983, Carpenito published the Bifocal Clinical Practice Model. In this model, nurses are accountable to treat two types of clinical judgments or diagnoses: nursing diagnoses and collaborative problems.

Nursing diagnoses are clinical judgments about individual, family, or community responses to actual or potential health problems/life processes. Nursing diagnoses provide the basis for selection of nursing interventions to achieve outcomes for which the nurse has accountability (NANDA, 1998, 2008).

Collaborative problems are certain physiological complications that nurses monitor to detect onset or changes in status. Nurses manage collaborative problems using physician-prescribed and

---

*The terminology for collaborative problems has been changed to Risk for Complications of (specify) from Potential Complications: (specify).

nurse-prescribed interventions to minimize the complications of the events (Carpenito-Moyet, 2010).

Nursing interventions are classified as nurse-prescribed or physician-prescribed. Nurse-prescribed interventions are those that the nurse can legally order for nursing staff to implement. Nurse-prescribed interventions treat, prevent, and monitor nursing diagnoses. Nurse-prescribed interventions manage and monitor collaborative problems. Physician-prescribed interventions represent treatments for collaborative problems that the nurse initiates and manages. Collaborative problems require both nursing-prescribed and physician-prescribed interventions. Box 1 represents these relationships.

The following illustrates the types of interventions associated with the collaborative problem Risk for Complications of Hypoxemia:

NP	1. Monitor for signs of acid–base imbalance.
NP/PP	2. Administer low flow oxygen as needed.
NP	3. Ensure adequate hydration.
NP	4. Evaluate the effects of positioning on oxygenation.
NP/PP	5. Administer medications as needed.

(NP: Nurse-prescribed; PP: Physician-prescribed)

Selection of Collaborative Problems

As mentioned earlier, collaborative problems are different from nursing diagnoses. The nurse makes independent decisions regarding both collaborative problems and nursing diagnoses. The decisions differ in that, for nursing diagnoses, the nurse prescribes the definitive treatment for the situation and is responsible for outcome achievement; for collaborative problems, the nurse monitors the client's condition to detect onset or status of physiological complications and manages the events with nursing- and physician-prescribed interventions. Collaborative problems are

Risk for Complications of Bleeding
Risk for Complications of Kidney Failure

The physiological complications that nurses monitor usually are related to disease, trauma, treatments, and diagnostic studies. The following examples illustrate some collaborative problems:

Situation	*Collaborative Problem*
Anticoagulant therapy	Risk for Complications of Bleeding
Pneumonia	Risk for Complications of Hypoxemia

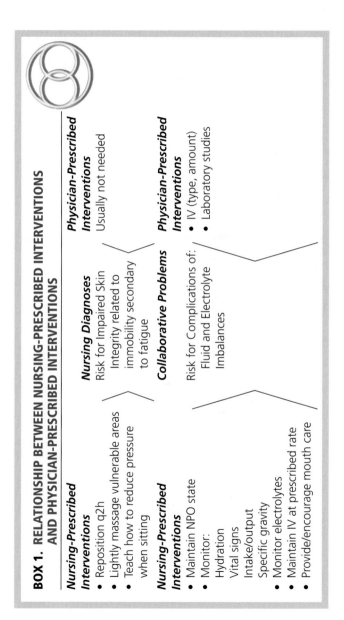

BOX 1. RELATIONSHIP BETWEEN NURSING-PRESCRIBED INTERVENTIONS AND PHYSICIAN-PRESCRIBED INTERVENTIONS

Nursing-Prescribed Interventions
- Reposition q2h
- Lightly massage vulnerable areas
- Teach how to reduce pressure when sitting

Nursing Diagnoses
Risk for Impaired Skin Integrity related to immobility secondary to fatigue

Physician-Prescribed Interventions
Usually not needed

Nursing-Prescribed Interventions
- Maintain NPO state
- Monitor:
  Hydration
  Vital signs
  Intake/output
  Specific gravity
- Monitor electrolytes
- Maintain IV at prescribed rate
- Provide/encourage mouth care

Collaborative Problems
Risk for Complications of: Fluid and Electrolyte Imbalances

Physician-Prescribed Interventions
- IV (type, amount)
- Laboratory studies

Outcome criteria or client goals are used to measure the effectiveness of nursing care. When a client is not progressing to goal achievement or has worsened, the nurse must reevaluate the situation. Box 2 represents the questions to be considered. If none of these options is appropriate, the situation may not be a nursing diagnosis.

Collaborative problems have nursing goals that represent the accountability of the nurse—to detect early changes and to co-manage with physicians. Nursing diagnoses have client goals that represent the accountability of the nurse—to achieve or maintain a favorable status after nursing care. Box 3 includes frequently used collaborative problems.

Some physiologic complications, such as pressure ulcers and infection from invasive lines, are problems that nurses can prevent. Prevention is different from detection. Nurses do not prevent paralytic ileus but, instead, detect its presence early to prevent greater severity or even death. Physicians cannot treat collaborative problems without nursing knowledge, vigilance, and judgment.

Formulate Nursing Diagnoses Correctly

Types of Nursing Diagnoses

A nursing diagnosis can be actual, risk, or a wellness or syndrome type.

- Actual: An actual nursing diagnosis describes a clinical judgment that the nurse has validated because of the presence of major defining characteristics.
- Risk: A risk nursing diagnosis describes a clinical judgment that an individual/group is more vulnerable to develop the problem than others in the same or a similar situation because of risk factors.
- Wellness: A wellness nursing diagnosis is a clinical judgment about an individual, family, or community in transition from a

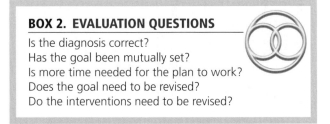

BOX 2. EVALUATION QUESTIONS

Is the diagnosis correct?
Has the goal been mutually set?
Is more time needed for the plan to work?
Does the goal need to be revised?
Do the interventions need to be revised?

BOX 3. CONDITIONS THAT NECESSITATE NURSING CARE

*Nursing Diagnoses**

1. Health Perception—Health Management

Contamination
Contamination, Risk for
Energy Field, Disturbed
Growth and Development, Delayed
   Adult Failure to Thrive
   Growth, Risk for Delayed
   Development, Risk for Delayed
Health Behavior, Risk-Prone
Health Maintenance, Ineffective
Self-Health Management, Ineffective
Self-Health Management, Ineffective Family
Self-Health Management, Ineffective Community
Self-Health Management, Readiness for Enhanced
Health-Seeking Behaviors
Immunization Status, Readiness for Enhanced
Injury, Risk for
   Risk for Suffocation
   Risk for Poisoning
   Risk for Trauma
Injury, Risk for Perioperative Positioning
Noncompliance
Surgical Recovery, Delayed

2. Nutritional—Metabolic

Adaptive Capacity, Decreased: Intracranial
Body Temperature, High Risk for Imbalanced
   Hypothermia
   Hyperthermia
   Thermoregulation, Ineffective
Breastfeeding, Readiness for Enhanced
Breastfeeding, Ineffective

(box continues on page 12)

BOX 3. CONDITIONS THAT NECESSITATE NURSING CARE
(Continued)

Breastfeeding, Interrupted
Deficient Fluid Volume
Electrolyte Imbalances, Risk for
Excess Fluid Volume
Fluid Volume Imbalance, Risk for
Glucose, Risk for Unstable Blood
Infection, Risk for
†Infection Transmission, Risk for
Jaundice, Neonatal
Latex Allergy
   Latex Allergy, Risk for
Liver Function, Risk for Impaired
Nutrition, Imbalanced: Less Than Body
   Requirements
Nutrition, Imbalanced: More Than Body
   Requirements
Nutrition, Imbalanced: Potential for More Than
   Body Requirements
   Dentition, Impaired
   Feeding Pattern, Ineffective Infant
   Swallowing, Impaired
Protection, Ineffective
   Tissue Integrity, Impaired
   Oral Mucous Membrane, Impaired
   Skin Integrity, Impaired

3. Elimination
Bowel Incontinence
Constipation
   Constipation, Risk for
   Perceived Constipation
Diarrhea
Urinary Elimination, Impaired
   Continuous Incontinence

BOX 3. CONDITIONS THAT NECESSITATE NURSING CARE
(Continued)

Functional Incontinence
Overflow Incontinence
Urge Incontinence
Urge Incontinence, Risk for
Stress Incontinence
†Maturational Enuresis

4. Activity—Exercise
Activity Intolerance
Activity Planning, Ineffective
Adaptive Capacity, Decreased Intracranial
Bleeding, Risk for
Cardiac Output, Decreased
Disuse Syndrome
Diversional Activity, Deficient
Home Maintenance Management, Impaired
Infant Behavior, Disorganized
Infant Behavior, Risk for Disorganized
Infant Behavior, Readiness for Enhanced Organized
Liver Function, Risk for Impaired
Mobility, Impaired Physical
    Bed Mobility, Impaired
    Transfer Ability, Impaired
    Walking, Impaired
    Wheelchair Mobility, Impaired
Peripheral Neurovascular Dysfunction, Risk for
Respiratory Function, Risk for Impaired
    Dysfunctional Ventilatory Weaning Response
    Ineffective Airway Clearance
    Ineffective Breathing Patterns
    Impaired Gas Exchange
    Ventilation, Inability to Sustain Spontaneous
Sedentary Lifestyle
Self-Care, Readiness for Enhanced

(box continues on page 14)

BOX 3. CONDITIONS THAT NECESSITATE NURSING CARE
(Continued)

†Self-Care Deficit Syndrome (Specify):
  (Feeding, Bathing, Dressing, Toileting,
  Instrumental)
Shock, Risk for
Tissue Perfusion, Ineffective
Vascular Trauma, Risk for
Wandering

5. Sleep—Rest
Disturbed Sleep Pattern
  Insomnia
  Sleep Deprivation
Sleep, Readiness for Enhanced

6. Cognitive—Perceptual
Aspiration, Risk for
Autonomic Dysreflexia
  Autonomic Dysreflexia, Risk for
†Comfort, Impaired
  Acute Pain
  Chronic Pain
  Pain
  Nausea
†Confusion
  Acute Confusion
  Acute Confusion, Risk for
  Chronic Confusion
Decision-Making, Readiness for Enhanced
Decisional Conflict
Environmental Interpretation Syndrome, Impaired
Deficient Knowledge: (Specify)
Disturbed Sensory Perception: (Specify) (Visual,
  Auditory, Kinesthetic, Gustatory, Tactile,
  Olfactory)
Thought Processes, Impaired
Unilateral Neglect

BOX 3. CONDITIONS THAT NECESSITATE NURSING CARE
(Continued)

7. Self-Perception
Anxiety
  Death Anxiety
Dignity, Risk for Compromised Human
Fatigue
Fear
Hope, Readiness for Enhanced
Hopelessness
Power, Readiness for Enhanced
Powerlessness
Disturbed Self-Concept
  Disturbed Body Image
  Disturbed Personal Identity
Disturbed Self-Esteem
  Chronic Low Self-Esteem
  Situational Low Self-Esteem
Self-Neglect

8. Role—Relationship
†Communication, Impaired
  Communication, Impaired Verbal
Family Processes, Interrupted
Family Processes, Dysfunctional: Alcoholism
Grieving
  Grieving, Anticipatory
  Grieving, Complicated
  Grieving, Risk for Complicated
Chronic Sorrow
Loneliness, Risk for
Parent-Infant-Child Attachment, Risk for Impaired
Parenting, Impaired
Parental Role Conflict
Relationship, Readiness for Enhanced
Role Performance, Ineffective
Social Interaction, Impaired

(box continues on page 16)

BOX 3. CONDITIONS THAT NECESSITATE NURSING CARE
(Continued)

Social Isolation
9. Sexuality—Reproductive
Childbearing Process, Readiness for Enhanced
    Maternal/Fetal Dyad, Risk for Disturbed
Sexual Dysfunction
Sexuality Patterns, Ineffective
10. Coping—Stress Tolerance
Adjustment, Impaired
Caregiver Role Strain
Coping, Ineffective Individual
    Defensive Coping
    Ineffective Denial
Coping, Disabled Family
Compromised Family Coping
Readiness for Enhanced Family Coping
Coping, Ineffective Community
Readiness for Enhanced Community Coping
Post-Trauma Syndrome
    Post-Trauma Syndrome, Risk for
    Rape-Trauma Syndrome
Relocation Stress Syndrome
Resilience, Impaired Individual
Resilience, Risk for Compromised
Resilience, Readiness for Enhanced
†Self-Harm, Risk for:
    †Self-Abuse, Risk for
    Self-Mutilation, Risk for
    Suicide, Risk for
Stress Overload
Violence, Risk for Other-Directed
11. Value—Belief
Moral Distress
Religiosity, Impaired
    Impaired Religiosity, Risk for

BOX 3. CONDITIONS THAT NECESSITATE NURSING CARE
(Continued)

Religiosity, Readiness for Enhanced
Spiritual Distress
  Spiritual Distress, Risk for
Spiritual Well-Being, Readiness for Enhanced

‡Collaborative Problems

Risk for Complications of Cardiac/Vascular Dysfunction

RC of Decreased Cardiac Output
RC of Dysrhythmias
RC of Pulmonary Edema
RC of Cardiogenic Shock
RC of Thromboembolic/Deep Vein Thrombosis
RC of Hypovolemia
RC of Peripheral Vascular Insufficiency
RC of Hypertension
RC of Congenital Heart Disease
RC of Angina
RC of Endocarditis
RC of Pulmonary Embolism
RC of Spinal Shock
RC of Ischemic Ulcers

Risk for Complications of Respiratory Dysfunction

RC of Hypoxemia
RC of Atelectasis/Pneumonia
RC of Tracheobronchial Constriction
RC of Pleural Effusion
RC of Tracheal Necrosis
RC of Ventilator Dependency
RC of Pneumothorax
RC of Laryngeal Edema

Risk for Complications of Renal/Urinary Dysfunction

RC of Acute Urinary Retention
RC of Renal Failure

(box continues on page 18)

BOX 3. CONDITIONS THAT NECESSITATE NURSING CARE
(Continued)

RC of Bladder Perforation
RC of Renal Calculi

Risk for Complications of Gastrointestinal/Hepatic/Biliary Dysfunction

RC of Paralytic Ileus/Small Bowel Obstruction
RC of Hepatic Failure
RC of Hyperbilirubinemia
RC of Evisceration
RC of Hepatosplenomegaly
RC of Curling's Ulcer
RC of Ascites
RC of Gastrointestinal Bleeding

Risk for Complications of Metabolic/Immune/Hematopoietic Dysfunction

RC of Hypoglycemia/Hyperglycemia
RC of Negative Nitrogen Balance
RC of Electrolyte Imbalances
RC of Thyroid Dysfunction
RC of Hypothermia (Severe)
RC of Hyperthermia (Severe)
RC of Sepsis
RC of Acidosis (Metabolic, Respiratory)
RC of Alkalosis (Metabolic, Respiratory)
RC of Hypo/Hyperthyroidism
RC of Allergic Reaction
RC of Donor Tissue Rejection
RC of Adrenal Insufficiency
RC of Anemia
RC of Thrombocytopenia
RC of Opportunistic Infection
RC of Polycythemia
RC of Sickling Crisis
RC of Disseminated Intravascular Coagulation

BOX 3. CONDITIONS THAT NECESSITATE NURSING CARE
(Continued)

Risk for Complications of Neurological/Sensory Dysfunction

RC of Increased Intracranial Pressure
RC of Stroke
RC of Seizures
RC of Spinal Cord Compression
RC of Meningitis
RC of Cranial Nerve Impairment (Specify)
RC of Paralysis
RC of Peripheral Nerve Impairment
RC of Increased Intraocular Pressure
RC of Corneal Ulceration
RC of Neuropathies

Risk for Complications of Muscular/Skeletal Impairments

RC of Osteoporosis
RC of Joint Dislocation
RC of Compartment Syndrome
RC of Pathological Fractures

Risk for Complications of Reproductive Disorders

RC of Fetal Distress
RC of Postpartum Bleeding
RC of Gestational Hypertension
RC of Hypermenorrhea
RC of Polymenorrhea
RC of Syphilis
RC of Prenatal Bleeding
RC of Preterm Labor

Risk for Complications of Multisystem

RC of Medication Therapy Adverse Effects
RC of Adrenocorticosteroid Therapy Adverse Effects
RC of Antianxiety Therapy Adverse Effects
RC of Antiarrhythmia Therapy Adverse Effects

(box continues on page 20)

BOX 3. CONDITIONS THAT NECESSITATE NURSING CARE
(Continued)

RC of Anticoagulant Therapy Adverse Effects

RC of Anticonvulsant Therapy Adverse Effects

RC of Antidepressant Therapy Adverse Effects

RC of Antihypertensive Therapy Adverse Effects

RC of Beta-Adrenergic Blocker Therapy Adverse Effects

RC of Calcium Channel Blocker Therapy Adverse Effects

RC of Angiotensin-Converting Enzyme Therapy Adverse Effects

RC of Antineoplastic Therapy Adverse Effects

RC of Antipsychotic Therapy Adverse Effects

*The Functional Health Patterns were identified in Gordon, M. (1994). *Nursing diagnosis: Process and application.* New York: McGraw-Hill, with minor changes by the author.

†These diagnoses are not currently on the NANDA list but have been included for clarity and usefulness.

‡Frequently used collaborative problems are represented on this list. Other situations not listed here could qualify as collaborative problems.

specific level of wellness to a higher level of wellness (NANDA, 1998).

- Syndrome: A syndrome diagnosis comprises a cluster of actual or risk nursing diagnoses that are predicted to present because of a certain situation or event.
- Possible nursing diagnosis is not a type of diagnosis as are actual, risk, and syndrome. Possible nursing diagnoses are a diagnostician's option to indicate that some data are present to confirm a diagnosis but are insufficient at this time.

Diagnostic Statements

The diagnostic statement describes the health status of an individual or group and the factors that have contributed to the status.

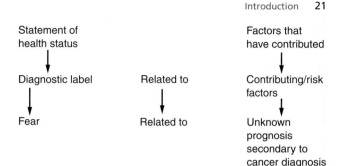

One-Part Statements

Wellness nursing diagnoses will be written as one-part statements: Readiness for Enhanced _____, e.g., Readiness for Enhanced Parenting. Related factors are not present for wellness nursing diagnoses because they would all be the same: motivated to achieve a higher level of wellness. Syndrome diagnoses, such as Rape-Trauma Syndrome, have no "related to" designations.

Two-Part Statements

Risk and possible nursing diagnoses have two parts. The validation for a risk nursing diagnosis is the presence of risk factors. The risk factors are the second part, as in:

Risk Nursing Diagnosis Related to Risk Factors

Possible nursing diagnoses are suspected because of the presence of certain factors.

The Following Are Examples of Two-Part Statements:

Risk for Impaired Skin Integrity related to immobility secondary to fractured hip

Possible Self-Care Deficit related to impaired ability to use left hand secondary to IV

Designating a diagnosis as possible provides the nurse with a method to communicate to other nurses that a diagnosis may be present. Additional data collection is indicated to rule out or confirm the tentative diagnosis.

Three-Part Statements

An actual nursing diagnosis consists of three parts.

Diagnostic label + contributing factors
+ signs and symptoms

The presence of major signs and symptoms (defining characteristics) validates that an actual diagnosis is present. This is the third part. It is not possible to have a third part for risk or possible diagnoses because signs and symptoms do not exist.

The Following Are Examples of Three-Part Statements:

Anxiety related to unpredictable nature of asthmatic episodes as evident by statements of "I'm afraid I won't be able to breathe"

Urge Incontinence related to diminished bladder capacity secondary to habitual frequent voiding evident by inability to hold off urination after desire to void and report of voiding out of habit, not need

The presence of a nursing diagnosis is determined by assessing the individual's health status and ability to function. To guide the nurse who is gathering this information, a Screening Assessment Tool is available at http://thepoint.lww.com under Carpenito's *Nursing Diagnosis: Application to Clinical Practice* (13th ed.). This guide directs the nurse to collect data according to the individual's functional health patterns. Functional health patterns and the corresponding nursing diagnoses are listed in Box 3. If significant data are collected in a particular functional pattern, the next step is to check the related nursing diagnoses to see whether any of them are substantiated by the data that are collected.

Client Validation

The process of validating a nursing diagnosis should not be done in isolation from the client or family. Individuals are the experts on themselves. During assessments and interactions, nurses are provided a small glimpse of their clients. Diagnostic hunches or inferences about data should be discussed with clients for their input. Clients are given opportunities to select what they want assistance with, which problems are important to them, and which ones are not.

Clinical Example

After the screening assessment has been completed, the nurse applies each of these questions to each functional or need area:

- Is there a possible problem in a specific area?
- Is the person at risk (or high risk) for a problem?
- Does the person desire to improve his/her health?

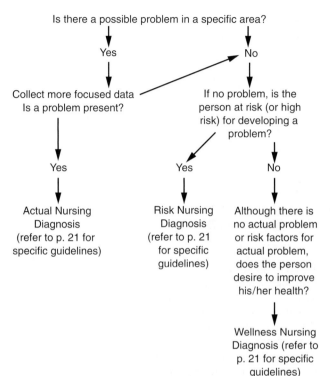

Is there a possible problem in a specific area?

Yes → Collect more focused data. Is a problem present?

No → If no problem, is the person at risk (or high risk) for developing a problem?

Collect more focused data / Is a problem present?

Yes → Actual Nursing Diagnosis (refer to p. 21 for specific guidelines)

Yes → Risk Nursing Diagnosis (refer to p. 21 for specific guidelines)

No → Although there is no actual problem or risk factors for actual problem, does the person desire to improve his/her health?

→ Wellness Nursing Diagnosis (refer to p. 21 for specific guidelines)

For example, after assessing a client's elimination pattern, the nurse would then analyze the data. Does this person have a possible problem with constipation or diarrhea? If yes, the nurse would then ask the person more focused questions to confirm the presence of the defining characteristics of constipation or diarrhea. If these defining characteristics are not present, then there is no actual diagnosis of Constipation or Diarrhea. Is there a risk diagnosis? To determine this, the nurse will assess for risk factors of constipation or diarrhea (listed under related/risk factors). If none of these are present, there is no risk for constipation or diarrhea.

Lastly, if there is no actual or at risk elimination nursing diagnosis, the nurse can ask whether the individual would like to improve his or her elimination patterns. If the answer is yes, the wellness diagnosis Potential for Enhanced Elimination is the appropriate choice.

Actual Nursing Diagnoses

Actual nursing diagnoses are written in two- or three-part statements:

1st part
Diagnostic Label

2nd part
related to *factors*
that have caused or
contributed

3rd part
as evident by *signs*
and symptoms in
the individual
that indicate the
diagnosis is present

Now that the defining characteristics have been confirmed to be present in the individual, you have:

Label: Constipation
Causative/contributing factors: related to inadequate fiber and
                                    fluid intake
Signs/symptoms: as evident by reports of dry,
  (defining characteristics)   hard stools, q 3–4 days

Clinical Example

As part of the screening assessment under nutrition you elicit:

Usual food intake   Usual fluid intake
BMI   Current weight
Appearance of skin, nails, hair

You then analyze the data to determine which data are within a normal range, and which are not:

- Are there sufficient servings of five food groups?
- Is there sufficient intake of calcium, protein, and vitamins?
- Is the fat intake <30% of total caloric intake?
- Does the person drink at least 6 to 8 cups of water besides coffee or soft drinks?
- Does the appearance of skin, hair, and nails reflect a healthy nutrition pattern?
- Is the person's weight within normal limits for height?

For example, in a specific person, Mr. Jewel, you find there is:

- Appropriate weight for height
- Insufficient fluid intake (4 8-oz. glasses of water/juice)
- Insufficient vegetable intake (two servings)
- Excess bread, cereal, rice, pasta intake (eight servings)
- Dry skin and hair

From your assessment, you have confirmed that a nursing diagnosis is present because the person has signs or reports symptoms that represent those listed as defining characteristics under that specific diagnosis. These are usually the person's complaints.

At this point you have two parts of the diagnostic statement—the first and third but not the second:

Imbalanced Nutrition: less than body requirement related to _____, as evident from dry skin and hair, dietary intake (low in fiber, vegetables, fluids, and high in CHO)

Now you want to determine what has caused or contributed to Mr. Jewel's imbalanced nutrition. Look at the list of related factors or risk factors under Imbalanced Nutrition. Do any relate to Mr. Jewel's situation? Does Mr. Jewel think his diet is inadequate? If he says no, "lack of knowledge" would be the third part of your diagnostic statement. If he says yes, but it is not important to him to change his habits at his age, you will need to talk with him. Perhaps he has a problem with constipation or energy. Maybe a change of diet could help. When you are assured that Mr. Jewel understands the reasons for a balanced diet, but see that he has decided to continue his present diet, record his decision and your attempts to influence that decision.

Select Priority Diagnoses

KEY CONCEPTS
Priority criteria
Use of consultants/referrals

Priority Criteria

Nurses cannot treat all the nursing diagnoses and collaborative problems that an individual client, family, or community has. Attempts to do this will result in frustration for the nurse and the client. By identifying a priority set—a group of nursing diagnoses and collaborative problems that take precedence over other nursing diagnoses or collaborative problems—the nurse can best direct resources toward goal achievement. It is useful to differentiate priority diagnoses from those that are important, but not priority.

Priority diagnoses are those nursing diagnoses or collaborative problems that, if not managed now, will deter progress to achieve outcomes or will negatively affect the client's functional status.

Non-priority diagnoses are those nursing diagnoses or collaborative problems for which treatment can be delayed to a later time without compromising present functional status. How does the nurse identify a priority set? In an acute-care setting, the client enters the hospital for a specific purpose, such as surgery or other treatments for acute illness.

- What are the nursing diagnoses or collaborative problems associated with the primary condition or treatments (e.g., surgery)?
- Are there additional collaborative problems associated with co-existing medical conditions that require monitoring (e.g., hypoglycemia)?
- Are there additional nursing diagnoses that, if not managed now, will deter recovery or affect the client's functional status (e.g., High Risk for Constipation)?
- What problems does the client perceive as priority?

Use of Consultants/Referrals

How are other diagnoses not on the diagnostic cluster selected for a client's problem list? Limited nursing resources and increasingly reduced client care time mandate that nurses identify important nursing diagnoses that can be addressed later and do not need to be included on the client's problem list. For example, for a client hospitalized after myocardial infarction who is 50 pounds overweight, the nurse would want to explain the effects of obesity on cardiac function and refer the client to community resources for a weight-reduction program after discharge. The discharge summary record would reflect the teaching and the referral; a nursing diagnosis related to weight reduction would not need to appear on the client's problem list.

Summary

Making accurate nursing diagnoses takes knowledge and practice. If the nurse uses a systematic approach to nursing diagnosis validation, then accuracy will increase. The process of making nursing diagnoses is difficult because nurses are attempting to diagnose human responses. Humans are unique, complex, and ever-changing; thus, attempts to classify these responses have been difficult.

References

Alfaro-LeFevre, R. (2002). *Applying nursing diagnosis and nursing process: A step-by-step guide* (5th ed.). Philadelphia: Lippincott Williams & Wilkins.

American Nurses Association. (1985). *A nursing social policy statement.* Washington, DC: ANA.

Carpenito, L. J. (1983). *Nursing diagnosis: Application to clinical practice.* Philadelphia: J. B. Lippincott.

Carpenito-Moyet, L. J. (2010). *Nursing diagnosis: Application to clinical practice* (13th ed.). Philadelphia: Lippincott Williams & Wilkins.

North American Nursing Diagnosis Association. (2008). National conference, Miami, FL.

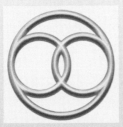

SECTION ONE

Nursing Diagnoses

ACTIVITY INTOLERANCE

DEFINITION

A reduction in one's physiologic capacity to endure activities to the degree desired or required (Magnan, 1987).

■■■■ **AUTHOR'S NOTE**

Activity Intolerance is a diagnostic judgment that describes a person with compromised physical conditioning. This person can engage in therapies that increase strength and endurance. Activity Intolerance is different than Fatigue. Fatigue is a pervasive, subjective drained feeling. Rest does not relieve fatigue but it will relieve tiredness. *For Activity Intolerance*, the goal is to increase tolerance to activity; in *Fatigue*, the goal is to assist the person to adapt to the fatigue, not to increase endurance.

DEFINING CHARACTERISTICS

Major (Must Be Present, One or More)

An altered physiologic response to activity

Respiratory
Dyspnea
Shortness of breath

Excessively increased rate
Decreased rate

Pulse
Weak
Excessively increased
Rhythm change

Decreased
Failure to return to pre-activity
    level after 3 min

Blood Pressure
Failure to increase with
    activity

Increased diastolic pressure
    >15 mm Hg

Minor (May Be Present)

Pallor or cyanosis
Confusion
Vertigo

RELATED FACTORS

Any factors that compromise oxygen transport, physical deconditioning, or create excessive energy demands that outstrip the
person's physical and psychological abilities can cause *Activity Intolerance*. Some common factors are listed below.

Pathophysiologic

Related to compromised oxygen transport system secondary to:
Cardiac

Congenital heart disease	Valvular disease
Cardiomyopathies	Dysrhythmias
Myocardial infarction	Angina
Congestive heart failure	

Respiratory

Chronic obstructive pulmonary disease	Bronchopulmonary dysplasia
	Atelectasis

Circulatory

Anemia	Hypovolemia
Peripheral arterial disease	

Related to increased metabolic demands secondary to:
Acute or Chronic Infection

Viral infection	Hepatitis
Mononucleosis	

Endocrine or Metabolic Disorders

Chronic Diseases

Renal	Inflammatory
Hepatic	Musculoskeletal
Cancer	Neurologic

Related to inadequate energy sources secondary to:

Obesity	Inadequate diet
Malnourishment	

Related to compromised oxygen transport secondary to:
Hypovolemia

Treatment-Related

Related to increased metabolic demands secondary to:

Surgery	Treatment schedule
Diagnostic studies	

Situational (Personal, Environmental)

Related to the deconditioning effects of bed rest
***Related to inactivity secondary to depression, insufficient
knowledge, inadequate social support, sedentary lifestyle***

Related to increased metabolic demands secondary to:
Assistive equipment (walkers, crutches, braces)
Extreme stress
Pain, dyspnea
Obesity
Environmental barriers (e.g., stairs)
Climatic extremes (especially hot, humid climates)

Related to decreased available oxygen secondary to atmospheric pressure (e.g., recent relocation to high-altitude living)

Related to Fear of Falling

Maturational

Older adults may experience decreased muscle strength and flexibility and sensory deficits. All these can undermine body confidence and may contribute directly or indirectly to *Activity Intolerance.*

NOC
Activity Tolerance

Goals

The person will progress activity to (specify level of activity desired).

Indicators
- Identify factors that aggravate activity intolerance.
- Identify methods to reduce activity intolerance.
- Maintain blood pressure within normal limits 3 minutes after activity.

NIC
Energy Management, Exercise Promotion, Sleep Enhancement, Mutual Goal Setting

Generic Interventions

Monitor the Person's Response to Activity.

1. Take resting pulse, blood pressure, and respirations.
2. Consider rate, rhythm, and quality (if signs are abnormal— e.g., pulse >100—consult physician/nurse practitioner about the advisability of increasing activity).
3. Take vital signs immediately after activity; take pulse for 15 seconds, and multiply by 4 instead of for 1 full minute.

4. Have person rest for 3 minutes; take vital signs again. Compare findings with resting vital signs.
5. Discontinue the activity if the client responds to the activity with:
   - Reports of chest pain, dyspnea, vertigo, or confusion
   - Decrease in pulse rate
   - Failure of systolic rate to increase
   - Decrease in systolic blood pressure
   - Increase in diastolic rate of 15 mm Hg
   - Decrease in respiratory rate
6. Reduce the intensity, frequency, or duration of the activity if:
   - The pulse takes longer than 3 to 4 minutes to return within 6 beats of the resting pulse rate.
   - The respiratory rate increase is excessive after the activity.
   - Other signs of hypoxia are present (e.g., confusion, vertigo).

Progress the Activity Gradually.

For a person who is or has been on prolonged bed rest, begin range of motion at least twice a day.

Plan rest periods according to the person's daily schedule (rest periods may occur between activities).

Promote a sincere "can do" attitude to provide a positive atmosphere to encourage increased activity; convey to clients the belief that they can improve their mobility status. Acknowledge progress.

Allow person to set activity schedule and functional activity goals (if the goal is too low, make a contract: e.g., "If you walk halfway up the hall, I will play a game of cards with you").

Increase tolerance for the activity by having the client perform the activity more slowly, for a shorter period with more rest pauses, or with more assistance.

Gradually increase exercise tolerance by increasing the time out of bed by 15 minutes each day, three times a day.

Allow person to gauge the rate of the ambulation.

Encourage person to wear comfortable walking shoes (slippers do not support the feet properly).

Teach Energy Conservation Methods for Activities.

Take rest periods during activities, at intervals during the day, and 1 hour after meals.

Sit rather than stand when performing activities, unless this is not feasible.

When performing a task, rest every 3 minutes for 5 minutes to allow the heart to recover.

Stop an activity if fatigue or signs of cardiac hypoxia are present (increased pulse, dyspnea, chest pain).

**Instruct the Person to Consult Physician and
Physiatrist for a Long-Term Exercise Program or
to Contact the American Heart Association for
Names of Cardiac Rehabilitation Programs.**

For Clients with Chronic Pulmonary Insufficiency:

Encourage conscious controlled-breathing techniques during
increased activity and times of emotional and physical stress
(techniques include pursed-lip and diaphragmatic breathing).

For pursed-lip breathing, the person should breathe in through
the nose, then breathe out slowly through partially closed lips
while counting to 7 and making a "poo" sound (often this is
learned naturally by a person with progressive lung disease).

Teach diaphragmatic breathing:

- Place your hands on the person's abdomen below the base of
  the ribs, and keep them there while the client inhales.
- To inhale, the person should relax the shoulders, breathe in
  through the nose, and push the stomach outward against the
  nurse's hands, holding breath for 1 to 2 seconds to keep the
  alveoli open.
- To exhale, the person should breathe out slowly through the
  mouth while the nurse applies slight pressure at the base of
  the ribs.
- Practice several times; then have the person place his or her
  own hands at the base of the ribs and practice independently.
- Instruct to practice this exercise a few times each hour.
- Encourage gradual increase in daily activity to prevent "pulmonary crippling."
- Encourage person to use adaptive breathing techniques to
  decrease the work of breathing.

Discuss physical barriers at home and at work (e.g., number of
stairs) and ways of alternating expenditure of energy with
rest pauses (place a chair in bathroom near sink to rest during
daily hygiene).

Explain the importance of supporting arm weight to reduce the
work of respiratory muscles (Breslin, 1992).

Teach how to increase unsupported arm endurance with lower
extremity exercises performed during exhalation (Breslin,
1992).

Refer to Community Nurse for Follow-Up If Needed.

👥 Pediatric Interventions

**Provide Age-Appropriate Games and
Activities that Are Quiet and Challenging.**

Sensory adventures (What does the hospital smell, sound, or look like?)

Telling and writing stories, creating collages, playing with puppets, playacting

👥 Maternal Interventions

Explain the Causes of Fatigue and Dyspnea in Mid- to Late Pregnancy.

Changes in center of gravity

Increased weight

Pressure of enlarged uterus on diaphragm

Teach Energy Conservation Methods (Refer to Generic Interventions).

INEFFECTIVE ACTIVITY PLANNING

DEFINITION

The state in which an individual has an inability to prepare for a set of actions fixed in time and under certain circumstances.

DEFINING CHARACTERISTICS

Verbalization of fear toward a task to be undertaken

Verbalization of worries toward a task to be undertaken

Excessive anxieties toward a task to be undertaken

Failure pattern of behavior

Lack of plan

Lack of resources

Lack of sequential organization

Procrastination

Unmet goals for chosen activity

RELATED FACTORS

Compromised ability to process information

Defensive flight behavior when faced with proposed solution

Hedonism

Lack of family support
Lack of friend support
Unrealistic perception of events
Unrealistic perception of personal competence

AUTHOR'S NOTE

This newly accepted NANDA-I nursing diagnosis can represent a problematic response that relates to many existing nursing diagnoses as Chronic Confusion, Self Care Deficit, Anxiety, Ineffective Denial, Ineffective Coping and Ineffective Self-health management. This author recommends that ineffective activity planning should be seen as a sign or symptom. The questions are:

- What activities are not being planned effectively? Self-care? Self-health management?
- What is preventing effective activity planning? Confusion? Anxiety? Fear? Denial? Stress Overload?

Examples are:

- Stress Overload related to unrealistic perception of events as evidenced by impaired ability to plan ….(specify activity}
- Ineffective Self-health management related to lack of plan, lack of resources, lack of social support as evidenced by impaired ability to plan…(specify activity)
- Anxiety related to compromised ability to process information and unrealistic perception of personal competence as evidenced by impaired ability to plan {specify activity}.

ADAPTIVE CAPACITY, DECREASED INTRACRANIAL

DEFINITION (NANDA)

A clinical state in which intracranial fluid dynamic mechanisms that normally compensate for increases in intracranial volumes are compromised, resulting in repeated disproportionate increases in intracranial pressure in response to a variety of noxious and non-noxious stimuli.

■■■ **AUTHOR'S NOTE**
This diagnosis represents increased intracranial pressure. It is a collaborative problem because it requires two disciplines to treat—nursing and medicine. In addition, it requires invasive monitoring for diagnosis. The collaborative problem Risk for Complications of Increased Intracranial Pressure represents this clinical situation.

DEFINING CHARACTERISTICS (NANDA)

Major (Must Be Present)

Repeated increases in intracranial pressure (ICP) of >10 mm Hg for >5 minutes after any of a variety of external stimuli.

Minor (May Be Present)

Disproportionate increase in ICP after one environmental or nursing maneuver stimulus
Elevated P_2 ICP waveform
Volume-pressure response test variation (volume–pressure ratio >2); pressure–volume index (<10)
Baseline ICP ≥10 mm Hg
Wide-amplitude ICP waveform

ANXIETY

Anxiety
Death Anxiety

DEFINITION

The state in which an individual or group experiences feelings of uneasiness (apprehension) and activation of the autonomic nervous system in response to a vague, nonspecific threat.

■■■ **AUTHOR'S NOTE**
Anxiety is a vague feeling of apprehension and uneasiness from a threat to one's value system or security pattern (May,

(continued)

AUTHOR'S NOTE *(Continued)*
1987). The person may be able to identify the situation (e.g., surgery, cancer), but in actuality the threat to self relates to the uneasiness and apprehension enmeshed in the situation. The situation is the source of, but is not itself, the threat.

In contrast, fear is the feeling of apprehension over a specific threat or danger to which one's security patterns alert one (e.g., flying, heights, snakes). When the threat is removed, the fearful feeling dissipates (May, 1987).

Fear can exist without anxiety, and anxiety can be present without fear. Clinically, both may coexist in a person's response to a situation. An individual who is facing surgery may be fearful of pain and anxious about a possible cancer diagnosis.

DEFINING CHARACTERISTICS

Major (Must Be Present)

Manifested by symptoms from three categories: physiologic, emotional, and cognitive; symptoms vary according to the level of anxiety.

Physiologic

Increased heart rate	Insomnia
Elevated blood pressure	Fatigue and weakness
Increased respiratory rate	Flushing or pallor
Diaphoresis	Dry mouth
Dilated pupils	Body aches and pains
Voice tremors/pitch changes	(especially chest, back, neck)
Trembling, twitching	Restlessness
Palpitations	Faintness/dizziness
Nausea or vomiting	Paresthesias
Frequent urination	Hot and cold flashes
Diarrhea	Anorexia

Emotional
Person Reports Feelings of:

Apprehension	Losing control
Helplessness	Tension or being "keyed up"
Nervousness	Inability to relax
Lack of self-confidence	Anticipation of misfortune

Person Exhibits:

Irritability/impatience	Criticism of self and others
Angry outbursts	Withdrawal
Crying	Lack of initiative

Tendency to blame others

Startle reaction

Self-deprecation

Poor eye contact

Cognitive

Inability to concentrate
    (inability to remember)

Lack of awareness of
    surroundings

Forgetfulness

Rumination

Orientation to past rather
    than to present or future

Blocking of thoughts

Hyperattentiveness

Preoccupation

Diminished learning ability

Confusion

RELATED FACTORS

Pathophysiologic

Any factor that interferes with the basic human needs for food,
    air, comfort, and security

Situational (Personal, Environmental)

*Related to actual or perceived threat to self-concept secondary
to:*

Change in status and prestige

Failure (or success)

Loss of valued possessions

Ethical dilemma

Lack of recognition from
    others

*Related to actual or perceived loss of significant others
secondary to:*

Death

Divorce

Cultural pressures

Moving

Temporary or permanent
    separation

*Related to actual or perceived threat to biologic integrity
secondary to:*

Dying

Assault

Invasive procedures

Disease

*Related to actual or perceived change in environment
secondary to:*

Hospitalization

Moving

Retirement

Safety hazards

Environmental pollutants

*Related to actual or perceived change in socioeconomic status
secondary to (e.g., unemployment, new job, promotion)*

Related to idealistic expectations of self and unrealistic goals

Maturational

Infant/Child
Related to separation
Related to changes in peer relationships
Related to unfamiliar environment or persons

Adolescent
Related to threat to self-concept secondary to (e.g., sexual development, peer relationship changes)

Adult
Related to threat to self-concept or role status secondary to:

Pregnancy	Career changes
Parenting	Effects of aging

Older Adult
Related to threat to self-concept or role status secondary to:

Sensory losses	Financial problems
Motor losses	Retirement changes

NOC

Anxiety Level, Coping, Impulse Control

Goals

The person will relate an increase in psychological and physiologic comfort.

Indicators
- Describe his or her own anxiety and coping patterns.
- Use effective coping mechanisms.

NIC

Anxiety Reduction, Impulse Control Training, Anticipatory Guidance

Generic Interventions

Assess Level of Anxiety: Mild, Moderate, Severe, Panic.

Provide Reassurance and Comfort.

Stay with person.
Do not make demands or ask the person to make decisions. Sit in front of person.
Emphasize that all people feel anxious from time to time.
Speak slowly and calmly, using short, simple sentences.

Be aware of your own concern, and avoid reciprocal anxiety.

Convey a sense of empathic understanding (e.g., quiet presence, touch, allowing crying, talking).

Remove Excess Stimulation (e.g., Take Person to Quieter Room); Limit Contact with Others—Clients or Family—Who Are Also Anxious.

When Anxiety Is Diminished Enough for Learning to Take Place, Assist Person in Recognizing the Anxiety to Initiate Learning or Problem-Solving.

Encourage person to keep a diary (e.g., when client felt anxious, what was he or she doing or thinking? Who was with him or her?)

Assist to analyze diary to identify triggers.

Explore what alternative behaviors might have been used if coping mechanisms were maladaptive (e.g., assertiveness training).

Teach Anxiety Interrupters to Use When Stressful Situations Cannot Be Avoided.

Look up.

Control breathing.

Lower shoulders.

Slow thoughts.

Alter voice.

Give directions to self (out loud, if possible).

Exercise.

"Scruff your face"—change facial expression.

Change perspective—imagine watching the situation from a distance.

Assist Person with Anger (Thomas, 1989).

Identify the presence of anger (e.g., feelings of frustration, anxiety, helplessness, irritability; verbal outbursts).

Recognize your reactions to client's behavior; be aware of your own feelings when working with angry individuals.

Do not interrupt; listen to grievance.

Encourage alternative problem-solving if expectations are not realistic or possible (e.g., "What can you do differently?").

Provide positive validation if possible.

Focus on what can be done, not on what was not done.

Explore consequences of explosive anger.

Elicit alternative behavior to violent behavior (e.g., "What could you do instead of punching the wall?").

Use "time-out" when needed (e.g., "I can see that we are not accomplishing anything. Let's try again when we are both less emotional.").

State limits clearly; tell person exactly what is expected (e.g., "I cannot allow you to scream" [throw objects, etc.]).

When stating an unacceptable behavior, give an alternative (e.g., suggest a quiet room, physical exertion, a chance for one-to-one communication).

Develop behavior modification strategies; discuss with all personnel involved for consistency.

Interact with person when he or she is not demanding or manipulative.

Explore Interventions that Decrease Anxiety (e.g., Music, Aromatherapy, Relaxation Exercises, Guided Imagery, Hydrotherapy, Thought-Stopping, Massage, Exercise) (Keegan, 2000).

Refer to Risk for Other-Directed Violence.

For Persons Identified as Having Chronic Anxiety and Maladaptive Coping Mechanisms, Refer for Psychiatric Evaluation.

👥 Pediatric Interventions

Explain Events Using Simple, Age-Appropriate Terms and Illustrations; Puppets; Dolls; and Sample Equipment.

Allow Child to Wear Underwear and Have Familiar Toys or Objects.

Assist Parents or Caregivers to Manage Their Anxiety When with Child.

Use the Following Nursing Interventions to Help Children Cope with Anxiety:

Establish a trusting relationship.
Minimize separation from parents.
Encourage expression of feelings.
Involve child in play.
Prepare child for new experiences (e.g., procedures, surgery).
Provide comfort measures.

Allow for regression.

Encourage parental involvement in care.

Allay parental apprehension, and provide parents with information (Hockenberry & Wilson, 2009).

Assist Child with Anger.

Encourage child to share anger (e.g., "How did you feel when you had your injection?" "How did you feel when Mary would not play with you?").

Tell child that being angry is okay (e.g., "I sometimes get angry when I can't have what I want.").

Encourage and allow child to express anger in acceptable ways (e.g., talking loud or running outside around the house).

👥 Maternal Interventions

Explore Fears and Concerns During Each Trimester (Reeder et al., 1997; Lugina et al., 2001).

First Trimester

Ambivalence, new role expectations, uncertainty about adequacy

Second Trimester

Success as a new mother

Third Trimester

Feels unattractive; fears for own well-being, performance during labor, and well-being of fetus

Help Her and Her Partner Identify Unrealistic Expectations.

Acknowledge Her Anxiety and the Normalcy of It.

Discuss These Concerns with the Woman Alone, Her Partner Alone, and Then Together as Indicated.

🄒 Geriatric Interventions

Explore the Person's Worries (e.g., Financial, Security, Health, Living Arrangements, Crime, Violence).

▶ Death Anxiety

DEFINITION

The state in which an individual experiences apprehension, worry, or fear related to death or dying.

■■■ ■ **AUTHOR'S NOTE**
The inclusion of *Death Anxiety* in the NANDA classification creates a diagnostic category with the etiology in the label. This opens the NANDA list to thousands of diagnostic labels with etiology, such as separation anxiety, divorce anxiety, infidelity anxiety, failure anxiety, and travel anxiety. Many diagnostic labels can take this same path: fear as claustrophobic fear, diarrhea as traveler's diarrhea, decisional conflict as end-of-life decisional conflict.

There is a possibility that the development of an End-of Life Syndrome, which could cluster a group of nursing diagnoses for individuals and families experiencing a terminal condition, would be clinically useful.

DEFINING CHARACTERISTICS

Worrying about the impact of one's own death on significant others

Feeling powerless over issues related to dying

Fear of loss of physical and/or mental abilities when dying

Anticipated pain related to dying

Deep sadness

Fear of the process of dying

Concerns of overworking the caregiver as terminal illness incapacitates self

Concern about meeting one's creator or feeling doubtful about the existence of a god or higher being

Total loss of control over any aspect of one's own death

Negative death images or unpleasant thoughts about any event related to death or dying

Fear of delayed demise

Fear of premature death because it prevents the accomplishment of important life goals

RELATED FACTORS

Impending death is the situation that causes this diagnosis. Additional factors can contribute to death anxiety.

Situational (Personal, Environmental)

Related to the recent diagnosis of a potentially terminal condition

Related to situational factors (anxiety)

Related to fear of being a burden

Related to fear of unmanageable pain

Related to fear of abandonment
Related to unresolved conflict (family, friends)
Related to fear that one's life lacked meaning
Related to social disengagement
Related to powerlessness and vulnerability

NOC

Dignified Life Closure, Fear Level

Goals

The person will report diminished anxiety or fear.

Indicators

- Share his or her feelings regarding dying.
- Identify two activities that increase control and self-knowledge.

NIC

Coping Enhancement, Dying Care, Emotional Support, Spiritual Support

Generic Interventions

Allow person to share his or her perceptions of the situation
(e.g., "Share with me what you are experiencing.").
Encourage person to share his or her conflicts and concerns (e.g.,
"If you could fix something before you die, what would it be?"
"What are you most concerned about?").
Explore person's relationship of spirituality and approaching
death:
- Afterlife beliefs
- Search for meaning
- Relationship with greater Other
Explore the person's interpretation of suffering (e.g.,
punishment, testing, bad luck, nature's course, will of greater
Other, denial, redemption).
Encourage telling life stories and reminiscing.
Discuss leaving a legacy (e.g., donation, personal articles, taped
message for survivors).
Encourage reflective activities (e.g., prayer, meditation, writing
a journal).
Encourage person to return the gift of love to others (e.g.,
listening, praying for others, sharing personal wisdom gained
from illness, creating legacy gifts) (Taylor, 2000).

Encourage friends and family to be emotionally and spiritually honest.

Explain advance directives and assist in process if desired.

Aggressively manage unrelieved symptoms (e.g., nausea, vomiting, pain).

Encourage person to reconstruct his or her worldview (Taylor, 2000):

- Allow to verbalize feelings about the meaning of death.
- Advise that there are no right or wrong feelings.
- Advise that his or her responses are choices.
- Acknowledge the struggles.

RISK FOR BLEEDING

DEFINITION (NANDA)

At risk for a decrease in blood volume that may compromise health.

RISK FACTORS (NANDA)

Aneurysm

Circumcision

Deficient knowledge

Disseminated intravascular coagulation

History of falls

Gastrointestinal disorders (e.g., gastric ulcer disease, polyps, and varices]

Impaired liver function (e.g., cirrhosis, hepatitis)

Inherent coagulopathies (e.g., thrombocytopenia}

Postpartum complications (e.g., uterine atony, retained placenta)

Pregnant-related complications (e.g., placenta previa. Molar pregnancy, abruption placenta)

Trauma

Treatment-related side effects (e.g., surgery, medications, administration of platelets, deficient blood products, chemotherapy)

■■■■ **AUTHOR'S NOTE**
This new NANDA-I diagnosis represents several collaborative problems.

Interventions/goals

Refer to Section 3 to the specific collaborative problem for example as Risk for Complications of Hypovolemia, Risk for Complications of Bleeding, Risk for Complications of GI Bleeding, Risk for Complications of Prenatal Bleeding, Risk for Complications of Postpartum Bleeding, or Risk for Complications of Anticoagulant Therapy

BODY TEMPERATURE, RISK FOR IMBALANCED

Body Temperature, Risk for Imbalanced
Hyperthermia
Hypothermia
Thermoregulation, Ineffective

■■■■ **AUTHOR'S NOTE**
Risk for Imbalanced Body Temperature includes those at risk for hyperthermia, hypothermia, or ineffective thermoregulation. If the person is at risk for only one of the diagnoses (e.g., hypothermia but not hyperthermia), then it is more useful to label the problem with the more specific diagnosis (*Risk for Hypothermia*). If the person is at risk for two or more of the diagnoses, then *Risk for Imbalanced Body Temperature* is more appropriate. The focus of nursing care for these diagnoses is to prevent abnormal body temperatures by identifying and treating those persons with a normal temperature who demonstrate risk factors that can be controlled by nursing-prescribed interventions (e.g., by removing or adding blankets or by controlling environmental temperature). If the alteration in body temperature is related to a pathophysiologic complication that requires nursing and medical interventions, then the problem should be labeled as a

(continued)

■■■ **AUTHOR'S NOTE** *(Continued)*
collaborative problem (e.g., Risk for Complication of Fever related to atelectasis or Risk for Complications of Severe Hypothermia related to hypothalamus injury). The focus of concern then becomes monitoring to detect and report significant temperature fluctuations and implementing collaborative interventions (e.g., a warming or cooling blanket) as ordered. (See also diagnostic considerations for *Hyperthermia* and *Hypothermia*.)

DEFINITION

The state in which an individual is at risk of failing to maintain body temperature within normal range 36.6 to 37.3 C or 90 to 99F (Smeltzer, Bare, Hinkle & Cheever, 2008).

RISK FACTORS
Major (Must Be Present, One or More)
Presence of risk factors (see Related Factors)

RELATED FACTORS
Treatment-Related
Related to cooling effects of:
Parenteral fluid infusion, blood transfusion
Dialysis
Cooling blanket
Operating suite

Situational (Personal, Environmental)
Related to:
Exposure to cold, rain, snow, wind; exposure to heat, sun, humidity extremes
Inappropriate clothing for climate
Inability to pay for shelter, heat, or air-conditioning
Extremes of weight
Consumption of alcohol
Dehydration/malnutrition
Newborn environmental exposure

Maturational
Related to ineffective temperature regulation secondary to extremes of age (e.g., newborn, older adult)

▶ Hyperthermia

DEFINITION

The state in which an individual has or is at risk of having a sustained elevation of body temperature >37.8° C (100° F) orally or 38.8° C (101° F) rectally because of external factors.

DEFINING CHARACTERISTICS

Major (Must be Present)

Temperature >37.8° C (100° F) orally or 38.8° C (101° F) rectally
Skin warm to touch
Tachycardia

Minor (May Be Present)

Flushed skin
Increased respiratory depth
Shivering/goose pimples
Feelings of warmth or coolness

Specific or generalized aches and pains (e.g., headache)
Malaise, fatigue, weakness
Loss of appetite
Sweating

RELATED FACTORS

Treatment-Related

Related to reduced ability to sweat secondary to (specify medication)

Situational (Personal, Environmental)

Related to:
Exposure to heat, sun   No access to air conditioning
Inappropriate clothing for climate

Related to decreased circulation secondary to:
Extremes of weight   Dehydration

Related to insufficient hydration for vigorous activity

Maturational

Related to ineffective temperature regulation secondary to age

NOC

Thermoregulation

Goals

The person will maintain body temperature.

Indicators
- Identify risk factors for hyperthermia.
- Reduce risk factors for hyperthermia.

NIC

Fever Treatment, Temperature Regulation, Environmental Management, Fluid Management

Generic Interventions (for Risk for Hyperthermia)

Teach the person the importance of maintaining an adequate fluid intake (≥2000 mL/d unless contraindicated by heart or kidney disease) to prevent dehydration.

Monitor intake and output.

See also *Deficient Fluid Volume.*

Assess whether clothing or bed covers are too warm for the environment or planned activity.

Teach the importance of increasing fluid intake during warm weather and exercise.

Recommended fluid replacement for moderate activities in hot weather (DeFabio, 2000):

78° to 84.9° F:	16 oz/hour
85° to 89.9° F:	24 oz/hour
>90° F:	32 oz/hour

Explain the need to avoid alcohol; caffeine; and large, heavy meals during hot weather.

Explain the need to wear loose-fitting clothing and to wear a hat or use an umbrella.

Avoid outdoor activity between 11 A.M. and 2 P.M. and to wear a hat or use an umbrella

Take cool baths or showers several times a day during heat waves. Do not use soap.

Teach the early signs of hyperthermia or heat stroke:
- Flushed skin
- Headache
- Fatigue
- Loss of appetite

Pediatric Interventions

Determine if fever is drug-related (e.g., anticholinergics, amphetamines, epinephrine, acetaminophen [large doses], antihistamines [large doses], phenothiazines).

Explain to parents that fever is a protective measure and not harmful unless high (e.g., >41.1° C [100° F]).

Caution not to sponge, which causes extreme chilling.

Expain appropriate clothing for infants and children in warm weather.

Ⓖ Geriatric Interventions

Refer to *Ineffective Thermoregulation*, Geriatric Interventions.

▶ Hypothermia

DEFINITION

The state in which an individual has or is at risk of having a sustained reduction of body temperature of <35.5° C (96° F) rectally because of increased vulnerability to external factors.

DEFINING CHARACTERISTICS*

Major (80% to 100%)

Reduction in body temperature <35.5° C (96° F) rectally
Cool skin
Pallor (moderate)
Shivering (mild)

Minor (50% to 79%)

Mental confusion, drowsiness, restlessness
Decreased pulse and respiration
Cachexia, malnutrition

RELATED FACTORS

Situational (Personal, Environmental)

Related to:

Exposure to cold, rain, snow, wind
Inappropriate clothing for climate
Inability to pay for shelter or heat

Related to decreased circulation secondary to:

Extremes of weight
Consumption of alcohol
Dehydration
Inactivity

---

*Adapted from Carroll, S. M. (1989). Nursing diagnosis: Hypothermia. In R. M. Carroll-Johnson (Ed), *Classification of nursing diagnoses: Proceedings of the eighth conference*. Philadelphia: J. B. Lippincott.

Maturational

Related to ineffective temperature regulation secondary to age

NOC
Thermoregulation

Goals

The person will maintain body temperature within normal limits.

Indicators
• Identify risk factors for hypothermia.
• Reduce risk factors for hypothermia.

NIC
Hypothermia Treatment, Temperature Regulation, Temperature Regulation: Intraoperative, Environmental Management

Generic Interventions (for Risk for Hypothermia)

Teach Client to Reduce Prolonged Exposure to Cold Environment.

Explain the importance of wearing a hat, gloves, and warm socks and shoes to prevent heat loss.

Encourage the person to limit going outside when temperatures are very cold.

Acquire an electric blanket, warm blankets, or down comforter for bed.

Teach client to wear close-knit undergarments to prevent heat loss.

Consult with Social Services to Identify Sources of Financial Assistance, Warm Clothing, Blankets.

Teach the Early Signs of Hypothermia: Cool Skin, Pallor, Blanching, Redness.

Explain the Need to Drink 8 to 10 Glasses of Water Daily.

Explain the Need to Avoid Alcohol in Very Cold Weather.

Teach Person to Wear Extra Clothing in the Morning When Metabolism Is at Lowest Point.

👫 Ⓖ **Pediatric/Geriatric Interventions**

Explain to Family Members that Newborns, Infants, and the Elderly Are More Susceptible to Heat Loss (See Also Ineffective Thermoregulation).

For Children and Elderly During Surgery, Unless Hypothermia Is Desired to Reduce Blood Loss, Consider the Following Interventions (Puterbough, 1991):

Increase ambient temperature of operating room (OR) before case.

Use a portable radiant heating lamp to provide additional heat during surgery.

Cover with warm blankets when arriving in OR.

When possible, use a warming mattress.

During prepping and surgery, keep as much of body surface covered as possible.

Warm prep set, blood, fluids, anesthesia, irrigants.

Replace wet gowns and drapes with dry ones.

Keep head well covered.

Continue heat-conserving interventions postoperatively.

▶ Thermoregulation, Ineffective

DEFINITION

The state in which an individual experiences or is at risk of experiencing an inability to maintain normal body temperature in the presence of adverse or changing external factors.

> **AUTHOR'S NOTE**
> This diagnosis is indicated when the nurse can maintain or assist a client in maintaining a body temperature within normal limits by manipulating external factors (e.g., clothing) and environmental conditions. Persons who are at high risk for this diagnosis are the elderly and neonates. For those with temperature fluctuations because of disease, infections, or trauma, see *Impaired Comfort*.

DEFINING CHARACTERISTICS
Major (Must Be Present)

Temperature fluctuations related to limited metabolic compensatory regulation in response to environmental factors.

RELATED FACTORS

Situational (Personal, Environmental)

Related to:

Fluctuating environmental
   temperatures
Cold or wet articles
Inadequate housing

Wet body surface
Inadequate clothing for
   weather (excessive,
   insufficient)

Maturational

*Related to limited metabolic compensatory regulation
secondary to age (e.g., neonate, older adult)*

NOC

Thermoregulation

Goals

The infant will have a temperature between 97.5° F and 98.6° F
   (36.4° C and 37° C).
The parent will explain techniques to avoid heat loss at home.

NIC

Temperature Regulation, Environmental Management,
Newborn Monitoring, Vital Sign Monitoring

Indicators

- List situations that increase heat loss.
- Demonstrate how to conserve heat during bathing.
- Demonstrate how to take infant's temperature.
- State appropriate attire for outdoor/indoor climates

👪 Pediatric Interventions

Reduce or Eliminate the Sources of Heat Loss in Infants.

Evaporation

After delivery, quickly dry skin and hair with a heated towel and
   place infant in a pre-warmed, heated environment.
When bathing, provide a warm environment or bathe under a
   heat source.
Wash and dry in sections to reduce evaporation.
Limit time in contact with wet clothing or blankets.

Convection

Avoid drafts (air conditioning, fans, windows, open portholes on
  isolette).

Place sides of radiant warmer bed up at all times

Use only portholes for infant access in isolette whenever possible

Conduction

Warm all articles for care (stethoscopes, scales, hands of
  caregivers, clothes, bed linens).

Place infant close to mother to conserve heat and promote
  bonding

Warm or cover any equipment that may come in contact with
  the infant's skin.

Radiation

Limit objects in the room that absorb heat (metal).

Place crib or bed as far away from walls (outside) or windows as
  possible.

Monitor Temperature of Infants

If Temperature Is Below Normal:

Wrap in two blankets.

Put on head cap.

Assess for environmental sources of heat loss.

If hypothermia persists for >1 hour, notify physician.

Assess for complications of cold stress: hypoxia, respiratory
  acidosis, hypoglycemia, fluid and electrolyte imbalances,
  weight loss.

If Temperature Is Above Normal:

Loosen blanket.

Remove cap, if on.

Assess environment for thermal gain.

If hyperthermia persists for >1 hour, notify physician.

Assess for Signs of Sepsis (Respiratory Function, Skin, Poor Feeding, Irritability, Signs of Localized Infections [Skin, Umbilicus, Circumcision, Eyes]).

Teach Caregiver Why Infant Is Vulnerable to Temperature Fluctuations (Cold and Heat).

Demonstrate how to conserve heat during bathing.

Instruct that it is not necessary to check temperature routinely
  at home.

Teach to check temperature if infant is hot, sick, or irritable.

Ⓖ Geriatric Interventions

Explain age-related changes that interfere with thermoregulation
(Miller, 2009):
- Cold (inefficient vasoconstriction, decreased cardiac output,
  decreased subcutaneous tissue, delayed and diminished shivering)
- Heat (delayed sweating response, diminished sweating response)

Explain that these changes will distort perception of
environmental temperatures.

Investigate even a slight elevation of temperature. Use tympanic
route for temperatures, not oral or axillary.

Teach how to prevent hypothermia and hyperthermia (refer to
Hypothermia, *Hyperthermia*).

BOWEL INCONTINENCE

DEFINITION

The state in which an individual experiences a change in normal
bowel habits characterized by involuntary passage of stool.

AUTHOR'S NOTE

This diagnosis represents a situation in which nurses have
multiple responsibilities. Clients experiencing bowel incontinence have various responses that disrupt functioning, such
as embarrassment and skin problems related to the irritative
nature of feces on skin.

For some spinal cord–injured persons, *Bowel Incontinence*
related to lack of voluntary control over rectal sphincter
would be descriptive.

DEFINING CHARACTERISTICS
Major (Must be Present)

Involuntary passage of stool

RELATED FACTORS

Pathophysiologic

Related to impaired rectal sphincter secondary to:
Diabetes mellitus
Anal or rectal surgery
Anal or rectal injury

Related to cognitive impairment

Related to overdistention of rectum secondary to chronic constipation or fecal impaction

Related to lack of voluntary sphincter control secondary to:

Progressive neuromuscular disorder	Spinal cord compression
	Multiple sclerosis
Spinal cord injury	Cerebrovascular accident

Related to impaired reservoir capacity secondary to:

Inflammatory bowel disease	Chronic rectal ischemia

Treatment-Related

Related to impaired reservoir capacity secondary to:

Colectomy	Radiation proctitis

Situational (Personal, Environmental)

Related to inability to recognize, interpret, or respond to rectal cues secondary to:

Depression	Cognitive impairment

NOC

Bowel Continence, Tissue Integrity: Skin & Mucous Membranes, Bowel Elimination

Goals

The person will evacuate a soft, formed stool every other day or every third day.

Indicators

- Relate bowel elimination techniques.
- Describe fluid and dietary requirements.

NIC

Bowel Incontinence Care, Bowel Training, Bowel Management, Skin Surveillance

Generic Interventions

Assess Previous Bowel Elimination Patterns, Diet, and Lifestyle.

Determine Present Neurologic and Physical Status and Functional Level.

Plan a Consistent, Appropriate Time for Elimination:

Daily bowel program for 5 days or until a pattern develops; then bowel program every other day, morning or evening.

For Persons with Intact Sacral Reflex Center:

Position in an upright or sitting position if functionally able. If not functionally able (quadriplegic), position in left side–lying position; use digital stimulation: gloves, lubricant, index finger (adults).

For the functionally able, use assistive devices: dil stick, digital stimulator, raised commode seat, and lubricant and gloves as appropriate.

For Persons with Upper Extremity Mobility and Those with Abdominal Musculature Innervation, Teach Bowel Elimination Facilitation Techniques as Appropriate.

Valsalva's maneuver
Forward bends
Sitting push-ups
Abdominal massage

For Persons with Absent Sacral Reflex Center:

Plan daily evacuation schedule, either morning or evening, with manual evacuation of rectal contents.

Position in upright or sitting position if functionally able.

Use assistive devices, raised commode seats, gloves, and lubricant as appropriate.

Teach bowel facilitation techniques:
- Valsalva's maneuver
- Forward bends
- Abdominal massage
- Sitting push-ups if person is functionally able

Maintain an Elimination Record with Bowel Schedule to Include Time, Stool Results, Method(s) Used, and Number of Involuntary Stools if Any.

Teach the Importance of High-Fiber Diet and Optimal Fluid Intake.

Cleanse Skin after Each Bowel Movement. Protect Intact Skin with an Ointment (e.g., Aluminum Paste). If Skin is Not Intact, Consult Clinical Nurse Specialist or Enterostomal Therapist.

Provide Physical Activity and Exercise Appropriate to Functional Level (e.g., Abdominal Exercises, Walking).

Teach Appropriate Use of Stool Softeners and Suppositories and Hazards of Enemas.

Teach Signs and Symptoms of Fecal Impaction and Constipation.

Provide Home Care Training for Those Who Can Be Functionally Independent with Bowel Program.

BREASTFEEDING, EFFECTIVE

DEFINITION

The state in which a mother-infant dyad exhibits adequate proficiency and satisfaction with the breastfeeding process.

AUTHOR'S NOTE

This diagnosis reportedly represents a wellness diagnosis. The newly proposed NANDA wellness diagnosis is defined as "a clinical judgment about an individual, family or community in transition from a specific level of wellness to a higher level of wellness" (NANDA, 2001). This definition does not describe a mother-infant dyad seeking higher-level breastfeeding. Instead, it describes "adequate proficiency and satisfaction with the breastfeeding process."

In the management of the breastfeeding experience, the nurse will find three situations:

Ineffective Breastfeeding
Risk for Ineffective Breastfeeding
Readiness for Enhanced Breastfeeding

Readiness for Enhanced Breastfeeding can be used to describe correct and satisfying breastfeeding of a mother and child in
(continued)

■■■ **AUTHOR'S NOTE** *(Continued)*
the early weeks. The interventions would focus on teaching basic breastfeeding.

If the nurse, most likely in a community or private practice, has a mother who reports proficiency and satisfaction with the breastfeeding process and desires additional learning to achieve even greater proficiency and satisfaction, the nursing diagnosis of *Readiness for Enhanced Breastfeeding* is appropriate. The focus of this learning and continued support would not be to prevent *Ineffective Breastfeeding* or to maintain adequate proficiency and satisfaction but rather to promote enhanced, higher-quality breastfeeding.

DEFINING CHARACTERISTICS (NANDA)

Mother is able to position infant at breast to promote a successful latch-on response.

Infant is content after feeding.

Regular and sustained suckling/swallowing occurs at the breast.

Infant weight patterns are appropriate for age.

Effective mother-infant communication patterns (infant cues, maternal interpretation and response).

Signs and symptoms of oxytocin release (let-down or milk ejection reflex)

Adequate infant elimination patterns for age

Eagerness of infant to nurse

Maternal verbalization of satisfaction with the breastfeeding process

BREASTFEEDING, INEFFECTIVE

DEFINITION

The state in which a mother, infant, or child experiences or is at risk of experiencing dissatisfaction or difficulty with the breastfeeding process.

DEFINING CHARACTERISTICS
Major (Must Be Present, One or More)

Actual or perceived inadequate milk supply
Infant's inability to attach correctly onto breast
No signs of oxytocin release
Signs of inadequate infant intake
Nonsustained suckling at the breast
Insufficient emptying of each breast at each feeding
Persistence of sore nipples beyond the first week of breastfeeding
Infant exhibiting fussiness and crying within the first hour after breastfeeding; unresponsive to other comfort measures
Infant arching and crying at the breast, resisting latching on

RELATED FACTORS
Physiologic

Related to difficulty of neonate to attach or suck secondary to:
Cleft lip/palate
Prematurity
Previous breast surgery
Inverted nipples
Inadequate let-down reflex
Maternal Stress

Situational (Personal, Environmental)

Related to maternal fatigue
Related to maternal anxiety
Related to maternal ambivalence
Related to multiple birth
Related to inadequate nutritional intake
Related to inadequate fluid intake
Related to history of unsuccessful breastfeeding
Related to nonsupportive partner/family
Related to lack of knowledge
Related to interruption in breastfeeding secondary to:
Ill mother
Ill infant

Related to work schedule and/or barriers in the work environment

NOC
Breastfeeding Establishment: Infant, Breastfeeding Establishment: Maternal, Breastfeeding Maintenance

Goals

- The mother will report confidence in establishing satisfying, effective breastfeeding.
- The mother will demonstrate effective breastfeeding independently.

Indicators

- Identify factors that deter breastfeeding.
- Identify factors that promote breastfeeding.
- Demonstrate effective positioning.

The infant shows signs of adequate intake

Indicators

- Has wet diapers
- Gaining weight
- Relaxed and feeding

NIC

Breastfeeding Assistance, Lactation Counseling

Maternal Interventions

Assess for Factors Contributing to Difficulty or Dissatisfaction (Refer to Related Factors).

If Dissatisfied, Explore Specifics. Encourage Mother to Share Her Concerns Openly. Evaluate Her Fatigue Level, Knowledge, Anxiety, Support System, and History of Breastfeeding.

Evaluate:

Mother's state (comfort, anxiety, position)
Infant's state (quiet, alert, crying, extremely hungry)
Let-down reflex
Baby at breast
Alignment
Areolar grasp
Areolar compression
Audible swallowing
Infant's intake and frequency of feedings
Infants output (six to eight diapers per day, bowel movement daily)

Teach Management of Sore Nipples:

Decrease nursing time to 5 to 10 minutes per side. Start baby on nontender side first. Allow for more frequent, short feedings.

Suggest alternate positions to rotate infant's grasps. Allow breasts to dry after each feeding.

Keep nursing pads dry.

Use breast cream only after breasts are dry.

Use breast shield as last measure, and remove after milk has let down.

Be sure infant's mouth is positioned correctly on the breast.

If Symptoms of Mastitis or Breast Abscess Develop (Increased Warmth, Tenderness, Redness), Instruct Mother to Contact Her Advanced Practice Nurse or Physician.

If Engorgement Occurs:

Massage breast before nursing by encircling breast with both hands and moving hands downward toward nipple. Use lotion if desired.

Use heat before nursing (hot shower, hot pack).

If needed, massage breast again while infant is sucking in shorter sucks at end of feeding.

Use ice packs between feedings.

Wear a good support bra.

Use mild analgesics as needed.

Respond to Concerns Regarding Confidence and "Not Enough Milk."

If Supplementary Feedings Are Used, Consider the Pouch and Tubing Device to Continue Breastfeeding and Prevent Nipple Confusion.

Support Mother's Decision to Continue with Breastfeeding or to Discontinue.

If Breastfeeding Is Interrupted (e.g., Illness, Maternal Employment):

- Allow mother to share her feelings.
- Determine whether breastfeeding can be resumed if desired.

Teach How to Express, Handle, Store, and Transport Breast Milk Safely.

- Can store milk for 8 hours at room temperature
- 3 days in the refrigerator
- 6 months in the freezer
- Microwaving breast milk will destroy its immune properties

Provide Breast Pump, or Make Mother Aware of Availability, If Needed.

Encourage Verbal Expression of Feelings.

Explore Feelings and Anticipation of Problems.
Older Child May Be Jealous of Contact with Baby.
Mother Can Use This Time to Read to Older Child.

Stress the Need for Rest:
Encourage mother to make herself and infant a priority.
Discuss temporary housekeeper.
Encourage mother to limit visits from relatives for first 4 weeks.

**Provide Opportunities for Significant
Others to Ask Questions.**

**Initiate Referrals as Indicated (Lactation
Specialist, La Leche League).**

BREASTFEEDING, INTERRUPTED

DEFINITION

A break in the continuity of the breastfeeding process as a result
of inability to put the baby to breast for feeding or inadvisability
of doing so.

AUTHOR'S NOTE

This diagnosis represents a situation, not a response. If one
examines the diagnosis *Ineffective Breastfeeding*, interrupted
breastfeeding is listed as "related to." Nursing interventions do not treat the interruption but treat the effects of
this interruption. The situation is interrupted breastfeeding; the responses can be varied. For example, if continued
breastfeeding or use of a breast pump is contraindicated, the
nurse will focus on the loss of this breastfeeding experience,
using the nursing diagnosis of *Grieving*. If breastfeeding
is continued with expression and storage of breast milk,
teaching, and support, the diagnosis will be *Risk for Ineffective
Breastfeeding related to continuity problems* secondary to, for
example, maternal employment. If difficulty is experienced,
the diagnosis would be *Ineffective Breastfeeding related to interruption* secondary to (specify) and lack of knowledge. Refer
to *Ineffective Breastfeeding* for interventions.

DEFINING CHARACTERISTICS
Major (Must Be Present)
Infant does not receive nourishment at the breast for some or all of feedings.

Minor (May Be Present)
Maternal desire to maintain lactation and provide (or eventually provide) her breast milk for her infant's nutritional needs

Separation of mother and infant

Lack of knowledge about expression and storage of breast milk

RELATED FACTORS
Maternal or infant illness

Prematurity

Maternal employment

Contraindications to breastfeeding (e.g., drugs, true breast milk jaundice)

Need to wean infant abruptly

CARDIAC OUTPUT, DECREASED

▶ Risk for Complications of Cardiac/Vascular Dysfunction

DEFINITION
The state in which an individual experiences a reduction in the amount of blood pumped by the heart, resulting in compromised cardiac function.

■■■■ AUTHOR'S NOTE
This diagnosis represents a situation in which nurses have multiple responsibilities. Individuals experiencing decreased cardiac output may present various responses that disrupt functioning, such as:

- *Activity Intolerance*
- *Disturbed Sleep Pattern*

(continued)

• They may be at risk for developing physiologic complications, such as:
• Dysrhythmias
• Cardiogenic shock
• Congestive heart failure

I recommend that the nurse not use *Decreased Cardiac Output* but instead select nursing diagnoses that are resonses to decreased cardiac output as *Activity Intolerance*. Disturbed Sleep Patterns, Anxiety. For the physiological complications of decreased cardiac output, refer to collaborative problems as Risk for Complications of Cardiovascular Dysfunction or Risk for Complications of Dysrhthmias.

DEFINING CHARACTERISTICS

Low blood pressure	Vertigo
Rapid pulse	Edema (peripheral, sacral)
Dyspnea	Restlessness
Angina	Cyanosis
Dysrhythmia	Oliguria
Fatigability	

CAREGIVER ROLE STRAIN

Caregiver Role Strain
Caregiver Role Strain, Risk for

DEFINITION

A state in which an individual is experiencing physical, emotional, social, and/or financial burden(s) in the process of giving care to another.

■■■■ **AUTHOR'S NOTE**
Health care policies that rely on caregiver sacrifice can be made to appear cost effective only if the emotional, social, physical, and financial costs incurred by the caregiver are

(continued)

▪▪▪▪ **AUTHOR'S NOTE** *(Continued)*
ignored" (Winslow & Carter, 1999, p. 285). These caregivers provide care for individuals of all ages, some across their entire life span (e.g., children with permanent disabilities). The care receivers have physical or mental disabilities. These disabilities can be temporary or permanent. Some disabilities are permanent but stable (e.g., blind child), whereas others signal progressive deterioration (e.g., Alzheimer's disease).

Caregiver Role Strain represents the burden of caregiving on the physical and emotional health of the caregiver and its effects on the family and social system of the caregiver and care receiver. *Risk for Caregiver Role Strain* can be a significant nursing diagnosis, because nurses can identify at-risk individuals and assist them to prevent this grave situation.

DEFINING CHARACTERISTICS

Expressed or Observed

Reports insufficient time or physical energy
Difficulty performing caregiving activities required
Caregiving responsibilities interfere with other important roles
    (e.g., work, spouse, friend, parent)
Apprehension about the future for the care receiver's health and
    ability to provide care
Apprehension about care receiver's care when caregiver is ill or
    deceased
Depressed feelings, anger
Feelings of exhaustion
Feelings of resentment

RELATED FACTORS

Pathophysiologic

Related to unrelenting or complex care requirements secondary to:

Debilitating conditions   Chronic mental illness
    (acute, progressive)   Unpredictable illness course
Progressive dementia   Addiction
Disability

Treatment-Related

Related to 24-hour care responsibilities
Related to time (activities, e.g., dialysis, transportation)

Situational (Personal, Environmental)

Related to unrealistic expectations of caregiver by care receiver

Related to pattern of ineffective coping

Related to compromised physical health

Related to unrealistic expectations of self

Related to history of poor relationship

Related to history of family dysfunction

Related to unrealistic expectations for caregiver by others (society, other family members)

Related to duration of caregiving required

Related to isolation

Related to insufficient respite

Related to insufficient recreation

Related to insufficient finances

Related to no or unavailable support

Maturational (Infant, Child, Adolescent)

Related to unrelenting care requirements secondary to:

Mental disabilities (specify)

Physical disabilities (specify)

NOC

Caregiver Well-Being, Caregiver Performance, Caregiver Emotional Health, Family Coping, Family Integrity, Family Resiliency, Caregiver-Patient Relationship

Goals

The caregiver will report a plan to decrease his or her burden.

Indicators

- Share frustrations regarding caregiving responsibilities.
- Identify one source of support.
- Identify two changes that, if made, would improve daily life.

The family will establish a plan for weekly support or help.

- Relate an intent to listen without giving advice.
- Convey empathy to caregiver regarding daily responsibilities.

NIC

Caregiver Support, Respite Care, Coping Enhancement, Family Mobilization, Mutual Goal Setting, Support System Enhancement, Anticipatory Guidance

Generic Interventions

Assess for Causative or Contributing Factors:

Poor insight into situation
Unrealistic expectations (caregiver, family)
Reluctance or inability to access help
Unsatisfactory caregiver–care receiver relationship
Insufficient resources (e.g., help, financial)
Social isolation
Insufficient leisure
Competing roles (spouse, parenting, work)

Evaluate Caregiver's and Others' Interpretation of the Situation. Re-evaluate Periodically (Winslow & Carter, 1999).

What information have they been told?
Do they expect the situation to continue as is, improve, or worsen?
Are they realistic?

Provide Empathy and Promote a Sense of Competency.

Discuss the Effects of Present Schedule and Responsibilities on:

Physical health
Emotional status
Relationships

Assist to Identify Activities for Which Assistance Is Desired:

Care receiver's needs (hygiene, food, treatments, mobility)
Meals
Transportation
Yard work
Respite (number of hours per week)
Laundry
House cleaning
Shopping, errands
Appointments (doctor, hairdresser)
House repairs
Money management

Discuss with the Family (Shields, 1992; Winslow & Carter, 1999):

The importance of regularly acknowledging the burden of the situation for the caregiver

The benefits of listening without giving advice
The importance of emotional support:
- Regular phone calls
- Cards, letters
- Visits

The need to give caregiver "permission" to enjoy self (e.g., vacations, day trips)
The need to provide caregiver with opportunities to respond to "How can I help you?"

Identify All Possible Sources of Volunteer Help: Family (Siblings, Cousins), Friends, Neighbors, Church, Community Groups.

Role-Play How to Ask for Help.

Identify Community Resources Available:

Support groups	Counseling
Social services	Transportation
Home-delivered meals	Day care

Ⓒ Geriatric Interventions

If appropriate, discuss if and when an alternative source of care (e.g., nursing home, senior housing) may be indicated.
If elder abuse is suspected, refer to *Disabled Family Coping*.

▶ Caregiver Role Strain, Risk for

DEFINITION

The state in which an individual is at high risk to experience physical, emotional, social, and/or financial burden(s) in the process of giving care to another.

AUTHOR'S NOTE
Refer to *Caregiver Role Strain*.

RISK FACTORS

Presence of risk factors (refer to Related Factors)

RELATED FACTORS

Primary caregiver responsibilities for a recipient who requires regular assistance with self-care or supervision because of physical or mental disabilities in addition to one or more of the following:

Related to unrelenting or complex care requirements secondary to:

Care receiver characteristics
Unable to perform self-care activities
Not motivated to perform self-care activities
Cognitive problems
Psychological problems
Unrealistic expectations of caregiver
Caregiver/spouse characteristics
Pattern of ineffective coping
Compromised physical health
Unrealistic expectations of self
Related to history of relationship conflicts
Related to history of family dysfunction
Related to unrealistic expectations for caregiver by others
(society, other family members)
Related to duration of caregiving required
Related to isolation
Related to insufficient respite
Related to insufficient recreation
Related to insufficient finances
Related to no or unavailable support

NOC

Refer to *Caregiver Role Strain*

Goals

The person will relate a plan on how to continue social activities despite caregiving responsibilities.

Indicators

- Identify activities that are important for self.
- Relate an intent to enlist the help of at least two people.

NIC

Refer to *Caregiver Role Strain*

Generic Interventions

Explain factors that contribute to caregiver role strain

Poor insight into situation
Unrealistic expectations (caregiver, family)
Reluctance or inability to access help
Unsatisfactory caregiver–care receiver relationship

Insufficient resources (e.g., help, financial)
Social isolation
Insufficient leisure
Competing roles (spouse, parenting, work)

Assist with Anticipating the Effects of the Caregiving Role.

Stress the Importance of Daily Health-Promotion Activities:

Rest-exercise balance
Effective stress management
Low-fat, high–complex carbohydrate diet
Supportive social networks
Appropriate screening practices for age
See *Health-Seeking Behaviors* for specific interventions.

Discuss the Need for Respite and Short-Term Relief.

Maintain a Good Sense of Humor; Associate with Others Who Laugh.

Caution About Spending Too Much Time Complaining, Which Is Depressing for All Involved and May Lead to Avoidance.

Advise to Initiate Phone Contacts or Visits with Friends or Relatives Rather Than Waiting for Others to Do It.

Emphasize the Importance of Respites to Prevent Isolating Behaviors That Foster Depression.

Discuss the Implications of Caring for Ill Family Member with All Family Members. Include:

Available resources (finances, environmental)
24-hour responsibility
Effects on other household members
Likelihood of progressive deterioration
Sharing of responsibilities (with other household members, siblings, neighbors)
Likelihood of exacerbating long-standing conflicts
Impact on lifestyle
Alternative or assistive options (e.g., community-based health care providers, life care centers, group living, nursing home)

Assist to Identify Activities for Which Assistance Is Desired:

Care receiver's needs
(hygiene, food, treatments,
mobility)
Meals
Transportation
Yard work
Respite (number of hours per
week)

Laundry
House cleaning
Shopping, errands
Appointments (doctor,
hairdresser)
House repairs
Money management

Identify Community Resources Available:

Support group
Social service
Home-delivered meals

Counseling
Transportation
Day care

COMFORT, IMPAIRED

Comfort, Impaired*
Acute Pain
Chronic Pain
Nausea

DEFINITION

The state in which an individual experiences an uncomfortable
sensation in response to a noxious stimulus.

AUTHOR'S NOTE

This diagnosis, *Impaired Comfort*, can represent a variety of
uncomfortable sensations, such as pruritus, immobility, or
nothing by mouth (NPO) status. When an individual experiences nausea and vomiting, the nurse should assess whether
Nausea or *Risk for Imbalanced Nutrition* is the appropriate
category. Short-lived episodes of nausea or vomiting (e.g.,
postoperatively) can be best described with *Nausea related to
nausea/vomiting secondary to effects of anesthesia or analgesics.*
When the nausea/vomiting is at risk of compromising

(continued)

*This diagnosis is not currently on the NANDA list but has been included for
clarity and usefulness.

■■■ **AUTHOR'S NOTE** *(Continued)*
nutritional intake, use *Risk for Imbalanced Nutrition: Less Than Body Requirements related to nausea and vomiting secondary to* (specify).

DEFINING CHARACTERISTICS

Major (Must Be Present)

The person reports or demonstrates discomfort (e.g., pain, nausea, vomiting, pruritus).

Minor (May Be Present)

Autonomic response to acute pain:
- Blood pressure increased
- Pulse increased
- Respirations increased
- Diaphoresis
- Dilated pupils

Guarded position
Facial mask of pain
Crying, moaning

RELATED FACTORS

Any factor can contribute to altered comfort. The most common are listed below.

Biopathophysiologic

Related to uterine contractions during labor
Related to trauma to perineum during labor and delivery
Related to involution of uterus and engorged breasts
Related to tissue trauma and reflex muscle spasms secondary to:

Musculoskeletal Disorders

Fractures	Arthritis
Contractures	Spinal cord disorders
Spasms	

Visceral Disorders

Cardiac	Intestinal
Renal	Pulmonary
Hepatic	

Vascular Disorders

Vasospasm	Phlebitis

Occlusion   Vasodilation (headache)
Cancer

Related to inflammation of:
Nerve   Joint
Tendon   Muscle
Bursa   Juxtoarticular structures

Related to fatigue, malaise, and/or pruritus secondary to
contagious disease:
Rubella   Mononucleosis
Chickenpox   Pancreatitis
Hepatitis

Related to effects of cancer on (specify)

Related to abdominal cramps, diarrhea, and vomiting
secondary to gastroenteritis, influenza, or gastric ulcers

Related to inflammation and smooth-muscle spasms secondary
to renal calculi or gastrointestinal infections

Treatment-Related

Related to tissue trauma and reflex muscle spasms secondary
to:
Surgery
Accidents
Burns
Diagnostic tests:
  • Venipuncture
  • Invasive scanning
  • Biopsy
Related to nausea and vomiting secondary to chemotherapy,
  anesthesia, or side effects of (specify)

Situational (Personal, Environmental)

Related to fever

Related to immobility/improper positioning

Related to overactivity

Related to pressure points (tight cast, elastic bandage)

Related to allergic response

Related to chemical irritants

Related to unmet dependency needs

Related to severe repressed anxiety

Maturational

Related to tissue trauma secondary to:
Infancy: Colic
Infancy and early childhood: Teething, ear pain
Middle childhood: Recurrent abdominal pain, growing pains
Adolescence: Headaches, chest pain, dysmenorrhea

▶ Acute Pain

DEFINITION

The state in which an individual experiences and reports the presence of severe discomfort or an uncomfortable sensation lasting from 1 second to <6 months.

> **AUTHOR'S NOTE**
> The NANDA list contains *Acute Pain* and *Chronic Pain*. For clarity and usefulness, the author has organized diagnoses associated with pain and discomfort under two levels:
>
> *Impaired Comfort*
> - *Acute Pain*
> - *Chronic Pain*

DEFINING CHARACTERISTICS

Self-report of pain quality and intensity
For patients unable to provide self-reports:

- Presence of pathological condition or procedure known to cause pain
- Physiological responses as:
    diaphoresis
    changes in blood pressure or pulse
    pupil dilation
    change in respiratory rate
    guarding
    grimacing
    moaning, crying
    restlessness
- Surrogate reports (family, caregivers)
- Response to an analgesic trial

RELATED FACTORS

Refer to *Impaired Comfort*.

NOC

Comfort Level, Pain Level, Pain Control

Goals

The person will relate relief after a satisfactory relief measure as evidenced by (specify).

Indicators
• Relate factors that increase pain.
• Relate interventions that are effective.
• Convey that others validate that the pain exists.

NIC

Pain Management, Medication Management, Emotional Support, Teaching: Individual, Hot/Cold Application, Simple Massage

Generic Interventions

Reduce Lack of Knowledge:

Explain causes of the pain to the person, if known.
Relate how long the pain will last, if known.
Explain diagnostic tests and procedures in detail by relating the discomforts and sensations that will be felt, and approximate the length of time involved (e.g., "During the intravenous pyelogram, you might feel a momentary hot flash through your entire body.").

Provide Accurate Information to Reduce Fear of Addiction.

Relate Your Acceptance of the Person's Response to Pain:

Acknowledge the presence of the pain.
Listen attentively concerning the pain.
Convey that you are assessing the pain because you want to understand it better (not determine if it is really present).

Discuss the Reasons Why an Individual May Experience Increased or Decreased Pain (e.g., Fatigue [Increased] or Presence of Distractions [Decreased]).

Encourage family members to share their concerns privately (e.g., fear that the person will use pain for secondary gains if they give the person too much attention).

Assess whether the family doubts the pain, and discuss the effects of this on the person's pain and on the relationship.

Encourage the family to give attention also when pain is not exhibited.

Provide the Person with Opportunities to Rest During the Day and with Periods of Uninterrupted Sleep at Night (Must Rest When Pain Is Decreased).

Discuss with the Person and Family the Therapeutic Uses of Distraction as Well as Other Methods of Pain Relief.

Teach a Method of Distraction During Acute Pain (e.g., Painful Procedure) That Is Not a Burden (e.g., Count Items in a Picture; Count Anything in the Room, Such as Patterns on Wallpaper; Count Silently to Self; Breathe Rhythmically; Listen to Music, and Increase the Volume as the Pain Increases).

Teach Noninvasive Pain-Relief Measures.

Relaxation

Instruct on techniques to reduce skeletal muscle tension, which will reduce the intensity of the pain.

Promote relaxation with a back rub, massage, or warm bath.

Teach a specific relaxation strategy (e.g., slow, rhythmic breathing or deep breath—clench fists—yawn).

Cutaneous Stimulation

Discuss the various methods of skin stimulation and their effects on pain.

Discuss the following methods and the precautions:
- Hot water bottle, warm tub
- Electric heating pad, moist heat pack
- Hot summer sun
- Thin plastic wrap over painful area to retain body heat (e.g., knee, elbow)
- Cold towels (wrung out)
- Cold-water immersion for small body parts
- Ice bag, cold gel pack, ice massage

Explain the therapeutic uses of menthol preparations and massage/back rub.

Provide Optimal Pain Relief with Prescribed Analgesics.

After Administering a Pain-relief Medication, Return in 30 Minutes to Assess Effectiveness.

Give Accurate Information to Correct Family Misconceptions (e.g., Addiction, Doubts about Pain).

Provide Individuals with Opportunities to Discuss Their Fears, Anger, and Frustrations in Private; Acknowledge the Difficulty of the Situation.

👥 Pediatric Interventions

Assess the Child's Pain Experience:

Determine the child's concept of the cause of pain, if feasible.
Ask the child to point to the area that hurts.
For younger children, use Oucher Scale of five faces from very happy (1) to crying (5).
For older children, ask to rate the pain using a scale of 0 to 5 (0 = no pain, 5 = worst pain).
Ask the child what makes the pain better and what makes it worse.
Assess if fear or loneliness is contributing to the pain.

Promote Security with Honest Explanations and Opportunities for Choice.

Tell the truth. Explain:
- How much it will hurt
- How long it will last
- What will help the pain

Do not threaten (e.g., *do not* tell the child, "If you don't hold still, you won't go home.").
Explicitly explain and reinforce to the child that pain is not a means of punishment.
Explain to the parents that the child may cry more openly when they are present but that their presence is important for promoting trust.
Explain to the child that the procedure is necessary so he or she can get better, and it is important to hold still so the procedure can be done quickly.
Discuss with the parents the importance of truth-telling. Instruct parents to:
- Tell the child when they are leaving and when they will return.

- Relate to the child that they cannot take away the pain but that they will be there (except in circumstances when parents are not permitted to remain).

Allow the parents opportunities to share their feelings about witnessing their child's pain and their helplessness.

Prepare the Child for a Painful Procedure:

Discuss the procedure with the parents; determine what they have told the child.

Explain the procedure in words suited to the child's age and developmental level.

Relate the discomforts that will be felt (e.g., what the child will feel, taste, see, or smell).

Encourage the child to ask questions before and during the procedure; ask the child to share with you what he or she thinks is going to happen and why.

Share with the child (who is old enough, between 3 and 12 years):

- You expect that the child will hold still and that such behavior will be pleasing to you.
- It is all right to cry or squeeze your hand if it hurts.

Arrange to have parents present for procedures (especially for children 18 months to 5 years).

Explain to the Child That He or She Can Be Distracted from the Procedure If He or She Wishes. (The Use of Distraction Without the Child's Knowledge of the Impending Discomfort Is Not Advocated Because the Child Will Learn to Mistrust):

Tell a story with a puppet.

Ask the child to name or count objects in a picture.

Ask the child to look at a picture, and to locate certain objects ("Where is the dog?").

Ask the child to tell you about a pet.

Ask the child to count your blinks.

Blow a party noisemaker.

Provide the Child with Privacy During the Painful Procedure; Use a Treatment Room Rather Than the Child's Bed.

Assist the Child with the Aftermath of Pain:

Tell the child when the painful procedure is over.

Pick up the small child to indicate that it is over.

Encourage the child to discuss the pain experience (draw or act out with dolls).

Encourage the child to perform the painful procedure under supervision using the same equipment on a doll.

Praise the child for endurance, and convey that the pain was handled well, regardless of the child's behavior (unless the child was violent to others).

Give the child a souvenir of the pain (Band-Aid, badge for bravery).

Teach the child to keep a record of painful experiences and to place a star next to those for which he or she held still (e.g., gold stars on a paper for each injection or venipuncture).

👥 Maternal Interventions

Assess Contractions and Discomfort (Onset, Frequency, Duration, Intensity, Description of Discomfort).

Determine the Presence of Other Discomforts Not Related to Labor (e.g., Chronic or Recent Illness).

Assess Goals and Expectations Regarding:
- Labor
- Pain relief methods
- Persons to be present
- Medications

Explain Pain Relief Methods Available:
- Relaxation techniques
- Breathing patterns
- Acupressure
- Massage
- Cold/heat applications
- Positioning
- Physical activities
- Distraction
- Medications

Determine What Types of Methods Are Desired. Encourage Client to Try Several Methods.

Coach Her with the Method, and Include Her Labor Support Person.

Stand and Walk as Much as Possible During First Stage.

Change Positions at Least Every Hour.

For Backaches, Try Squatting, Kneeling, or an All-Fours Position (Hands and Knees).

Encourage Use of Heat (Bath, Showers, Heating Pad) for Lower Abdomen, Groin, Back, Perineum, or Thigh Pain.

For Back Pain, Apply Cold Pack to Back or Neck (20 to 30 Minutes).

If Mother Panics During Transition, Be Firm and Direct:
- "I'm here, and I'm in charge."
- "I'm here for you."
- Make her look at you.
- Hold her wrist.
- Exaggerate your coaching breathing.

Assist Her with the Aftermath of Labor:
- Praise her for her hard work.
- Allow her to relive difficult moments.
- Explain why pain increased.
- Acknowledge support person's help.

▶ Chronic Pain

DEFINITION

The state in which an individual experiences pain that is persistent or intermittent and lasts for >6 months.

DEFINING CHARACTERISTICS

Major (Must Be Present)

The person reports that pain has existed for >6 months (may be the only assessment data present).

Minor (60% to 79%)

Disruption of social and family relationships
Irritability
Physical inactivity or immobility
Depression
Rubbing of painful part
Anxiety
"Beaten" look
Self-focusing
Skeletal muscle tension
Somatic preoccupation

Agitation
Fatigue
Decreased libido
Restlessness

RELATED FACTORS

Refer to *Impaired Comfort*.

NOC

Comfort Status, Pain Level, Pain Control, Depression
Level

Goals

The person will relate improvement of pain and an increase in
daily activities as evidenced by (specify).

Indicators

* Relate that others validate that the pain exists.
* Practice selected noninvasive pain relief measures to manage
  the pain.

The child will demonstrate coping mechanism for pain and methods of controlling pain, as evidenced by an increase in play and
usual activities of childhood, and (specify).

* Communicate improvement in pain verbally, by pain assessment scale, or by behavior (specify).
* Maintain usual family role and relationships throughout pain
  experience, as evidenced by (specify).

NIC

Pain Management, Medication Management, Exercise
Promotion, Mood Management, Coping Enhancement

Generic Interventions

Refer to *Acute Pain*.

Assess the Effects of Chronic Pain on the Individual's Life.

Performance (job, role responsibilities)
Social interactions
Finances
Activities of daily living (sleeping, eating, mobility, sex)

Cognition/mood (concentration, depression)
Family unit (response of members)

Explore Expectations of Course of Pain, Treatment, and Side Effects; Clarify if Unrealistic.

Discuss the Effectiveness of Combining Physical and Psychological Techniques and Pharmacotherapy.

Discuss with the Individual and Family the Various Treatment Modalities Available (Family Therapy, Group Therapy, Behavior Modification, Biofeedback, Hypnosis, Acupuncture, Exercise Program, Cognitive Strategies).

Discuss the Suffering Caused by the Pain Experience: Decreased Endurance, Poor Appetite, Interrupted Sleep, Diminished Enjoyment, Anxiety, Fear, Difficulty Concentrating, and Diminished Social and Sexual Relationships

👥 Pediatric Interventions

Assess Pain Experiences by Using Developmentally Appropriate Assessment Scales and by Assessing Behavior.

Set Goals for Pain Management with Child and Family (Short- and Long-Term), and Evaluate Regularly.

Promote the "Normal" Aspects of the Child's Life: Play, School, Relationships with Family, Physical Activity.

Promote a Trusting Environment for the Child and Family:

Believe the child's pain.
Encourage the child's perception that interventions are attempts to help.
Have the child, family, and nurse participate in controlling pain.

Use Interdisciplinary Team for Pain Management as Necessary (e.g., Nurse, Physician, Child Life Therapist, Mental Health Therapist, Occupational Therapist, Physical Therapist, Nutritionist).

▶ Nausea

DEFINITION

The state in which an individual experiences an unpleasant, wavelike sensation in the back of the throat, epigastric area, or throughout the abdomen that may or may not lead to vomiting.

DEFINING CHARACTERISTICS

Usually precedes vomiting, but may be experienced after vomiting or when vomiting does not occur

Accompanied by pallor, cold and clammy skin, increased salivation, tachycardia, gastric stasis, and diarrhea

Accompanied by swallowing movements affected by skeletal muscles

Reports "nausea" or "sick to my stomach"

RELATED FACTORS

Biopathophysiologic

Related to gastrointestinal irritation secondary to:

Acute gastroenteritis
Irritable bowel syndrome
Migraine headaches
Infections (e.g., food poisoning)
Renal calculi

Peptic ulcer disease
Pancreatitis
Pregnancy
Drug overdose
Motion sickness

Treatment-Related

Related to effects of medications (e.g., chemotherapy, theophylline, digitalis, or antibiotics)
Related to effects of anesthesia

NOC

Comfort Status, Hydration, Nutritional Status

Goals

The person will report decreased nausea.

Indicators

- Name foods or beverages that do not increase nausea.
- Describe factors that increase nausea.

NIC

Medication Management, Nausea Management, Fluid/
Electrolyte Management, Nutrition Management

Generic Interventions

**Explain the Cause of the Nausea
and the Duration if Known.**

**Encourage the Client to Eat Small, Frequent
Meals and to Eat Slowly. Cool, Bland Foods
and Liquids Are Usually Well Tolerated.**

**Eliminate Unpleasant Sights and
Odors from the Eating Area.**

Instruct the Client to Avoid the following:

- Hot or cold liquids
- Foods containing fat and fiber
- Spicy foods
- Caffeine

**Encourage the Client to Rest in a Semi-Fowler's
Position after Eating and to Change Position Slowly.**

Teach Techniques to Reduce Nausea:

- Restrict fluid with meals.
- Avoid the smell of food preparation and other noxious stimuli.
- Loosen clothing before eating.
- Sit in fresh air or use a fan.
- Avoid lying flat for at least 2 hours after eating.

**Determine Etiology of Nausea and Consult with
Nurse Practitioner or Physician for Treatment:**

- Cough
- Constipation
- Urinary tract infection
- Reflux disease
- Electrolyte imbalances
- Candidiasis
- Increased intracranial pressure
- Pharmaceutical agent
- Anxiety

**Teach How to Use Antiemetic Medications
Aggressively Prior to and After
Chemotherapy (Eckert, 2001).**

COMMUNICATION, IMPAIRED

Communication, Impaired*
Communication, Impaired Verbal

DEFINITION

The state in which an individual experiences or is at high risk to experience difficulty exchanging thoughts, ideas, desires, wants, or needs with others.

AUTHOR'S NOTE

Impaired Communication and *Impaired Verbal Communication* are diagnoses to describe people who desire to communicate but who are encountering problems. *Impaired Communication* may not be useful to describe a person for whom communication problems are a manifestation of a psychiatric illness or coping problem. If nursing interventions are focusing on reducing hallucinations, fear, or anxiety, the diagnosis of *Fear*, *Anxiety*, or *Disturbed Thought Processes* is more appropriate.

DEFINING CHARACTERISTICS

Major (Must Be Present, One or More)

Impaired ability to speak or hear
Inappropriate or absent speech or response

Minor (May Be Present)

Incongruence between verbal
    and nonverbal messages
Stuttering
Dysarthria
Aphasia
Slurring
Word-finding problems
Weak or absent voice
Statements of not
    understanding or being
    misunderstood

---

*This diagnosis was developed by Rosalinda Alfaro-LeFevre and is not currently on the NANDA list; it has been included for clarity or usefulness.

RELATED FACTORS

Pathophysiologic

Related to disordered, unrealistic thinking secondary to schizophrenic disorder, delusional disorder, psychotic or paranoid disorder

Related to impaired motor function of muscles of speech secondary to: or

Related to ischemia of temporal or frontal lobe secondary to:

Expressive or receptive aphasia
Cerebrovascular accident
Oral, facial trauma
Alzheimer's disease
Brain damage (e.g., birth/head trauma)
Central nervous system (CNS) depression/increased intracranial pressure
Tumor (head, neck, or spinal cord)
Chronic hypoxia/decreased cerebral blood flow
Quadriplegia
CNS diseases (e.g., myasthenia gravis, multiple sclerosis, muscular dystrophy)
Vocal cord paralysis

Related to impaired ability to produce speech secondary to:

Respiratory impairment (e.g., shortness of breath)
Laryngeal edema/infection
Oral deformities
Cleft lip or palate
Malocclusion or fractured jaw
Missing teeth
Dysarthria

Related to auditory impairment

Treatment-Related

Related to impaired ability to produce speech secondary to:

Endotracheal intubation
Tracheostomy/tracheotomy/laryngectomy
Surgery of the head, face, neck, or mouth
Pain (especially of the mouth or throat)

Situational (Personal, Environmental)

Related to decreased attention secondary to fatigue, anger, anxiety, or pain

Related to access to hearing aid or malfunction of hearing aid

Related to psychological barrier (e.g., fear, shyness)

Related to lack of privacy
Related to loss of recent memory recall
Related to lack of interpreter

Maturational

Infant/Child
Related to inadequate sensory stimulation

Older Adult (Auditory Losses)
Related to hearing impairment
Related to cognitive impairments secondary to (specify)

NOC

Communication, Communication: Expressive, Communication: Receptive

Goals

The person will report improved satisfaction with ability to communicate.

Indicators

- Demonstrate increased ability to understand.
- Demonstrate improved ability to express self.
- Use alternative methods of communication, as indicated.

NIC

Communication Enhancement: Hearing Deficit, Communication Enhancement: Speech Deficit, Active Listening, Socialization Enhancement

Generic Interventions

Use Factors that Promote Hearing and Understanding.

Talk distinctly and clearly, facing the person.
Minimize unnecessary sounds in the room.
- Have only one person talk.
- Be aware of background noises (e.g., close the door, turn off the television or radio).

Repeat, then rephrase, a thought if the person does not seem to understand the whole meaning.
Use touch and gestures to enhance communication.
If the person can understand only sign language, have an interpreter present as often as possible.

If the person is in a group (e.g., diabetes class), place him or her in front of the room near the teacher.

Approach the person from the side on which hearing is best (e.g., if hearing is better with left ear, approach the person from the left).

If the person can lip-read, look directly at the person, and talk slowly and clearly.

Assess functioning of hearing aids (e.g., batteries).

Provide Alternative Methods of Communication.

Use pad and pencil, alphabet letters, hand signals, eye blinks, head nods, bell signals.

Make flash cards with pictures or words depicting frequently used phrases (e.g., "Wet my lips," "Move my foot," glass of water, bedpan).

Encourage the person to point and to use gestures and pantomime.

Provide a Non-rushed Environment.

Use normal loudness level, and speak unhurriedly in short phrases.

Encourage the person to take plenty of time talking and to enunciate words carefully with good lip movements.

Decrease external distractions.

Delay conversation when the person is tired.

Use Techniques to Increase Understanding.

Use uncomplicated one-step commands and directives.

Encourage the use of gestures and pantomime.

Match words with actions; use pictures.

Terminate conversation on a note of success (e.g., move back to an easier item).

Use same words with same task.

Make a Concerted Effort to Understand When the Person is Speaking.

Allow enough time to listen if the person speaks slowly.

Rephrase the person's message aloud to validate it.

Respond to all attempts at speech even if they are unintelligible (e.g., "I do not know what you are saying. Can you try to say it again?").

Ignore mistakes and profanity.

Do not pretend you understand if you do not.

Allow the person time to respond; do not interrupt. Supply words only occasionally.

Teach Techniques to Improve Speech.

Ask the person to slow speech down and to say each word clearly; provide an example.

Encourage the person to speak in short phrases.

Suggest a slower rate of talking or taking a breath before beginning to speak.

Encourage the person to take time and concentrate on forming the words.

Ask the person to write the message or to draw a picture if verbal communication is difficult.

Ask questions that can be answered with a "yes" or "no."

Focus on the present; avoid topics that are controversial, emotional, abstract, or lengthy.

Verbally Address the Problem of Frustration about Inability to Communicate, and Explain that Patience is Needed for the Nurse and the Person Who is Trying to Talk.

Give the Person Opportunities to Make Decisions about Care (e.g., "Do You Want a Drink?" "Would You Rather Have Orange Juice or Prune Juice?").

Teach Techniques to Significant Others and Repetitive Approaches to Improve Communications.

If a Translator is Needed, Refer to Impaired Verbal Communication.

If the Person is Hearing-Impaired, Refer to Geriatric Interventions.

Ⓒ Geriatric Interventions

If the person can hear with a hearing aid, make sure that it is on and functioning.

If the person can hear with one ear, speak slowly and clearly into the good ear. (It is more important to speak distinctly than to speak loudly.)

If the person can read and write, provide pad and pencil at all times (even when going to another department).

If the person can understand only sign language, have an interpreter with him or her as much as possible.

Write and speak all important messages.

Validate the person's understanding by asking questions that require more than "yes" or "no" answers. Avoid asking, "Do you understand?"

Assess if cerumen impaction is impairing hearing.

▶ Communication, Impaired Verbal

DEFINITION

The state in which an individual experiences or is at high risk to experience a decreased ability to speak but can understand others.

DEFINING CHARACTERISTICS

Major (Must Be Present)

Inability to speak words but can understand others *or*
Articulation or motor planning deficits

Minor (May Be Present)

Shortness of breath

RELATED FACTORS

See *Impaired Communication*.

NOC

Communication: Expressive

Goals

The person will demonstrate improved ability to express self.

Indicators

• Relate decreased frustration with communication.
• Use alternative methods as indicated.

NIC

Active Listening, Communication Enhancement: Speech Deficit

Generic Interventions

Identify a method by which the person can communicate basic needs.
Provide alternative methods of communication:
  • Use pad and pencil, alphabet letters, hand signals, eye blinks, head nods, bell signals.
  • Make flash cards with pictures or words depicting frequently used phrases (e.g., "Wet my lips," "Move my foot," glass of water, bedpan).

- Encourage the person to point and to use gestures and pantomime.
- Consult with speech pathologist for assistance in acquiring flash cards.

For individuals with dysarthria:

- Reduce environmental noise.
- Encourage the person to make a conscious effort to slow speech down and to speak louder (e.g., "Take a deep breath between sentences.").
- Ask the person to repeat words that are unclear.
- If the person is tired, ask questions that require only short answers.
- If speech is unintelligible, teach the person to use gestures, written messages, and communication cards.

Do not alter your speech, tone, or type of message, because the person's ability to understand is not affected; speak on an adult level.

Verbally address the problem of frustration about inability to communicate, and explain that patience is needed for the nurse and the person who is trying to talk.

Write the method of communication that is used on the person's care plan.

Teach significant others techniques and repetitive approaches to improve communication.

Encourage the family to share feelings concerning communication problems.

Seek consultation with a speech pathologist early in treatment regimen.

For individuals with language barriers (Giger & Davidhizar, 2009):

- Communicate in an unhurried, caring manner. Be polite and formal.
- Speak in a low, moderate voice. Listen carefully; validate mutual understanding.
- Use gestures and pictures.
- Keep the message simple; do not use medical or technical terms.
- If an interpreter is needed:
- Clarify what language is spoken at home.
- Attempt to use same gender and similar age as client.
- Avoid interpreters from rival tribe, nation.
- Ask to translate verbatim.

Use telephone translating system when necessary.

CONFUSION*

Confusion
Acute Confusion
Acute Confusion, Risk for
Chronic Confusion

DEFINITION

The state in which the individual experiences or is at risk of experiencing a disturbance in cognition, attention, memory, and orientation of an undetermined origin or onset.

AUTHOR'S NOTE
This author has added *Confusion* to the diagnostic list to provide the nurse with an option when the origin, onset, or duration of the confusion is unknown. By providing this diagnostic option, the nurse can refrain from too quickly labeling the confusion as acute or chronic. Careful assessment is indicated. Until data collection is complete, the diagnosis can be written as *Confusion related to unknown etiology as evidenced by* (specify supporting data).

DEFINING CHARACTERISTICS
Major (Must Be Present, One or More)
Disturbances of:

Consciousness
Attention
Perception

Memory
Orientation
Thinking

Minor (May Be Present)
Misperceptions
Hypervigilance
Agitation

*This diagnosis is not currently on the NANDA list but has been included for clarity and usefulness.

▶ Acute Confusion

DEFINITION

The state in which there is an abrupt onset of a cluster of global, fluctuating disturbances in consciousness, attention, perception, memory, orientation, thinking, sleep-wake cycle, and psychomotor behavior

DEFINING CHARACTERISTICS

Major (Some Must Be Present)

Abrupt onset of:

Reduced ability to focus	Hypervigilance
Disorientation	Restlessness
Incoherence	Fear
Anxiety	Excitement

Symptoms worse at night or when fatigued

Minor (May Be Present)

Illusions	Hallucinations
Delusions	Misperception of stimuli

RISK FACTORS

Presence of risk factors (see Related Factors)

RELATED FACTORS

Pathophysiologic

Related to abrupt onset of cerebral hypoxia or disturbance in cerebral metabolism secondary to (Miller, 2009):

Fluid and Electrolyte Disturbances

Dehydration	Hypercalcemia
Volume depletion	Hyponatremia/hypernatremia
Acidosis/alkalosis	Hypoglycemia/hyperglycemia
Hypokalemia	

Nutritional Deficiencies

Folate or vitamin B_{12} deficiency	Niacin deficiency
Anemia	Magnesium deficiency

Cardiovascular Disturbances

Myocardial infarction	Heart block
Congestive heart failure	Temporal arteritis
Dysrhythmias	

Respiratory Disorders

Chronic obstructive
    pulmonary disease

Pulmonary embolism

Tuberculosis

Pneumonia

Infections

Sepsis

Meningitis, encephalitis

Urinary tract infection

Metabolic and Endocrine Disorders

Hypothyroidism

Hypopituitarism

Parathyroid disorders

Hypoadrenocorticism

Postural hypotension

Hypothermia/hyperthermia

Hepatic or renal failure

Central Nervous System Disorders

Multiple infarctions

Parkinson's disease

Neurosyphilis

Alzheimer's disease

Head trauma

Tumors

Seizures and postconvulsive
    states

Normal pressure
    hydrocephalus

Treatment-Related

Related to a disturbance in cerebral metabolism secondary to:

Surgery

Therapeutic drug intoxication (e.g., neuroleptics, narcotics)

General anesthesia

Side effects of medication:

Diuretics

Digitalis

Propranolol

Atropine

Oral hypoglycemics

Anti-inflammatory agents

Anticholinergics

Phenothiazines

Opiates

Barbiturates

Methyldopa

Disulfiram

Lithium

Phenytoin

Antianxiety agents

Over-the-counter cold, cough,
    and sleeping preparations

Situational (Personal, Environmental)

Related to disturbance in cerebral metabolism secondary to:

Withdrawal from alcohol

Withdrawal from sedatives, hypnotics

Heavy metal or carbon monoxide intoxication

Related to pain, bowel impaction, immobility, or depression

Related to chemical intoxications or medications (specify):

Alcohol

Amphetamines

Heroin

Cocaine

Hallucinogenics

NOC

Cognitive Orientation, Safe Home Environment, Stress Level, Self-Control, Information Processing

Goals

The person will have diminished episodes of delirium.

Indicators
- Is less agitated.
- Participates in activities of daily living.
- Is less combative.

NIC

Delirium Management, Cognitive Stimulation, Calming Technique, Reality Orientation, Environmental Management: Safety, Fall Prevention, Surveillance: Safety

Generic Interventions

Assess for Causative and Contributing Factors.

Ensure that a thorough diagnostic workup has been completed.

Laboratory:
- Complete blood count, electrolytes, chemistry
- B_{12} and folate, thiamine
- Rapid plasma reagin (RPR)
- TSH, T_4
- Drug levels: alcohol, barbiturates
- Serum thyroxine and serum free thyroxine
- Serum glucose tolerance test
- Urinalysis

Diagnostic:
- Electroencephalogram
- Computed tomography scan
- Electrocardiogram
- Chest x-ray, skull x-ray
- Spinal tap
- Psychiatric evaluation

Promote Communication that Contributes to the Person's Sense of Integrity.

Examine attitudes about confusion (in self, caregivers, significant others). Provide education to family, significant other(s), and caregivers regarding the situation and methods of coping.

Maintain standards of empathic, respectful care.

Attempt to obtain information that will provide useful and meaningful topics for conversations (likes, dislikes; interests, hobbies; work history). Interview early in the day.

Encourage significant others and caregivers to speak slowly with low voice pitch and at an average volume (unless hearing deficits are present), as one adult to another, with eye contact, and as if expecting person to understand.

Provide respect and promote sharing:
- Pay attention to what the person is saying.
- Pick out meaningful comments, and continue talking.
- Address the person by name, and introduce yourself each time a contact is made; use touch if welcomed.
- Use name the person prefers; avoid "Pops" or "Mom."
- Convey to the person that you are concerned and friendly (through smiles, an unhurried pace).

Use memory aids, if appropriate.

Provide Sufficient and Meaningful Sensory Input.

Keep person oriented to time and place.

Encourage family to bring familiar objects from home (e.g., photographs with nonglare glass, blanket).

Discuss current events, seasonal events (snow, water activities); share your interests (travel, crafts).

Assess if person can perform an activity with hands (e.g., latch rugs, wood crafts).

When teaching a task or activity (e.g., eating), break it into small, brief steps by giving only one instruction at a time.

Promote a Well Role.

Discourage the wearing of nightclothes during the day.

Encourage self-care and grooming activities.

Promote socialization during meals.

Plan an activity each day.

Encourage participation in decision-making.

Do Not Endorse Confusion.

Do not argue with person.

Never agree with confused statements.

Direct person back to reality; do not allow him or her to ramble.

Adhere to the schedule; if changes are necessary, advise person of them.

Avoid talking to coworkers about other topics in person's presence.

Provide simple explanations that cannot be misinterpreted.

Remember to acknowledge your entrance with a greeting and your exit with a closure. ("I will be back in 10 minutes.")

Avoid open-ended questions.

Replace five- or six-step tasks with two- or three-step tasks.

Promote Safety.

Ensure that the person carries identification.

Adapt the environment so the person can pace or walk if desired.

Keep the environment uncluttered.

Keep medications, cleaning solutions, and other toxic chemicals in inaccessible places.

If the person cannot manipulate the call button, use another method (e.g., bell, extension from bed call system).

Discourage Use of Restraints; Explore Alternatives

If the person's behavior disrupts treatment (e.g., nasogastric tube, urinary catheter, intravenous line), reevaluate whether treatment is appropriate.

Evaluate if restlessness is associated with pain. If analgesics are used, adjust dosage to reduce side effects.

Put the person in a room with others who can help watch him or her.

Enlist aid of family or friends to watch the person during confused periods.

Give the person something to hold (e.g., a stuffed animal).

▶ Risk for Acute Confusion

DEFINITION

A state in which the individual is at risk for reversible disturbances of consciousness, attention, cognition, and perception that develop over a short period of time.

RISK FACTORS

Refer to Related Factors under Acute Confusion

NOC

Refer to *Acute Confusion.*

Goal

The individual will demonstrate continued level of orientation, attention and cognition.

Interventions

Refer to *Acute Confusion*.

▶ Chronic Confusion

DEFINITION

A state in which the individual experiences an irreversible, long-standing, and/or progressive deterioration of intellect and personality.

DEFINING CHARACTERISTICS

Major (Must Be Present, One or More)

Progressive or long-standing:

Cognitive or Intellectual Losses

Loss of memory
Loss of time sense

Inability to make choices, decisions

Inability to Problem-Solve, Reason

Altered perceptions
Loss of language abilities

Poor judgment

Affective or Personality Losses

Loss of affect
Diminished inhibition
Loss of tact, control of temper
Loss of recognition
   (others, environment, self)

Increasing self-preoccupations
Psychotic features
Antisocial behavior
Loss of energy reserve

Cognitive or Planning Losses

Loss of general ability to plan
Impaired ability to set goals, plan

Progressively Lowered Stress Threshold

Purposeful wandering
Violent, agitated, or anxious behavior
Purposeless behavior
Withdrawal or avoidance behavior
Compulsive repetitive behavior

RELATED FACTORS

Pathophysiologic (Hall, 1991)

Related to progressive degeneration of the cerebral cortex secondary to:

Alzheimer's disease

Multi-infarct disease (MID)

Combination of senile dementia of Alzheimer's type and MID

Related to disturbance in cerebral metabolism, structure, or integrity secondary to:

Pick's disease

Creutzfeldt-Jakob disease

Toxic substance injection

Degenerative neurologic disease

Brain tumor

Huntington's chorea

End-stage diseases:

- AIDS
- Cancer
- Cardiac failure
- Cirrhosis
- Renal failure
- Chronic obstructive pulmonary disease

Psychiatric disorders

NOC

Cognitive Ability, Cognitive Orientation, Stress Level, Distorted Thought Self-Control, Safe Home Environment

Goals

The person will participate to maximum level of independence in a therapeutic milieu.

Indicators

- Has decreased frustration
- Has diminished episodes of combativeness
- Has decreased use of restraints
- Increases hours of sleep at night
- Stabilizes or gains weight

NIC

Dementia Management, Cognitive Stimulation, Reality Orientation, Surveillance: Safety, Emotional Support, Environmental Management, Fall Prevention, Calming Technique

Generic Interventions

Refer to Interventions Under **Acute Confusion**.

Observe the Person to Determine Baseline Behaviors (Hall, 1994):

Client's best time of day
Response time to a simple question
Amount of distraction tolerable
Judgment ability
Insight into own disability
Signs/symptoms of depression
Usual routine

Promote a Sense of Integrity (Miller, 2009):

Adapt communication to the ability level of the person. It may be necessary to use very simple sentences and to present one idea at a time.

Avoid "baby talk" and a condescending tone of voice.

If the person does not understand, repeat the sentence using the same words.

Use positive statements; avoid "don'ts."

Unless a safety issue is involved, do not argue with the person.

Avoid general questions such as, "What would you like to do?" Instead ask, "Do you want to go for a walk or work on your rug?"

Be sensitive to the feelings the person is trying to express.

Avoid questions you know he or she cannot answer.

If possible, demonstrate to reinforce verbal communication.

Use touch to gain attention or show concern, unless a negative response is elicited.

Maintain good eye contact and pleasant facial expressions.

Determine which sense dominates the person's perception of the world (auditory, kinesthetic, olfactory, or gustatory).

Communicate through the preferred sense.

Promote Safety.

Ensure that the person carries identification.

Adapt the environment so that the person can pace or walk if desired.

Keep the environment uncluttered.

Keep medications, cleaning solutions, and other toxic chemicals in inaccessible places.

If person cannot manipulate the call button, use another method (e.g., bell, extension from bed call system).

Discourage Use of Restraints; Explore Alternatives (Quinn, 1994).

If person's behavior disrupts treatment (e.g., nasogastric tube, urinary catheter, intravenous line), re-evaluate whether treatment is appropriate.

Intravenous therapy:
- Camouflage the tubing with loose gauze.
- If dehydration is a problem, institute a regular schedule for offering oral fluids.
- Use sites that are least restrictive.

Urinary catheters:
- Evaluate causes of incontinence; institute specific treatment depending on type. Refer to *Impaired Urinary Elimination*.
- Place urinary collection bag at end of bed with catheter between legs rather than draped over legs. Velcro bands can hold catheter against leg.

Gastrointestinal tubes:
- Check frequently for pressure against nares.
- Camouflage gastrostomy tube with a loosely applied abdominal binder.
- If the person is pulling out tubes, use mitts instead of wrist restraints.

Evaluate if restlessness is associated with pain. If analgesics are used, adjust dosage to reduce side effects.

Put person in a room with others who can help watch him or her.

Enlist aid of family or friends to watch the person during confused periods.

Give the person something to hold (e.g., stuffed animal).

Ensure Physical Comfort and Maintenance of Basic Health Needs (e.g., Elimination, Nutrition, Bathing, Toileting, Hygiene, Grooming, Safety). Refer to Individual Nursing Diagnoses to Assist a Cognitively Impaired Person with Self-Care.

Use Various Modalities to Promote Stimulation.

Music Therapy
Provide soft, familiar music during meals.
Play music to individuals that they preferred in their younger years.

Recreation Therapy
Encourage arts and crafts (knitting and crocheting).

Suggest creative writing.

Provide puzzles.

Organize group games.

Remotivation Therapy

Topics for remotivation sessions are based on suggestions from group leaders and the interest of the group. Examples are pets, bodies of water, canning fruits and vegetables, transportation, holidays (Janssen & Giberson, 1988).

Use associations and analogies:

"If ice is cold, then fire is . . . ?"

"If day is light, then night is . . . ?"

Sensory Training

Stimulate vision (with brightly colored items of different shapes; pictures, color decorations, kaleidoscopes).

Stimulate smell (with flowers, coffee, cologne).

Stimulate hearing (ring a bell, play records).

Stimulate touch (sandpaper, velvet, steel wool pads, silk, stuffed animals).

Stimulate taste (spices, salt, sugar, sour substances).

Reminiscence Therapy (Burnside & Haight, 1994)

Consider instituting reminiscence therapy on a one-to-one or group basis. Discuss purpose and goals with client care team. Prepare yourself well before initiating. Refer to Burnside and Haight (1994) for specific protocols for one-to-one and group reminiscence.

Implement Techniques to Lower the Stress Threshold in Individuals in Middle or Later Stages of Dementia (Hall & Buckwalter, 1987; Miller, 2009).

Reduce competing or excessive stimuli.

Plan and maintain a consistent routine.

Focus on the person's ability level.

Reduce fatigue and anxiety.

Allow for wandering.

Be alert to the individual's expressions of fatigue or increasing anxiety, and immediately reduce stimuli.

Discuss the Proposed Benefits of Selected Nutrients: Zinc, Choline, Lecithin, Selenium, Magnesium, Beta Carotene, Folic Acid, and Vitamins C and E (Miller, 2009).

CONSTIPATION

Constipation
Perceived Constipation
Risk for Constipation

DEFINITION

The state in which an individual experiences stasis of the large intestine, resulting in infrequent (two or less weekly) elimination and/or hard, dry feces.

DEFINING CHARACTERISTICS

Major (Must Be Present, One or More)

Hard, formed stool *and/or*
Defecation fewer than three times a week
Prolonged and difficult defecation

Minor (May Be Present)

Decreased bowel sounds
Reported feeling of rectal fullness
Reported feeling of pressure in rectum
Straining and pain on defecation
Palpable impaction
Feeling of inadequate emptying

RELATED FACTORS

Pathophysiologic

***Related to defective nerve stimulation, weak pelvic floor
muscles, and immobility secondary to:***
• Spinal cord lesions
• Spinal cord injury
• Spina bifida
• Dementia
• Cerebrovascular accident, stroke
• Neurologic diseases (multiple sclerosis, Parkinson's disease)

Related to decreased metabolic rate secondary to:
• Obesity
• Pheochromocytoma

- Diabetic neuropathy
- Hypopituitarism
- Uremia
- Hypothyroidism
- Hyperparathyroidism

Related to decreased response to urge to defecate secondary to:
Affective disorders
Related to pain on defecation (e.g., hemorrhoids, back injury)
Related to decreased peristalsis secondary to hypoxia (cardiac, pulmonary)
Related to failure to relax anal sphincter or high resting pressure in the anal canal secondary to:
Multiple vaginal deliveries
Chronic straining

Treatment-Related

Related to side effects of (specify):
- Antacids (calcium, aluminum)
- Iron
- Barium
- Aluminum
- Aspirin
- Phenothiazines
- Calcium
- Anticholinergics
- Anesthetics
- Narcotics (codeine, morphine)
- Diuretics
- Antiparkinsonian agents

Related to effects of anesthesia and surgical manipulation on peristalsis
Related to habitual laxative use
Related to mucositis secondary to radiation

Situational (Personal, Environmental)

Related to decreased peristalsis secondary to: e.g., immobility, pregnancy, stress, lack of exercise
Related to irregular evacuation patterns
Related to cultural or health beliefs
Related to lack of privacy
Related to inadequate fiber in diet
Related to fear of rectal or cardiac pain
Related to faulty appraisal

Related to inadequate fluid intake
Related to inability to perceive bowel cues

NOC
Bowel Elimination, Hydration, Symptom Control

Goals

The person will report bowel movements at least every 2 to 3 days.

Indicators
- Describe components of effective bowel movements.
- Explain rationale for lifestyle change(s).

NIC
Bowel Management, Fluid Management, Constipation/
Impaction Management Nutritional Counseling

Generic Interventions

Teach the Importance of a Balanced Diet.

Review list of foods high in bulk:
- Fresh fruits with skins
- Bran, dried beans
- Nuts and seeds
- Whole-grain breads and cereals
- Cooked fruits and vegetables
- Fruit juices

Include approximately 800 g of fruits and vegetables (about four pieces of fresh fruit and large salad) for normal daily bowel movement.

Gradually increase amount of bran as tolerated (may add to cereals, baked goods, etc.). Explain the need for fluid intake with bran.

Encourage Daily Intake of at Least 2 L of Fluids—8 to 10 Glasses—Unless Contraindicated. Limit Coffee to Two to Three Cups per Day.

Recommend a Glass of Warm Water to Be Taken 30 Minutes Before Breakfast; This May Act as Stimulus to Bowel Evacuation.

Establish a Regular Time for Elimination.
Use a Commode Chair or Toilet
Instead of Bedpan, If Possible.

Assist Person to Normal Semisquatting
Position to Allow Optimal Use of Abdominal
Muscles and Effect of Force of Gravity.

Teach How to Massage Along Lower
Abdomen Gently While on Toilet.

Teach the Importance of Responding
to Urge to Defecate.

If Fecal Impaction Is Present, Instill Warm
Mineral Oil, and Retain It for 20 to 30
Minutes. Using a Well-Lubricated Glove,
Break Up Hard Stool, and Remove Pieces.

Monitor for Vagal Stimulation (Dizziness, Slow Pulse).

Explain the Hazards of Enema and Non–
Bulk-Producing Laxative Use (Refer
to Perceived Constipation).

Explain How to Use Bulk-Producing Laxatives
(e.g., Psyllium Hydrophilic Mucilloid [Metamucil,
Effersyllium Citrucel, FiberCon]).

Emphasize the Need for Regular Exercise.

Suggest walking.
If walking is prohibited:
- Teach client to lie in bed or sit on chair, and bend one knee at a time to chest (10 to 20 times each knee) three or four times a day.
- Teach client to sit in chair or lie in bed, and turn torso from side to side (10 to 20 times) 6 to 10 times a day.

Reduce Rectal Pain, if Possible, by Instructing
Person in Corrective Measures:

Gently apply a lubricant to anus to reduce pain on defecation.
Apply cool compresses to area to reduce itching.
Take sitz bath or soak in tub of warm water (43° to 46°C) for 15-minute intervals if soothing.
Take stool softeners or mineral oil as an adjunct to other approaches.
Consult with physician concerning use of local anesthetics and antiseptic agents.

Protect the Skin from Contamination.

Evaluate the surrounding skin area.

Cleanse properly with nonirritating agent (e.g., use gentle motion; use soft tissues following defecation).

Suggest a sitz bath following defecation.

Gently apply protective emollient or lubricant.

Initiate Health Teaching If Indicated.

Teach methods to prevent rectal pressure, which contributes to hemorrhoids.

Avoid prolonged sitting and straining at defecation.

Soften stools (e.g., low-roughage diet, high fluid intake).

Pediatric Interventions

Discuss some causes of constipation in infants and children (underfeeding; high-protein, low-carbohydrate diet; lack of roughage; dehydration).

If bowel movements are infrequent with hard stools:

With infants, add corn syrup to feeding or fruit to diet. Avoid apple juice or sauce.

With children, add bran cereal, prune juice, fruits, and vegetables.

Persistent constipation should be evaluated medically.

Maternal Interventions

Explain the risks of constipation in pregnancy and postpartum (Reeder et al., 1997):

- Decreased gastric motility
- Prolonged intestinal time
- Pressure of enlarging uterus
- Distended abdominal muscles (postpartum)
- Relaxation of intestines (postpartum)

Explain aggravating factors for hemorrhoid development (straining at defecation, constipation, prolonged standing, wearing constrictive clothing).

If the woman has a history of constipation, discuss how to use bulk-producing laxatives to keep stool soft. Advise patient to avoid other types of laxatives (e.g., stimulants, mineral oil).

Postdelivery, assess bowel sounds, presence of abdominal distention, hemorrhoids, perineal swelling, and if passing flatus.

Postdelivery, provide relief from pain of hemorrhoids, episiotomy, or perineal lacerations.

Consider the need for stool softeners, laxative, or rectal
   suppository. Promote defecation 2 to 3 days postdelivery.

Geriatric Interventions

Discuss that individual bowel patterns vary (e.g., three times a
   day to three times a week).
Discuss medication that can contribute to constipation
   (anticholinergics, narcotics, iron sulfate, psychotropic
   medications, aluminum and calcium antacids, tricyclic
   antidepressants, overuse of antidiarrheals).

▶ Perceived Constipation

DEFINITION

The state in which an individual self-prescribes the daily use
of laxatives, enemas, or suppositories to ensure a daily bowel
movement.

DEFINING CHARACTERISTICS (MCLANE & MCSHANE, 1986)

Major (80% to 100%)

Expectation of a daily bowel movement with the resulting
   overuse of laxatives, enemas, and/or suppositories
Expected passage of stool at the same time every day

RELATED FACTORS

Pathophysiologic

*Related to faulty appraisal secondary to: e.g., obsessive-
compulsive disorders, central nervous system (CNS)
deterioration, depression*

Situational (Personal, Environmental)

Related to inaccurate information secondary to: e.g., cultural
   beliefs, family beliefs

NOC

Bowel Elimination, Health Beliefs: Perceived Threat

Goals

The person will verbalize acceptance of bowel movements every
2 or 3 days.

Indicators

- Do not use laxatives regularly.
- Relate the causes of constipation.
- Describe the hazards of laxative use.
- Relate an intent to increase fiber, fluid, and exercise in daily life as instructed.

NIC

Bowel Movement Health Education, Behavior Modification, Nutrition Counseling

Generic Interventions

Explore with person his or her bowel patterns and expectations.

Gently explain that bowel movements are needed every 2 to 3 days, not daily.

Explain the hazards of regular laxative, enema, or suppository use:

- Temporary relief
- Impaired nutrient metabolism: riboflavin, calcium, magnesium, zinc, potassium
- Water deficiency
- Malabsorption of fat-soluble vitamins A, D, E, and K
- Diarrhea-constipation cycle
- Possible interactions with other medications (e.g., diuretics, digoxin [Lanoxin])

Teach the importance of a balanced diet (refer to *Constipation*).

Encourage intake of at least 6 to 10 glasses of water (unless contraindicated).

Recommend drinking a glass of warm water 30 minutes before breakfast; this may act as a stimulus to bowel evacuation.

Establish a regular time for elimination.

Emphasize the need for regular exercise.

Suggest walking.

If walking is prohibited:

- Teach client to lie in bed or sit on chair, and bend one knee at a time to chest (10 to 20 times each knee) three or four times a day.
- Teach client to sit in chair or lie in bed, and turn torso from side to side (20 to 30 times) 6 to 10 times a day.

Emphasize that normal bowel function is possible without laxatives, enemas, or suppositories.

▶ Risk for Constipation

DEFINITION

The state in which an individual is at high risk of experiencing stasis of the large intestine, resulting in infrequent elimination and/or hard, dry feces.

RISK FACTORS

Refer to *Constipation*.

Goals

The person will report continued satisfactory bowel movements every 1 to 3 days.

Indicators

Identify the effects of fluid, fiber, and activity on bowel elimination.

Generic Interventions

Refer to *Constipation*.

CONTAMINATION: INDIVIDUAL

Contamination: Individual
Contamination: Individual, Risk for

DEFINITION

Exposure to environmental contaminants in doses sufficient to cause adverse health effects.

DEFINING CHARACTERISTICS

Defining characteristics are dependent on the causative agent. Causative agents include pesticides, chemicals, biologics, waste, radiation, and pollution.

Pesticide Exposure Effects

Pulmonary

Anaphylactic reaction, asthma, irritation to nose and throat, burning sensation in throat and chest, pulmonary edema, shortness of breath, pneumonia, upper airway irritation, dyspnea, bronchitis, pulmonary fibrosis, COPD, bronchiolitis, airway hyper-reactivity, damage to mucous membranes of the respiratory tract

Neurologic

Reye's-like syndrome, confusion, anxiety, seizures, decreased level of consciousness, coma, muscle fasciculation, skeletal muscle myotonia, peripheral neuropathy, pinpoint pupils, blurred vision, headache, dizziness, CNS excitation, depression, paresthesia

Gastrointestinal

Nausea, vomiting, diarrhea, flu-like symptoms

Dermatologic

Chloracne

Cardiac

Cardiac dysrhythmia, tachycardia, bradycardia, conduction block, hypotension

Hepatic

Liver dysfunction

Chemical Exposure Effects

Pulmonary

Irritation of nose and throat, dyspnea, bronchitis, pulmonary edema, cough

Neurologic

Headache, ataxia, confusion, seizures, lethargy, unconsciousness, coma, lacrimation, ataxia, vertigo, mood changes, delirium, hallucinations, nystagmus, diplopia, psychosis, CNS depression, tremors, weakness, paralysis, memory changes, encephalopathy, hearing loss, Parkinson-like syndrome, euphoria, narcosis, syncope, hyperthermia

Renal

Acetonuria, renal failure

Gastrointestinal

Hyper/hypoglycemia, nausea, vomiting, ulceration of the GI tract, metabolic acidosis

Dermatologic

Dermatitis, irritation of the skin and mucous membranes, mucosal burns of eyes, nose, pharynx and larynx, conjunctivitis, hyperpigmentation of skin and nails, dermal burns

Immunologic

Altered blood clotting, bone marrow depression

Reproductive
Shortening of menstrual cycle

Cardiac
Hypotension, chest pain

Ophthalmic
Pupil changes, blurred vision, severe eye pain, corneal irritation, temporary or permanent blindness

Hepatic
Jaundice, hepatomegaly, hepatitis, pancreatitis

Biological Exposure Effects

Bacteria

Anthrax
Fever, chills, drenching sweats, profound fatigue, minimally productive cough, nausea and vomiting, and chest discomfort

Cholera (Vibrio cholerae)
Profuse watery diarrhea, vomiting, leg cramps, dehydration, and shock

Salmonellosis (salmonella)
Fever, abdominal cramps, diarrhea (sometimes bloody), localized infection, sepsis

E. coli (Escherichia coli 0157:H7)
Severe bloody diarrhea, and abdominal cramps, no fever

Viruses

Smallpox (Variola virus)
High fever, head and body aches, vomiting, skin rash with bumps and raised pustules that crust, scab, form a pitted scar

Ebola hemorrhagic fever (Ebola filovirus)
Headache, fever, joint and muscle aches, sore throat, and weakness followed by diarrhea, vomiting and stomach ache; rash, red eyes, and skin rash

Lassa fever (Lassa virus)
Fever, retrosternal pain, sore throat, back pain, cough, abdominal pain, vomiting, diarrhea, conjunctivitis, facial swelling, proteinuria, mucosal bleeding

Toxins

Ricin
Respiratory distress, fever, cough, nausea, and tightness in chest, heavy breathing, pulmonary edema, cyanosis, hypotension, respiratory failure, hallucinations, seizures, blood in urine

Staphylococcal enterotoxin B

Fever, headache, myalgia, malaise, diarrhea, sore throat, sinus congestion, rhinorrhea, hoarseness, conjunctivitis

Radiation Exposure Effects

Oncologic

Skin cancer, thyroid cancer, leukemia

Immunologic

Impaired response to immunizations, bone marrow suppression, autoimmune diseases

Genetic

DNA mutations, teratogenic effect including smaller head or brain size, poorly formed eyes, abnormally slow growth, mental retardation.

Neurologic

CNS damage, malfunctions of the peripheral nervous system, neuroautoimmune changes, disturbances in neuroendocrine control

Dermatologic

Burns, skin irritation, dryness, inflammation, erythema, and dry or moist desquamation, itching, blistering, ulceration

Systemic radiation poisoning

Nausea, fatigue, weakness, hair loss, changes in blood chemistries, hemorrhage, diminished organ function, death

Ophthalmic

Cataracts, degeneration of the macula

Cardiovascular

Changes in cardiovascular control, irregular heartbeat, changes in the electrocardiogram, development of atherosclerosis, hypertension, and ischemia

Pulmonary

Disturbances in respiratory volume, increase in the number of allergic illnesses, atypical cells in the bronchial mucosa

Gastrointestinal

Pathologic changes in the digestive system, inflammation of the duodenum, spontaneously hyperplastic mucous membranes

Waste Exposure Effects

Coliform bacteria

Diarrhea, abdominal cramps

Giardia lamblia (protozoa)
Diarrhea, abdominal cramps, nausea, weight loss

Cryptosporidium (protozoa)
Diarrhea, headache, abdominal cramps, nausea, vomiting, low fever

Hepatitis A (enteric virus)
Lassitude, anorexia, weakness, nausea, fever, jaundice

Helminths (parasitic worms)
Diarrhea, vomiting, gas, stomach pain, loss of appetite, fever

Pollution Exposure Effects

Pulmonary
Coughing, wheezing, labored breathing, pulmonary and nasal congestion, exacerbated allergies, asthma exacerbation, pain when breathing, lung cancer

Cardiac
Chest pain

Neurologic
Headaches, developmental delay

Reproductive
Reduced fertility

Ophthalmic
Eye irritation

RELATED FACTORS

Pathophysiologic

Presence of bacteria, viruses, toxins
Nutritional factors (obesity, vitamin and mineral deficiencies)
Pre-existing disease states
Gender (females have greater proportion of body fat, which
    increases chance of accumulating more lipid-soluble toxins
    than men; pregnancy)
Smoking related complications (e.g., COPD, PAD)

Treatment-Related

Recent vaccinations
Insufficient or absent use of decontamination protocol
Inappropriate or no use of protective clothing

Situational

Flooding, earthquakes, and other natural disasters
Sewer line leaks
Industrial plant emissions; intentional or accidental discharge of
    contaminants by industries or businesses
Physical factors: Climatic conditions such as temperature, wind;
    geographic area
Social factors: Crowding, sanitation, poverty, personal and
    household hygiene practices, lack of access to health care
Biologic factors: Presence of vectors (mosquitoes, ticks, rodents)
Bioterrorism
Occupation
Dietary practices

Environmental

Contamination of aquifers by septic tanks
Intentional/accidental contamination of food and water supply
Concomitant or previous exposures
Exposure to heavy metals or chemicals, atmospheric pollutants,
    radiation, bioterrorism, disaster
Use of environmental contaminants in the home (pesticides,
    chemicals, environmental tobacco smoke)
Playing in outdoor areas where environmental contaminants are
    used
Type of flooring surface

Maturational

Developmental characteristics of children
Children less than 5 years
Older adults
Gestational age during exposure

NOC

Anxiety Level, Fear Level, Grief Resolution, Health
Beliefs: Perceived Threat, Immunization Behavior,
Infection Control, Knowledge: Health Resources,
Personal Safety Behavior, Community Risk Control, Safe
Home Environment. See *Contamination: Community* for
other possible NOC outcomes

Goal

Individual adverse health effects of contamination will be
minimized.

NIC

Community Disaster Preparedness, Environmental Management, Anger Control Assistance, Anxiety Reduction, Grief Work Facilitation, Crisis Intervention, Counseling, Health Education, Health Screening, Immunization/Vaccination Management, Infection Control, Resiliency Promotion, Risk Identification. See also appropriate NIC interventions based on patient's defining characteristics.

Generic Interventions

Help Individuals Cope with Contamination Incident; Use Groups that Have Survived Terrorist Attacks as Useful Resource for Victims.

Provide Accurate Information on Risks Involved, Preventive Measures, Use of Antibiotics and Vaccines.

Assist to Deal with Feelings of Fear, Vulnerability, and Grief.

Encourage Them to Talk to Others About Their Fears.

Assist Victims to Think Positively and to Move to the Future.

Specific Interventions

Employ Skin Decontamination with Dermal Exposures.

Clinical Effects on Body Systems Vary with Exposure to Specific Agents. Monitor Carefully and Provide Supportive Care.

Employ Appropriate Isolation Precautions: Universal, Airborne, Droplet, and Contact Isolation.

Monitor Individual for Therapeutic Effects, Side Effects, and Compliance with Post-exposure Drug Therapy.

Decontamination Procedure

Primary decontamination of exposed personnel is agent specific:
- Remove contaminated clothing.
- Use copious amounts of water and soap or diluted (0.5%) sodium hypochlorite.

Secondary decontamination (from clothing or equipment of those exposed)—use proper physical protection

▶ Contamination: Individual, Risk for

DEFINITION

Accentuated risk of exposure to environmental contaminants in doses sufficient to cause adverse health effects.

RISK FACTORS

See Related Factors under *Contamination: Individual*

NOC

Community Risk Control, Community health Status, Health Beliefs: Perceived Threat, Knowledge: Health Resources, Knowledge: Health Behavior; See *Contamination: Individual* for Other Possible NOC Outcomes

Goal

Individual will remain free of adverse effects of contamination.

NIC

Community Disaster Preparedness, Environmental Risk Protection, Environmental Management: Safety, Health Education, Health Screening, Immunization/Vaccination Management, Risk Identification, Surveillance: Safety

Generic Interventions

Provide Accurate Information on Risks Involved and Preventive Measures.

Assist to Deal with Feelings of Fear and Vulnerability.

Encourage Them to Talk to Others About Their Fears.

Specific Interventions

Conduct Surveillance for Environmental Contamination.

Notify Agencies Authorized to Protect the Environment of Contaminants in the Area.

Assist Individuals in Relocating to Safer Environment.

Modify the Environment to Minimize Risk.

CONTAMINATION: FAMILY

Contamination: Family
Contamination: Family, Risk for

DEFINITION

Exposure to environmental contaminants in doses sufficient to cause adverse health effects.

DEFINING CHARACTERISTICS

See Defining Characteristics for *Contamination: Individual* and *Community*

RELATED FACTORS

See Related Factors for *Contamination: Individual* and *Community*

NOC

See *Contamination: Individual* and *Community* for Possible NOC Outcomes

Goal

Family adverse health effects of contamination will be minimized.

NIC

See *Contamination: Individual* and *Community* for Possible NIC Outcomes; See Also Appropriate NIC Interventions Based on Family's Defining Characteristics

Interventions

See *Contamination: Individual* and *Community* for possible interventions

▶ Contamination: Family, Risk for

DEFINITION

Accentuated risk of exposure to environmental contaminants in doses sufficient to cause adverse health effects.

RISK FACTORS

See Related Factors under *Contamination: Individual*

NOC

See *Risk for Contamination: Individual* for Possible NOC Outcomes

Goal

Family will remain free of adverse effects of contamination.

NIC

See *Risk for Contamination: Individual* for Interventions

Interventions

See *Risk for Contamination: Individual* for Interventions

CONTAMINATION: COMMUNITY

Contamination: Community
Contamination: Community, Risk for

DEFINITION

Exposure to environmental contaminants in doses sufficient to cause adverse health effects.

DEFINING CHARACTERISTICS

Clusters of patients seeking care for similar signs or symptoms:
  • Signs and symptoms are dependent on the causative agent. Causative agents include pesticides, chemicals, biologics,

waste, radiation, and pollution. See *Contamination: Individual* for specific contaminant-related health effects.

Large numbers of patients with rapidly fatal illnesses
Sick, dying or dead animals or fish; absence of insects
Measurement of contaminants exceeding acceptable levels

RELATED FACTORS
Pathophysiologic
Presence of bacteria, viruses, toxins

Treatment-Related
Insufficient or no use of decontamination protocol
Inappropriate or no use of protective clothing

Situational
Acts of bioterrorism; flooding, earthquakes, natural disasters
Sewer line leaks
Industrial plant emissions; intentional or accidental discharge of contaminants by industries or businesses
Physical factors: Climatic conditions such as temperature, wind; geographic area
Social factors: Crowding, lack of sanitation, poverty, lack of access to health care
Biologic factors: Presence of vectors (mosquitoes, ticks, rodents)

Environmental
Contamination of aquifers by septic tanks
Intentional/accidental contamination of food and water supply
Exposure to heavy metals or chemicals, atmospheric pollutants, radiation, bioterrorism, disaster; concomitant or previous exposures

Maturational
Community dynamics (participation, power and decision making structure, collaborative efforts)

NOC
Community Competence, Community Disaster Readiness, Community Health Status, Community Risk Control: Communicable Disease, Community Risk Control: Lead Exposure, Grief Resolution, Community Risk Control: Violence, Infection Severity; See *Contamination: Individual* for Other Possible NOC Outcomes

Goal

Community utilizes health surveillance data system to monitor for contamination incidents.

Community will participate in mass casualty and disaster readiness drills.

Community will utilize disaster plan to evacuate and triage affected members.

Community exposure to contaminants will be minimized.

Community health effects associated with contamination will be minimized.

NIC

Environmental Management, Environmental Risk Protection, Community Health Development, Bioterrorism Preparedness, Communicable Disease Management, Community Disaster Preparedness, Crisis Intervention, Health Education, Health Policy Monitoring, Infection Control, Surveillance: Community, Triage: Disaster, Triage: Emergency Center

Generic Interventions

Monitor for Contamination Incidents Using Health Surveillance Data.

Provide Accurate Information on Risks Involved, Preventive Measures, Use of Antibiotics and Vaccines.

Encourage Community Members to Talk to Others About Their Fears.

Provide General Supportive Measures (Food, Water, Shelter).

Specific Interventions

Prevention: Identify Community Risk Factors and Develop Programs to Prevent Disasters from Occurring.

Preparedness: Plan for Communication, Evacuation, Rescue, and Victim Care; Schedule Mass Casualty and Disaster-Readiness Drills.

Response: Identify Contaminants in the Environment.

Educate community about the environmental contaminant.

Collaborate with other agencies (local health department, EMS, state and federal agencies).

Rescue, triage, stabilize, transport, and treat affected community members.

Recovery: Act to Repair, Rebuild, or Relocate Mental Health Services to Assist in Psychological Recovery (Adapted from Allender & Spradley, 2006).

Decontamination Procedure

Primary decontamination of exposed personnel is agent specific:

- Remove contaminated clothing.
- Use copious amounts of water and soap or diluted (0.5%) sodium hypochlorite.

Secondary decontamination (from clothing or equipment of those exposed)—use proper physical protection.

Employ Appropriate Isolation Precautions: Universal, Airborne, Droplet, and Contact Isolation.

▶ Contamination: Community, Risk for

DEFINITION

Community: Accentuated risk of exposure to environmental contaminants in doses sufficient to cause adverse health effects.

RISK FACTORS

See Related Factors under *Contamination: Community*

NOC

Community Disaster Readiness, Community Health Status, Community Risk Control: Communicable Disease; see *Contamination: Community* for other possible NOC outcomes

Goal

Community utilizes health surveillance data system to monitor for contamination incidents.

Community will participate in mass casualty and disaster readiness drills.

Community will remain free of contamination-related health effects.

NIC

Environmental Management, Environmental Risk Protection, Community Health Development, Bioterrorism Preparedness, Communicable Disease Management, Community Disaster Preparedness, Health Education, Health Policy Monitoring, Surveillance: Community

Generic Interventions

Monitor for Contamination Incidents Using Health Surveillance Data.

Provide Accurate Information on Risks Involved and Preventive Measures.

Encourage Community Members to Talk to Others About Their Fears.

Specific Interventions

Identify Community Risk Factors and Develop Programs to Prevent Disasters from Occurring.

Notify Agencies Authorized to Protect the Environment of Contaminants in the Area.

Modify the Environment to Minimize Risk.

COPING, INEFFECTIVE

Coping, Ineffective
Defensive Coping
Ineffective Denial

DEFINITION

The state in which the individual experiences or is at risk of experiencing an inability to manage internal or environmental stressors adequately because of inadequate resources (physical, psychological, behavioral, or cognitive).

■■■ **AUTHOR'S NOTE**
This diagnosis can be used to describe a variety of situations in which an individual does not adapt effectively to stressors. Examples can be isolating behaviors, aggression, and destructive behavior. If the response is inappropriate use of the defense mechanisms of denial or defensiveness, the diagnosis *Ineffective Denial* or *Defensive Coping* can be used instead of *Ineffective Coping*.

DEFINING CHARACTERISTICS (VINCENT, 1985)
Major (Must Be Present, One or More)
Verbalization of inability to cope or ask for help *or*
Inappropriate use of defense mechanisms *or*
Inability to meet role expectations
Destructive behavior toward self or others

Minor (May Be Present)
Chronic worry, anxiety
Reported difficulty with life stressors
Ineffective social participation
Verbal manipulation
Inability to meet basic needs
Nonassertive response patterns
Change in usual communication pattern

RELATED FACTORS
Pathophysiologic
Related to chronicity of condition or complex self-care regimens
Related to changes in body appearance
Related to biochemical changes in brain
Related to faulty thinking secondary to:
Bipolar disorder
Schizoid disorder
Personality disorder
Attention-deficit disorder
Affective disorders
Neurologic brain changes

Intake of mood-altering substance
Mental retardation

Treatment-Related

Related to separation from family and home (e.g., hospitalization, confinement to a nursing home)
Related to disfigurement caused by surgery
Related to altered appearance owing to drugs, radiation, or other treatment

Situational (Personal, Environmental)

Related to increased food consumption in response to stressors

Related to changes in physical environment secondary to:

War	Poverty
Natural disaster	Homelessness
Relocation	Inadequate finances
Seasonal work (migrant worker)	

Related to disruption of emotional bonds secondary to:

Death	Foster home
Separation or divorce	Orphanage
Desertion	Educational institution
Relocation	Institutionalization
Jail	

Related to sensory overload secondary to:
Factory environment
Urbanization: crowding, noise pollution, excessive activity

Related to inadequate psychological resources secondary to:
Poor self-esteem
Excessive negative beliefs about self
Negative role-modeling
Helplessness
Lack of motivation to respond

Related to ineffective problem-solving skills
Related to disorganized family system
Related to poor impulse control and frustration tolerance

Maturational

Child or Adolescent
Related to:
Inconsistent methods of discipline
Fear of failure
Childhood trauma

Parental substance abuse
Parental rejection
Repressed anxiety
Panic level of anxiety
Poor impulse control
Poor social skills
Peer rejection

Adolescent

Related to inadequate psychological resources to adapt to:

Physical and emotional changes   Sexual awareness
Independence from family   Educational demands
Relationships   Career choices

Young Adult

Related to inadequate psychological resources to adapt to:

Career choices   Marriage
Educational demands   Parenthood
Leaving home

Middle Adult

Related to inadequate psychological resources to adapt to:

Physical signs of aging   Problems with relatives
Career pressures   Social status needs
Child-rearing problems   Aging parents

Older Adult

Related to inadequate psychological resources to adapt to:

Physical changes   Retirement
Changes in financial status   Response of others to older
Changes in residence   persons

NOC

Coping, Self-Esteem, Social Interaction Skills

Goals

The person will make decisions and follow through with appropriate actions to change provocative situations in personal environment.

Indicators

- Verbalize feelings related to emotional state.
- Identify his or her coping patterns and the consequences of the behavior that results.
- Identify personal strengths and accept support through the nursing relationship.

NIC

Coping Enhancement, Counseling, Emotional Support, Active Listening, Assertiveness Training, Behavior Modification

Generic Interventions

Assess Individual's Present Coping Status.

Determine onset of feelings and symptoms and their correlation with events and life changes.

Assess ability to relate facts.

Listen carefully, and observe facial expressions, gestures, eye contact, body positioning, tone and intensity of voice.

Determine risk of client inflicting self-harm, and intervene appropriately (see *Risk for Self-Harm*).

Offer Support as Person Talks.

Reassure that the feelings he or she has must be difficult.

When person is pessimistic, attempt to provide a more hopeful, realistic perspective.

If Person Is Angry (Thomas, 1998):

Maintain an environment with low levels of stimuli.

Explore why the person is angry.

Do not argue or become defensive.

Focus on what can be done rather than what has not been done.

Offer options to increase sense of control.

Acknowledge that everyone gets angry, but certain actions are not acceptable.

If violence is a risk, refer to *Risk for Violence*.

Encourage a Self-Evaluation of His or Her Own Behavior.

"Did that work for you?"

"How did it help?"

"What did you learn from that experience?"

Assist the Person to Solve Problems in a Constructive Manner.

What is the problem?

Who or what is responsible for the problem?

What are the options? (Make a list.)

What are the advantages and disadvantages of each option?

Discuss Possible Alternatives (e.g., Talk about the Problem with Those Involved, Try to Change the Situation, or Do Nothing and Accept the Consequences).

Assist the Individual to Identify Problems that Cannot Be Controlled Directly and Help Him or Her to Practice Stress-Reducing Activities for Control (e.g., Exercise Program, Yoga).

Instruct the Person in Relaxation Techniques; Emphasize the Importance of Setting 15 to 20 Minutes Aside Each Day to Practice Relaxation.

Mobilize the Person into a Gradual Increase in Activity.

Find Outlets that Foster Feelings of Personal Achievement and Self-Esteem.

Provide opportunities to learn and use stress management techniques (e.g., jogging, yoga).

Establish a Network of Persons Who Understand the Situation.

For depression-related problems beyond the scope of nurse generalists, refer to appropriate professionals (marriage counselor, psychiatric nurse therapist, psychologist, psychiatrist).

Prepare for Problems that May Occur After Discharge.

Medications—schedule, cost, misuse, side effects
Increased anxiety
Sleep problems
Eating problems—access, decreased appetite
Inability to structure time
Family/significant other conflicts
Follow-up—forgetting, access, difficulty organizing time

🚺🚹 Pediatric Interventions

Establish eye contact before giving instructions.
Set firm, responsible limits.
State rules simply; do not lecture.
Maintain regular routine.
Advise parents to avoid disagreeing with each other in child's presence.
Maintain a calm, simple environment.
If hyperactive, provide for periods of activity using large muscles.
Provide immediate and constant feedback.

Advise parents to consult with educational professionals for educational programming.

▶ Defensive Coping

DEFINITION

The state in which an individual repeatedly presents falsely positive self-evaluation as a defense against underlying perceived threats to positive self-regard.

DEFINING CHARACTERISTICS (NORRIS & KUNES-CONNELL, 1987)

Major (80% to 100%)

Denial of obvious problems/weaknesses
Projection of blame/responsibility
Rationalization of failures
Hypersensitivity to slight criticism
Grandiosity

Minor (50% to 79%)

Superior attitude toward others
Difficulty in establishing or maintaining relationships
Hostile laughter or ridicule of others
Difficulty in testing perceptions against reality
Lack of follow-through or participation in treatment or therapy

RELATED FACTORS

See *Chronic Low Self-Esteem*, *Powerlessness*, and *Impaired Social Interaction*.

NOC

Acceptance: Health Status, Self-Esteem, Social Interaction Skills

Goals

The person will report or demonstrate less defensive behavior.

Indicators

• Identify defensive responses.
• Establish realistic goals in concert with caregivers.
• Work effectively toward achieving these goals.

NIC

Coping Enhancement, Emotional Support, Self-Awareness Enhancement, Environment Management, Presence Active Listening

Generic Interventions

Reduce Demands on the Individual if Stress Levels Increase.

Establish a Dialogue Stance that Will Reduce Defensiveness and Increase Effective Actions:

Maintain a neutral, matter-of-fact tone with a consistent positive regard. Ensure that all staff relate in a consistent fashion with consistent expectations.

Focus on simple here-and-now, goal-directed topics when encountering the client's defenses.

Encourage the client to express goals, and establish agreement with the client in at least one or two areas.

Do not defend or dwell on the client's negative projections or displacements.

Disengage from disagreement.

Do not challenge distortions or unrealistic/grandiose self-expressions. Try instead to redirect the conversation toward more neutral topics or more realistic topics about which some agreement has already been established.

Encourage the person to evaluate his or her own progress.

Identify for the person actions that have interfered with achieving established goals.

Practice role-playing less defensive responses to difficult situations.

Evaluate interactions, progress, and approach with other team members to ensure overall consistency within the treatment milieu.

Work to Establish a Therapeutic Relationship with the Client to Decrease the Need to Defend and Permit a More Direct Addressing of Underlying, Related Factors (See **Chronic Low Self-Esteem**).

Validate the client's reluctance to trust in the beginning.

Engage the client in diversional, non–goal-directed, noncompetitive activities (e.g., relaxation therapy, games, outing).

Encourage self-expression of neutral themes, positive reminiscences, and so forth.

Encourage other means for self-expression (e.g., writing or art) if verbal interaction is difficult or if another means is an area of personal strength.

Listen passively to some grandiose or negative self-expression to reinforce your "positive regard."

▶ Ineffective Denial

DEFINITION

The state in which the individual minimizes or disavows symptoms or a situation to the detriment of his or her health.

AUTHOR'S NOTE

This type of denial differs from the denial in response to a loss. The denial in response to an illness or loss is necessary to maintain psychological equilibrium and is beneficial. *Ineffective Denial* is not beneficial when the individual will not participate in regimens to improve health or the situation (e.g., denial of substance abuse). If the cause of the *Ineffective Denial* is not known, *Ineffective Denial related to unknown etiology* can be used; for example, *Ineffective Denial related to unknown etiology as manifested by repetitive refusal to admit that barbiturate use is a problem.*

DEFINING CHARACTERISTICS

Major (Must Be Present, One or More)

Delays seeking or refuses health care attention to the detriment of health

Does not perceive personal relevance of symptoms or danger

Minor (May Be Present)

Does not admit fear of death or invalidism

Minimizes symptoms

Displaces source of symptoms to other areas of the body

Unable to admit impact of disease on life pattern

Makes dismissive gestures or comments when speaking of distressing events

Displaces fear of impact of the condition

Displays inappropriate affect

RELATED FACTORS

Pathophysiologic

Related to inability to consciously tolerate the consequences of any chronic or terminal illness (e.g., HIV, cancer)

Treatment-Related

Related to prolonged treatment with no positive results

Situational/Psychological

Related to inability to tolerate consciously the consequences of, for example, drug use, alcohol use, smoking, obesity

Related to long-term self-destructive patterns of behavior and lifestyle choices (Varcolaris, 2007)

Related to dependence on substance use

Related to feelings of increased anxiety/stress; need to escape personal problems, anger, and frustration

Related to feelings of omnipotence

Related to culturally permissive attitudes toward alcohol/drug use

Biologic/Genetic

Related to family history of alcoholism

NOC

See *Ineffective Coping*

Goals

The person will use alternative coping mechanism instead of denial.

Indicators

- Acknowledges the source of anxiety or stress.
- Uses problem-focused coping skills.

NIC

See *Ineffective Coping*

Generic Interventions

Provide opportunities to share fears and anxieties.

Focus on present response.

Assist in lowering anxiety level (see *Anxiety* for additional interventions).

Avoid confronting person on use of denial.

Carefully explore with person his or her interpretation of the situation:

- Reflect self-reported cues used to minimize the situation (e.g., "a little," "only").
- Identify recent detrimental behavior, and discuss the effects of this behavior on health.

Emphasize strengths and past successful coping.

Provide positive reinforcement for any expressions of insight.

Do not accept rationalization or projection. Be polite, caring, but firm.

If substance abuse is present:

- Review observations and findings with client and family.
- Present evidence of damage (physical, social, financial, spiritual, familial).
- Establish goals.
- Provide self-help manuals or other pamphlets.
- Acquire commitment to keep daily log of alcohol/drug use.

At next visit:

- Review log.
- Review progress.
- Refer those who are dependent and desire to continue abstinence.
- Explain why women are more affected by alcohol than are men.

COPING, INEFFECTIVE COMMUNITY

DEFINITION

The state in which a community's patterns of activities for adaptation and problem-solving are unsatisfactory for meeting the demands or needs of the community.

AUTHOR'S NOTE

This diagnosis is useful for nurses who practice with aggregates.

(continued)

████ **AUTHOR'S NOTE** *(Continued)*

An aggregate is a group of persons "who have in common one or more personal or environmental characteristics" (Williams, 1977). Therefore, an aggregate can be the population of a small town, high school girls, or Hispanic men with hypertension.

This diagnosis may be more frequently used as a risk diagnosis than an actual one. Nurses practicing with community aggregates would identify risk factors that could cause *Ineffective Community Coping*. The focus would be on assisting the community to prevent the diagnosis.

DEFINING CHARACTERISTICS

Major (Must Be Present, One or More)

Failure of community to meet its own expectations
Unresolved community conflicts
Expressed difficulty in meeting demands for change
Expressed vulnerability

Minor (May Be Present)

Angry	Bitter
Indifferent	Apathetic
Helpless	Hopeless
Overwhelmed	

RISK FACTORS

Presence of risk factors (see Related Factors)

RELATED FACTORS

Situational (Personal, Environmental)

Related to lack of knowledge of resources
Related to inadequate communication patterns
Related to inadequate community cohesiveness
Related to inadequate problem-solving
Related to inadequate community resources
Related to inadequate law enforcement services
Related to overwhelming community destruction secondary to:

Flood	Hurricane
Earthquake	Epidemic

Related to traumatic effects of airplane crash, large fire, industrial disaster, or environmental accident

Related to threat to community safety (e.g., murder, rape, kidnapping, robberies)
Related to sudden rise in community unemployment

Maturational

Related to inadequate resources for children, adolescents, working parents, or older adults

NOC
Community Competence, Community Health Status, Community Risk Control

Goals

The community will engage in effective problem-solving.

Indicators
• Identify problem.
• Access information to improve coping.
• Use communication channels to access assistance.

NIC
Community Health Development, Environmental Risk Protection, Program Development, Risk Identification

Generic Interventions

Assess for causative or contributing factors:
  • Lack of knowledge of available resources
  • Inadequate problem-solving
  • Inadequate communication links
  • Overwhelming, multiple stressors
  • Threat to community safety

Provide opportunities (e.g., schools, churches, synagogues, town hall) for community members to face and discuss the situation and demonstrate acceptance of their anger, withdrawal, or denial.

Do not offer false reassurance. Emphasize their ability to cope effectively.

Explore techniques that may improve coping. Elicit suggestions from group.

Discuss resources that can be accessed. Prepare the group to accept outside help:
  • Emergency shelter, funds, food, clothes
  • Counseling

- Transportation
- Health care

Plan how to access isolated persons in the community.

Establish a method to access information and support (e.g., local health department, hospital, churches, synagogues, community center).

Initiate referrals as indicated:

- Counseling
- Public assistance

COMPROMISED FAMILY COPING

DEFINITION (NANDA)

The state in which a usually supportive primary person (family member or close friend) is providing insufficient, ineffective, or compromised support, comfort, assistance, or encouragement that may be needed by the client to manage or master adaptive tasks related to his or her health challenge.

AUTHOR'S NOTE

This nursing diagnosis describes situations that are similar to the diagnosis *Interrupted Family Processes*. Until clinical research differentiates this category from the preceding ones, use *Interrupted Family Processes*.

DEFINING CHARACTERISTICS (NANDA)

Subjective

Client expresses or confirms a concern or complaint about a significant other's response to his or her health problem.

Significant other describes preoccupation with personal reactions (e.g., fear, anticipatory grief, guilt, anxiety) to client's illness, disability, or other situational or developmental crises.

Significant other describes or confirms an inadequate understanding or knowledge base that interferes with effective assistive or supportive behaviors.

Objective

Significant other attempts assistive or supportive behaviors with less-than-satisfactory results.

Significant other withdraws or enters into limited or temporary
personal communication with the client in times of need.

Significant other displays protective behavior disproportionate
(too little or too much) to the client's abilities or need for
autonomy.

RELATED FACTORS

See *Interrupted Family Processes*.

DISABLED FAMILY COPING

DEFINITION

The state in which a family demonstrates, or is at risk to demonstrate, destructive behavior in response to an inability to manage internal or external stressors due to inadequate resources (physical, psychological, or cognitive).

> **AUTHOR'S NOTE**
> The diagnosis *Disabled Family Coping* describes a family that has a history of demonstrating destructive overt or covert behavior or that has adapted detrimentally to a stressor. This diagnosis differs from *Interrupted Family Processes*, which describes a family that usually functions constructively but is challenged by a stressor that has altered or may alter its functioning. Sustained *Interrupted Family Processes* may progress to *Disabled Family Coping*. This diagnosis requires long-term care by a nurse specialist. The interventions in this book are for nurses in a short-term relationship.

DEFINING CHARACTERISTICS

Major (Must Be Present, One or More)

Abusive or neglectful care of client

Partner violence

Neglectful relationships with other family members

Minor (May Be Present)

Distortion of reality regarding the client's health problem

Intolerance	Rejection
Abandonment	Desertion
Agitation	Depression
Aggression	Hostility

Impaired restructuring of family unit

RELATED FACTORS

Related to impaired ability to fulfill role responsibilities secondary to any acute or chronic illness

Situational (Personal, Environmental)

Related to impaired ability to manage stressors constructively secondary to:

Substance abuse; mental illness
Negative role-modeling
History of ineffective relationship with own parents
History of abusive relationships with parents
Related to unrealistic expectations of another family member

NOC

Family Coping, Abuse Protection, Abuse Cessation

Goals

The person will set short-term and long-term goals for change.

Indicators
* Appraise coping behaviors that are unhealthy for family members.
* Relate expectations for self and family.
* Relate community resources available.

NIC

Referral, Emotional Support, Abuse Protection Support (specify child, elder, domestic partner), Counseling

Generic Interventions

Assist Family to Evaluate Past and Present Family Functioning.

Provide All Family Members an Opportunity to Discuss Their Appraisal of the Situation.

Discourage Blaming, but Allow Ventilation of Anger.

Clarify Feelings of Members.

Assist Family with Appraisal of the Situation.

What is wrong? Causes?
Who has contributed to the problem? Options?
What are the advantages/disadvantages of each option?
What activity could be added to the family?

If Indicated, Ask Members to Consider the Problem from the Perspective of Another Family Member.

If a Member Is Ill, Assist Family to Have More Realistic Expectations.

If Domestic Abuse Is Suspected:

Know your state's laws regarding domestic abuse (e.g., mandatory reporting).
Provide an opportunity to validate abuse and talk about feelings.
Be direct and nonjudgmental:
- "How do you handle stress?"
- "How does your partner or caregiver handle stress?"
- "How do you and your partner argue?"
- "Are you afraid of your partner?"
- "Have you ever been hit, pushed, or injured by your partner?"

Encourage a realistic appraisal of the situation; dispel guilt and myths:
- "Violence is not normal for most families."
- "Violence may stop, but it usually becomes increasingly worse."
- "Alcohol and drugs do not cause violence."
- "The victim is not responsible for the violence."
- "You do not deserve this."
- "You have a right to be protected."

Provide options, but allow family members to make a decision at their own pace.
Discuss the importance of a "safety plan." For specifics of a safety plan, refer to a hotline or programs specific for domestic violence.
Provide a list of community agencies available to victim and abuser (emergency and long-term):
- Hotlines
- Legal services
- Shelters
- Counseling agencies

Discuss the availability of the social service department for assistance.

Consult with the legal resources in the community, and familiarize the victim with the state laws regarding:

- Eviction of abuser
- Counseling
- Temporary support
- Protection orders
- Criminal law
- Types of police interventions

Document findings and dialogue for possible future court use.

👫 Pediatric Interventions

Report Suspected Cases of Child Abuse.

Know Your State's Child Abuse Laws and Procedures for Reporting Child Abuse (e.g., Bureau of Child Welfare, Department of Social Services, Child Protective Services).

Maintain an Objective Record:

Description of injuries

Record conversations with parents and child using quotations

Description of behaviors, not interpretation (e.g., avoid "angry father"; instead, write "Father screamed at child, 'If you weren't so bad, this wouldn't have happened.' ")

Description of parent-child interactions (e.g., shies away from mother's touch)

Nutritional status

Growth and development compared with age-related norms

Provide the Child with Acceptance and Affection.

Assist Child with Grieving if Foster Home Placement Is Necessary.

Allow Opportunities for Child to Ventilate Feelings.

Provide Interventions that Promote Parents' Self-Esteem and Sense of Trust.

Tell them it was good that they brought the child to the hospital.

Promote their confidence by presenting a warm, helpful attitude and acknowledging any competent parenting activities.

Provide opportunities for parents to participate in their child's care (e.g., feeding, bathing).

Refer Abusive Parents to Community Agencies and Professionals for Counseling.

Disseminate Information to the Community (e.g., Parent-School Organizations, Radio, Television, Newspaper) About the Problem of Child Abuse.

Ⓒ Geriatric Interventions

Identify Suspected Cases of Elder Abuse; Observe For:

Failure to adhere to therapeutic regimens
Evidence of malnutrition, dehydration
Bruises, swelling, lacerations, burns, bites
Pressure ulcers
Caregiver not allowing nurse to be alone with elder

If Abuse Is Suspected (Anetzberger, 1987):

Know your state's laws regarding elder abuse.
Consult with supervisor for procedures.
Maintain an objective record, including:
  • Description of injuries
  • Conversations with elder and caregivers
  • Description of behaviors
  • Nutritional, hydration status
Consider the elder's right to choose to live at risk of harm, providing he or she is capable of making that choice.
Do not initiate an action that could increase the elder's risk of harm or antagonize the abuser.
Respect the elder's right to secrecy and the right for self-determination.

Disseminate Information to Community Regarding Prevention.

DECISIONAL CONFLICT

DEFINITION

The state in which an individual or group experiences uncertainty about a course of action when the choice involves risk, loss, or challenge.

DEFINING CHARACTERISTICS (HILTUNEN, 1987)

Major (80% to 100%)

Verbalization of uncertainty about choices
Verbalization of undesired consequences of alternative actions being considered
Vacillation between alternative choices
Delayed decision-making

Minor (50% to 79%)

Verbalized feeling of distress while attempting a decision
Physical signs of distress or tension (e.g., increased heart rate, increased muscle tension, restlessness) whenever the decision comes within focus of attention
Questioning personal values and beliefs while attempting to make a decision

RELATED FACTORS

Many situations can contribute to *Decisional Conflict*, particularly those that involve complex medical interventions of great risk. Any decisional situation can precipitate conflict for an individual; thus, the examples listed below are not exhaustive but reflect situations that may be problematic and possess factors that increase the difficulty.

Treatment-Related

Related to risks versus benefits of (specify test, treatment):
Surgery

Tumor removal
Cataract
Laminectomy
Orchiectomy
Cosmetic surgery

Joint replacement
Hysterectomy
Transplant
Cesarean section

Diagnostics
   Amniocentesis   X-rays
   Ultrasonography
Chemotherapy
Radiation
Dialysis
Mechanical ventilation
Enteral feedings
Intravenous hydration
Use of medications during labor
HIV antiviral therapy

Situational (Personal, Environmental)

Related to risks versus benefits of:

Personal
Marriage   Institutionalization
Separation   (child, parent)
Divorce   Breastfeeding versus
Parenthood   bottle-feeding
Birth control   Abortion
Artificial insemination   Sterilization
Adoption   Nursing home placement
Circumcision   Transport from rural facilities
Foster home placement   In vitro fertilization

Work/Task
Career change   Business investments
Relocation   Professional ethics

Related to lack of relevant information
Related to confusing information
Related to:

Disagreement within support systems
Inexperience with decision-making
Unclear personal values/beliefs
Conflict with personal values/beliefs
Resignation
Family history of poor prognosis
Hospital environment—loss of control
Ethical dilemmas of:
  • Quality of life
  • Cessation of life-support systems
  • "Do not resuscitate" orders
  • Termination of pregnancy
  • Organ transplant

Maturational

Adolescent
Related to risks versus benefits of:

Peer pressure
Sexual activity
Alcohol/drug use
Illegal/dangerous situations
College

Career choice
Use of birth control
Whether to continue a
    relationship

Adult
Related to risks versus benefits of:

Career change
Retirement

Relocation

Older Adult
Related to risks versus benefits of:

Retirement

Nursing home placement

NOC
Decision Making, Information Processing, Participation:
Health Care Decisions

Goals

The person will make an informed choice.

Indicators
- Relate the advantages and disadvantages of choices.
- Share fears and concerns regarding choices and responses of others.
- Define what would be most helpful to support the decision-making process.

NIC
Decision-Making Support, Mutual Goal Setting, Learning
Facilitation, Health System Guidance, Anticipatory
Guidance, Patient Rights Protection, Value Clarification,
Anxiety Reduction

Generic Interventions

Establish a trusting and meaningful relationship that promotes
    mutual understanding and caring.
Facilitate a logical decision-making process:

- Assist the person in recognizing what the problem is, and clearly identify that a decision needs to be made.
- Explore what the outcomes of not deciding would be.
- Have the person make a list of all the possible alternatives or options.
- Help identify the probable outcomes of the various alternatives.
- Help the person to face fears.
- Correct misinformation.
- Aid in evaluating the alternatives based on actual or potential threats to beliefs/values.
- Encourage the person to make a decision.

Encourage the person's significant others to be involved in the entire decision-making process.

Assist the individual in exploring personal values and relationships that may have an impact on the decision.

Support the individual making informed decision, even if decision conflicts with own values. Consult spiritual leader.

Actively reassure the person that the decision is his or hers to make and that he or she has the right to do so.

Do not allow others to undermine the person's confidence in making own decision.

Collaborate with family members to clarify the process.

Pediatric Interventions

Include children and adolescents in decision-making process.

Geriatric Interventions

Ensure that older adult is involved in decisions.

Facilitate communication among the elder, family, and professionals.

If needed, use simple explanations, and provide the pros and cons of the decision.

DIARRHEA

DEFINITION

The state in which an individual experiences or is at risk of experiencing frequent passages of liquid stool or unformed stool.

DEFINING CHARACTERISTICS

Major (Must Be Present, One or More)

Loose, liquid stools *and/or*
Increased frequency of stools (more than three times a day)

Minor (May Be Present)

Urgency
Cramping/abdominal pain
Increased frequency of bowel sounds
Increased fluidity or volume of stools

RELATED FACTORS

Pathophysiologic

Related to malabsorption or inflammation secondary to:

Gastritis
Peptic ulcer
Diverticulitis
Ulcerative colitis
Crohn's disease

Colon cancer
Spastic colon
Celiac disease (sprue)
Irritable bowel

Related to lactase deficiency

Related to increased peristalsis secondary to increased metabolic rate (hyperthyroidism)

Related to dumping syndrome

Related to infectious process secondary to:

Trichinosis
Dysentery
Cholera
Malaria
Cryptosporidium

Shigellosis
Typhoid fever
Infectious hepatitis
Microsporidia

Related to excessive secretion of fats in stool secondary to liver dysfunction

Related to inflammation and ulceration of gastrointestinal mucosa secondary to high levels of nitrogenous wastes (renal failure)

Treatment-Related

Related to malabsorption or inflammation secondary to surgical intervention of the bowel

Related to side effects of (specify):

Thyroid agents
Laxatives

Cancer chemotherapeutic
   agents

Antacids	Analgesics
(magnesium hydroxide)	Cimetidine
Stool softeners	Iron sulfate
Antibiotics	Antivirals (HIV)

Related to high-solute tube feedings

Situational (Personal, Environmental)

Related to stress or anxiety
Related to irritating foods (fruits, bran cereals)
Related to change in water or food secondary to travel
Related to change in bacteria in water
Related to bacteria, virus, or parasite to which no immunity is present
Related to increased caffeine consumption

Maturational

Infant: Related to breast milk

NOC

Bowel Elimination, Electrolyte and Acid/Base Balance, Fluid Balance, Hydration, Symptom Control

Goals

The person will report less diarrhea.

Indicators
• Describe contributing factors when known.
• Explain rationale for interventions.

NIC

Bowel Management, Diarrhea Management, Electrolyte Management, Nutrition Management, Enteral Tube Feeding

Generic Interventions

Assess for Causative or Contributing Factors: Tube Feedings, Dietary Indiscretions/Contaminated Foods, Food Allergies, Foreign Travel, Fecal Impaction.

Reduce Diarrhea.

Discontinue solids.
Ingest clear liquids (fruit juices, Gatorade, broth).

Avoid milk products, fat, high-fiber foods (whole-grain products, fresh fruits and vegetables).

Gradually add semisolids and solids (crackers, yogurt, rice, bananas, applesauce).

Increase Oral Intake to Maintain a Normal Urine Specific Gravity (Pale Yellow Urine).

Encourage Fluids High in Potassium and Low in Sugar (Water, Apple Juice, Flat Ginger Ale).

Caution Against Use of Very Hot or Very Cold Liquids.

Explain to Client and Significant Others the Interventions Required to Prevent Future Episodes.

If Related to Tube Feedings (Fuhrman, 1999):

Change to continuous-drip tube feedings.

Administer more slowly if signs of gastrointestinal intolerance occur.

If refrigerated, warm in hot water to room temperature.

Dilute strength of feeding temporarily.

Follow tube feeding with specified amount of water to ensure hydration.

Teach Precautions to Take When Traveling to Foreign Lands (Bennett, 2002).

Avoid foods served cold, salads, milk, fresh cheese, cold cuts, and salsa.

Drink carbonated or bottled beverages; avoid ice.

Peel fresh fruits and vegetables.

Consult with primary health care provider for treatment of traveler's diarrhea by prophylactic use of bismuth subsalicylate (e.g., Pepto-Bismol), 30 to 60 mL qid during travel and 2 days after return, or antimicrobials. Avoid opiate-containing antidiarrheals (e.g., Lomotil, Imodium).

Explain How to Prevent Transmission of Infection (Handwashing; Proper Storing, Cooking, and Handling of Food; Foods at Picnics).

👫 Pediatric Interventions

For Breastfed Infants:

Discontinue solids.

Offer clear liquid supplements.

Continue breastfeeding.

For Formula-Fed Infant or Milk-Fed Child:

Discontinue formula, milk products, and solid foods.

Avoid high-carbohydrate fluids (e.g., soft drinks, gelatin, fruit juices, caffeinated drinks, chicken or beef broth).

Use oral rehydration solutions (e.g., Pedialyte, Lytren, Infalyte, Resol) (Larson, 2000). Provide 60 to 80 mL/kg over a 2-hour period for mild to moderate diarrhea.

Gradually add plain solids (Jell-O, bananas, rice, cereal, crackers).

Gradually return to regular diet (except milk products) after 36 to 48 hours; after 3 to 5 days, gradually add milk products (half-strength skim milk to full-strength skim milk to half-strength whole milk to full-strength whole milk).

Gradually introduce formula (half-strength formula to full-strength formula).

Explain the BRAT Diet (Bananas, Rice, Applesauce, Tea, and Toast) to Counter the Effects of Diarrhea.

Ⓖ Geriatric Interventions

Determine if impaction is present; if so, remove it (refer to *Constipation* for specific interventions).

Monitor closely for hypovolemia and electrolyte imbalances (potassium, sodium).

DIGNITY, RISK FOR COMPROMISED HUMAN

DEFINITION

The state in which an individual is at risk for actual or perceived loss of respect and honor.

▰▰▰ AUTHOR'S NOTE

This nursing diagnosis was accepted by NANDA I in 2006. As approved, it is problematic. Most of the risk factors listed

(continued)

■■■ **AUTHOR'S NOTE** (*Continued*)
are defining characteristics (signs/symptoms), not risk factors, for example, perceived dehumanizing treatment, perceived humiliation, exposure of body, perceived invasion of privacy, perceived intrusion by clinical personnel, and disclosure of confidential information. This author has reworded them as risk factors.

This nursing diagnosis presents a new application for nursing practice. All persons are at risk for this diagnosis. Providing respect and honor to all persons, families, and communities is a critical core element of professional nursing. Prevention of Compromised Human Dignity must be a focus of all nursing interventions. It is the central concept of a caring profession. This diagnosis can also apply to prisoners, who as part of their penalty will be deprived of some rights, e.g., privacy and movement. Prisoners, however should always be treated with respect and not be tortured or humiliated. Nurses have the obligation to honor and "do no harm" in all settings in which they practice. This author recommends that this diagnosis be developed and integrated into a Standard of Care of the Nursing Department for all clients and families. The outcomes and interventions apply to all individuals, families and groups. This Department of Nursing Standards of Practice could also include *Risk for Infection, Risk for Infection Transmission, Risk for Falls*, and *Risk for Compromised Family Coping*.

RELATED FACTORS

Situational (Personal, Environmental)

Related to multiple factors associated with hospitalization, institutionalization, supervised group living environments, or any health care environment
Examples of factors are:
Unfamiliar procedures
Intrusions for clinical procedures
Multiple, unfamiliar personnel
Assistance needed for personal hygiene
Painful procedures
Unfamiliar terminology

Related to the nature of restrictions and environment of incarceration

NOC

Abuse Protection, Comfort Level, Dignified Life Closure, Information Processing, Knowledge: Illness Care, Self-Esteem, Spiritual Well-Being

Goals

The individual will report respectful and considerate care.

Indicators
Respect for privacy
Consideration of emotions
Feelings are anticipated.
Given options and control
Asked for permission
Given explanations
Minimization of body part exposure
No involvement of unnecessary personnel during stressful
    procedures

NIC

Patient Rights Protection, Anticipatory Guidance, Counseling, Emotional Support, Preparatory Sensory Information, Family Support, Humor, Mutual Goal Setting, Teaching: Procedure/Treatment, Touch

Interventions

Determine if the agency has a policy for prevention of
    Compromised Human Dignity. (Note: This type of policy or
    standard may be titled differently.)*
Review the policy; does it include (Walsh & Kowanko, 2002):
    Protection of privacy and private space
    Acquiring permission continuously
    Providing time for decision-making
    Advocating for the client
    Clear guidelines regarding the number of personnel, e.g.,
        students, nurses, physicians (residents, interns) that can be

---

*Whether a health care facility has a policy to protect client dignity, each nurse has an obligation to protect the human dignity of all persons. When performing an embarrassing procedure, engage the person in a conversation. Act as if the situation is matter-of-fact for you to reduce embarrassment. Use humor if appropriate. Talk to the person even if he or she is unresponsive.

present when confidential and/or stressful information is discussed or exposing procedures are needed

Reducing exposure of the body and the gaze of others

Providing care to each client and family as you would expect or demand for your family, partner, child, friend, or colleague

Explain the procedure to the person. During painful or embarrassing procedures, explain what he or she will feel.

Determine whether unnecessary personnel are present before a vulnerable or stressful event is initiated, e.g., code, and a painful or embarrassing procedure. Advise them that they are not needed.

Allow the person an opportunity to share his or her feelings after a difficult situation.

Expose the person as little as possible for the least possible time.

Maintain privacy for the individual's information and emotional responses.

Role model and advocate to maintain client dignity after death.

Discuss with involved personnel any incident that was disrespectful to the client or family. Report repeated incidents or any incident that is a violation of a client's dignity to the appropriate person.

When extreme measures are planned for or are being provided for an individual that are futile, refer to *Moral Distress*.

Practice expecting that honoring and protecting the dignity of individuals/groups is "not a value but a way of being" (Sodenberg et al., 1998).

DISUSE SYNDROME

DEFINITION

The state in which an individual is experiencing or at risk for deterioration of body systems or altered functioning as a result of prescribed or unavoidable musculoskeletal inactivity.

◼◼◼ AUTHOR'S NOTE

Disuse Syndrome represents an individual experiencing or at risk for the adverse effects of immobility. Syndrome nursing

(continued)

▓▓▓▓■■■■ **AUTHOR'S NOTE** *(Continued)*
diagnoses should not be written as *Risk*, because clustered
under them are risk and actual diagnoses. This author recommends using *Disuse Syndrome* without the Risk. *Syndrome*
identifies an individual as vulnerable to certain complications
and experiencing altered functioning in a health pattern. In
most situations, syndrome diagnoses do not require causative
or contributing factors (e.g., *Disuse Syndrome related to spinal
cord injury*). When the causative or contributing factors to
Disuse Syndrome are personal, environmental, or maturational, it may be useful to specify the related factors.

If an individual who is immobile manifests the signs and
symptoms of *Impaired Skin Integrity* or another diagnosis, the
specific diagnosis should be used. The nurse should continue
to use *Disuse Syndrome* so that deterioration of the other
body systems does not occur.

DEFINING CHARACTERISTICS

Presence of a Cluster of Actual or Risk Nursing Diagnoses Related to Inactivity:

Risk for Impaired Skin Integrity
Risk for Constipation
Risk for Impaired Respiratory Function
Risk for Impaired Peripheral Tissue Perfusion
Risk for Infection
Risk for Activity Intolerance
Risk for Impaired Physical Mobility
Risk for Injury
Risk for Disturbed Sensory Perception
Powerlessness
Disturbed Body Image

RELATED FACTORS (OPTIONAL)

Pathophysiologic

Related to:

Decreased sensorium
Unconsciousness
Neuromuscular impairment

Multiple sclerosis
Parkinsonism
Guillain-Barré syndrome

Muscular dystrophy
Partial or total paralysis
Spinal cord injury

Musculoskeletal conditions

Fractures	Rheumatic diseases

End-stage disease

AIDS	Cardiac disease
Renal disease	Cancer

Psychiatric/mental health disorders

Major depression	Severe phobias
Catatonic state	

Treatment-Related

Related to:

Surgery (amputation, skeletal)	Prescribed immobility
Mechanical ventilation	Invasive vascular lines
Traction/casts/splints	

Situational (Personal, Environmental)

Related to depression, fatigue, debilitated state, or pain

Maturational

Newborn, Infant, Child, or Adolescent

Related to:

Down syndrome	Osteogenesis imperfecta
Legg-Calvé-Perthes disease	Cerebral palsy
Spina bifida	Risser turnbuckle jacket
Autism	Juvenile arthritis
Mental/physical disability	

Older Adult

Related to:

Decreased motor agility	Presenile dementia
Muscle weakness	

NOC

Endurance, Immobility Consequences: Physiological, Immobility Consequences: Psycho-Cognitive, Mobility Level

Goals

The person will not experience complications of immobility.

Indicators

• Display intact skin/tissue integrity; maximum pulmonary function; maximum peripheral blood flow; full range of motion; bowel, bladder, and renal functioning within normal limits.

- Use social contacts and activities when possible.
- Explain rationale for treatments.
- Make decisions regarding care when possible.
- Share feelings regarding immobile state.

NIC

Activity Therapy, Energy Management, Mutual Goal Setting, Exercise Therapy, Fall Prevention, Pressure Ulcer Prevention, Body Mechanism Connection, Skin Surveillance, Positioning, Coping Enhancement, Decision-Making Support

Generic Interventions

Assist to reposition, turning frequently from side to side (hourly if possible).

Encourage deep breathing and controlled coughing exercises five times every hour.

Auscultate lung fields every 8 hours.

Maintain usual pattern of bowel elimination. Refer to *Constipation* for specific interventions.

Prevent pressure ulcers:

- Use repositioning schedule that relieves vulnerable area most often.
- Turn the person or instruct the person to turn or shift weight every 30 minutes to 2 hours.
- Keep bed as flat as possible to reduce shearing forces; limit Fowler's position to 30 minutes at a time.
- Use foam blocks or pillows to provide a bridging effect.
- Use enough personnel to lift person up in bed or chair.

Observe for erythema and blanching, and palpate for warmth and tissue sponginess with each position change.

Do not massage reddened areas.

Refer to *Impaired Skin Integrity* for additional interventions.

Elevate extremity above the level of the heart (may be contraindicated if severe cardiac or respiratory disease is present).

Perform range-of-motion exercises (frequency to be determined by condition of the individual).

Position the person in alignment to prevent complications.

Provide a daily intake of fluid of 2000 mL or greater (unless contraindicated); refer to *Deficient Fluid Volume* for specific interventions.

Provide weight bearing when possible (e.g., tilt table).

Encourage the person to share feelings and fears regarding restricted movement.

Encourage the person to wear own clothes rather than pajamas.
Include the individual in planning schedule for daily routine.
Be creative; vary the physical environment and daily routine
    when possible.
Provide opportunities for the individual to control decisions.

👫 Pediatric Interventions

Provide the child with play appropriate for condition.
Encourage the child to share feelings regarding immobilization.
Encourage the child to keep a diary of experiences.
If possible, provide the child with lunch mates (e.g., staff, other
    children).

DEFICIENT DIVERSIONAL ACTIVITY

DEFINITION

The state in which an individual or group experiences or is at risk
of experiencing decreased stimulation from or interest in activities
that promote enjoyment of life.

DEFINING CHARACTERISTICS

Major (Must Be Present)

Observed or statements of boredom/depression from inactivity

Minor (May Be Present)

Frequent expression of unpleasant thoughts or feelings
Yawning or inattentiveness, flat affect
Body language (shifting of body away from speaker)
Restlessness/fidgeting
Weight loss or gain

RELATED FACTORS

Pathophysiologic

*Related to difficulty accessing or participating in enjoyable
activities secondary to communicable disease, pain, mobility
problems, disabling disorder (specify) (e.g., MS, arthritis,
cancer, severe hearing/vision losses)*

Situational (Personal, Environmental)

Related to unsatisfactory social behaviors

Related to no peers or friends

Related to monotonous environment

Related to confinement

Related to lack of motivation

Related to difficulty accessing or participating in enjoyable activities secondary to:

Excessive long hours of work

No time for leisure activities

Career changes (e.g., teacher to homemaker, retirement)

Children leaving home ("empty nest")

Multiple role responsibilities

Maturational

Infant/Child

Related to lack of appropriate stimulation, toys, peers

Older Adult

Related to difficulty accessing or participating in enjoyable activities secondary to:

Sensory motor deficits   Lack of peer group

Lack of transportation   Limited finances

Fear of crime   Confusion

NOC

Leisure Participation, Social Involvement

Goals

The person will report participating in at least one enjoyable activity each day.

Indicators

• Relate improved satisfaction with current activity level.

• Identify enjoyable activities that can enhance quality of life.

NIC

Recreation Therapy, Socialization Enhancement, Self-Esteem Enhancement

Generic Interventions

Stimulate motivation by showing interest and encouraging sharing of feelings and experiences.

Help the person to work through feelings of anger and grief.

Vary daily routine when possible (e.g., give bath in the afternoon so that the person can watch a special show or talk with a visitor who drops in).

Include the individual in planning daily schedule.

Plan time for visitors.

Be creative; vary the physical environment when possible.

Place the person near a window or take outside, if possible.

Discuss previously enjoyed hobbies. Consult with recreational or occupational therapist.

Provide reading material, radio, television, and books on tape.

Plan an activity daily to give person something to look forward to, and always keep your promises.

Discourage the use of television as the primary source of recreation unless it is highly desired.

Consider using a volunteer to spend time reading to the person or helping with an activity.

If appropriate, enlist the person to help others with an activity.

In an institutional setting:

Encourage participation in recreational therapy.

Praise involvement.

Allow the person to choose which recreational activities are of interest.

Focus on capabilities, not deficits.

Consider using reminiscence, music, or pet therapy.

Organize book discussions.

Pediatric Interventions

Provide an environment with accessible playthings that suit the child's developmental age, and ensure that they are well within reach.

Encourage family to bring in child's favorite playthings, including items from nature that will help to keep the real world alive (e.g., goldfish; leaves in the fall).

DYSREFLEXIA, AUTONOMIC

Autonomic Dysreflexia
Risk for Autonomic Dysreflexia

DEFINITION

The state in which an individual with a spinal cord injury at T6 or above experiences or is at risk of experiencing a potential life-threatening uninhibited sympathetic response of the nervous system to a noxious stimulus.

AUTHOR'S NOTE
This is a situation that the nurse or client can prevent or treat. If the nurse's initial treatment does not relieve the symptoms, medical treatment is imperative. An individual does not experience Dysreflexia as a continued state but rather is at risk for it, so if it is experienced, it must be abated. Thus, *Risk for Autonomic Dysreflexia* better describes the clinical situation than does *Autonomic Dysreflexia*.

DEFINING CHARACTERISTICS

Major (Must Be Present, One or More)

Individual with Spinal Cord Injury at T6 or Above with:

Paroxysmal hypertension (sudden periodic elevated blood pressure in which systolic pressure is >140 mm Hg and diastolic is >90 mm Hg)
Bradycardia (pulse rate <60) or tachycardia (>100 beats/min)
Diaphoresis (above the injury)
Red splotches on the skin (above the injury)
Pallor (below the injury)
Headache (a diffuse pain in different portions of the head and not confined to any nerve distribution area)
Apprehension

Minor (May Be Present)

Chilling
Conjunctival congestion

Horner's syndrome (contraction of the pupil, partial ptosis of the
    eyelid, enophthalmos, and sometimes loss of sweating over
    the affected side of the face)
Paresthesia
Pilomotor reflex
Blurred vision
Nasal congestion
Chest pain
Metallic taste in the mouth

RELATED FACTORS
Pathophysiologic
Related to visceral stretching and irritation secondary to:

Bowel

Constipation	Fecal impaction
Acute abdominal condition	Hemorrhoids
Gastric ulcers	Anal fissure

Bladder

Distended bladder	Infection
Urinary calculi	

Cutaneous

Pressure ulcers	Insect bites
Burns	Ingrown toenails
Sunburn	Blister

Reproductive

Menstruation	Epididymitis
Pregnancy or delivery	Uterine contraction
Vaginal infection	Vaginal dilation

Related to stimulation of skin (abdominal, thigh)
Related to spastic sphincter
Related to deep vein thrombosis

Treatment-Related
Related to visceral stretching secondary to:
Removal of fecal impaction
Clogged or nonpatent catheter
Visceral stretching and irritation secondary to surgical incision
Catheterization, enema

Situational (Personal, Environmental)
Related to lack of knowledge of prevention or treatment
Related to visceral stretching secondary to:
Sexual activity

Menstruation
Boosting
Pregnancy or delivery
Submergence in cold water

NOC

Neurological Status, Neurological Status: Autonomic,
Vital Signs Status

Goals

The individual/family will prevent or respond to early signs/
symptoms.

Indicators
- State factors that cause dysreflexia.
- Describe the treatment for dysreflexia.
- Relate when emergency treatment is indicated.

NIC

Dysreflexia Management, Vital Signs Monitoring,
Emergency Care, Medication Administration

Generic Interventions

If signs of dysreflexia occur:
- Stand person up, or sit person up, or raise head of bed.
- Lower legs.
- Loosen all constrictive clothing, appliances.

Check for distended bladder.
If catheterized:
- Check catheter for kinks or compression.
- Irrigate with only 30 mL saline very slowly.
- Replace catheter if it will not drain.

If not catheterized, insert catheter using an anesthetic ointment
    and remove 500 mL, then clamp for 15 minutes; repeat cycle
    until bladder is drained.
For fecal impaction:
- First apply dibucaine hydrochloride ointment (Nupercainal)
    to the anus and 1 inch (2.54 cm) into the rectum.
- Gently check rectum with a well-lubricated glove.
- Insert rectal suppository, or gently remove impaction.

Assess for other causes:
- Skin stimulation: spray lesion with a topical anesthetic agent.

- Other stimuli: these include cold draft, objects that pressure skin.
- Bladder infection: send urine for culture.

Continue to monitor blood pressure every 3 to 5 minutes.

Immediately consult physician for pharmacologic treatment if hypertension or noxious stimuli are not eliminated.

Teach signs and symptoms and treatment of dysreflexia to person and family.

Teach when immediate medical intervention is warranted.

Explain what situations can trigger dysreflexia (menstrual cycle, sexual activity, bladder or bowel routines).

Advise consultation with physician for long-term pharmacologic management if individual is very vulnerable.

Document how frequently episodes occur and precipitating factor(s).

Provide with printed instructions to guide actions during crisis or to show other health care personnel (e.g., dentists, gynecologists) (Kavchak-Keyes, 2000).

Advise athletes with high spinal cord injury about the danger of boosting (binding their legs, distending bladder to increase norepinephrine levels) (McClain, 1999).

▶ Risk for Autonomic Dysreflexia

DEFINITION

The state in which an individual with a spinal cord injury at T7 or above is at risk of experiencing a potential for a life-threatening uninhibited sympathetic response of the nervous system to a noxious stimulus.

RISK FACTORS

Refer to Related Factors in *Autonomic Dysreflexia*.

RELATED FACTORS

Refer to Related Factors in *Autonomic Dysreflexia*.

Goals

Refer to *Autonomic Dysreflexia*.

Generic Interventions

Teach signs and symptoms and treatment of dysreflexia to person and family.

Teach when immediate medical intervention is warranted.

Explain what situations can trigger dysreflexia (menstrual cycle, sexual activity, bladder or bowel routines).

Teach to observe for early signs of bladder infections and skin lesions (pressure ulcers, ingrown toenails).

Advise consultation with physician for long-term pharmacologic management if individual is very vulnerable.

DISTURBED ENERGY FIELD

DEFINITION

The state in which a disruption of the flow of energy surrounding a person's being results in a disharmony of the body, mind, and/or spirit.

AUTHOR'S NOTE

This addition to the NANDA list is unique for two reasons. It represents a specific theory (human energy field theory), and the interventions used require specialized instruction and supervised practice. Meehan (1991) recommends:

- At least 6 months' experience in professional practice in an acute care setting
- Guided learning by a nurse with at least 2 years' experience
- Conformance with practice guidelines
- Thirty hours of instruction in the theory and practice
- Thirty hours of supervised practice with relatively healthy individuals
- Successful completion of written and practice evaluations

This diagnosis may be considered unconventional by some. Perhaps each nurse needs to be reminded that there are many theories, philosophies, and frameworks of nursing practice, just as there are many definitions of clients and practice settings; some nurses practice on street corners with homeless persons, whereas others practice in an office attached to their home. Nursing diagnoses should not represent only the practices of nurses in the mainstream practice setting (acute care, long-term care, and home health). Rather

(continued)

■■■ **AUTHOR'S NOTE** *(Continued)*
than criticize a diagnosis as having little applicability to
one's own practice, perhaps we should celebrate the diversity
among us. Fundamentally, nurses are all connected as each
of us and all of us seek to improve the condition of clients,
families, groups, and communities.

DEFINING CHARACTERISTICS

Perception of changes in patterns of the energy flow, such as:

Temperature Change

Warmth	Coolness

Visual Changes

Image	Color

Disruption of the Field

Vacant	Hole
Spike	Bulge

Movement

Wave	Spike
Tingling	Dense
Flowing	

Sounds

Tone	Words

RELATED FACTORS

Pathophysiologic

*Related to slowing or blocking of energy flows secondary to:
illness (specify), injury, or pregnancy*

Treatment-Related

*Related to slowing or blocking of energy flows secondary to:
immobility, labor and delivery, or perioperative experience*

Situational (Personal, Environmental)

*Related to the slowing or blocking of energy flows secondary to
pain, anxiety, fear, or grieving*

Maturational

*Related to age-related developmental difficulties or crises
(specify)*

NOC

Spiritual Well-Being, Well-Being

Goals

The person will report relief of symptoms after therapeutic touch.

Indicators
- Report increased sense of relaxation.
- Report a decrease in pain, using a scale of 0 to 10 before and after therapies.
- Have slower, deeper respirations.

NIC

Therapeutic Touch, Spiritual Support

Generic Interventions

The following phases of therapeutic touch are learned separately but are rendered concurrently.

The presentation of these interventions is for the purpose of describing the process for nurses who do not practice therapeutic touch. This discussion may help nurses support colleagues who practice therapeutic touch and initiate referrals. As discussed previously, preparing for therapeutic touch requires specialized instruction that is beyond the scope of this book.

Explain therapeutic touch, and obtain verbal permission.

Prepare the client and environment for therapeutic touch:
- Provide as much privacy as possible.
- Give the person permission to stop the therapy at any time.

Allow the person to assume a comfortable position (e.g., lying or sitting on a bed or couch).

Shift from a direct focus on the environment to an inner focus, which is perceived as the center of life within the nurse (centering).

Assess by scanning the person's energy field for openness and symmetry (Krieger, 1979).
- Move hands, palms toward the person, at a distance of 2 to 4 inches over the person's body from head to feet, in a smooth, light movement.
- Sense the cues to energy imbalance (e.g., warmth, coolness, tightness, heaviness, tingling, emptiness).

Facilitate a rhythmic flow of energy by moving hands more
    vigorously from head to toe (unruffling/clearing).
Focus intent on the specific repatterning of areas of imbalance
    and impeded flow. Using your hands as focal points, move the
    hands in gentle, sweeping movements from head to feet one
    time.
Encourage the person to provide feedback.
Document the procedure and the feedback.

ELECTROLYTE IMBALANCES, RISK FOR

▶ Risk for Complications of Electrolyte Imbalances

DEFINITION (NANDA)

At risk for a change in serum electrolyte levels that may compromise health.

RISK FACTORS

Diarrhea, vomiting
Fluid Imbalance (e.g., dehydration, water intoxication)
Impaired regulatory mechanisms (e.g., renal dysfunction,
    endocrine dysfunction)
Treatment-related side effects (e.g., medications, drains)

AUTHOR'S NOTE
This new NANDA-I diagnosis represents a collaborative
problem. If the nurse is preventing hypokalemia as a side
effect of diuretic, *Risk for Ineffective Self-Health Management*
can be used to teach prevention strategies.

Interventions/Goals

Refer to Section 3 for goals and interventions for Risk for Complications of Electrolyte Imbalances

ENVIRONMENTAL INTERPRETATION SYNDROME

DEFINITION (NANDA)

Consistent lack of orientation to person, place, time, or circumstances for more than 3 to 6 months, necessitating a protective environment.

■■■ **AUTHOR'S NOTE**
Environmental Interpretation Syndrome describes an individual who needs a protective environment because of consistent lack of orientation to person, place, time, or circumstances. This diagnosis is described under *Chronic Confusion, Wandering,* and *Risk for Injury*. Interventions focus on maintaining maximum level of independence and preventing injury. Until clinical research differentiates this diagnosis from the aforementioned diagnoses, use *Chronic Confusion, Wandering,* or *Risk for Injury*, depending on the data presented.

DEFINING CHARACTERISTICS (NANDA)

Major (Must Be Present, One or More)

Consistent disorientation in known and unknown environments
Chronic confusional states

Minor (May Be Present)

Loss of occupation or social functioning from memory decline
Slow in responding to questions

Inability to concentrate
Inability to reason
Inability to follow simple directions or instructions

RELATED FACTORS

Dementia (Alzheimer's disease, multi-infarct dementia, Pick's disease, AIDS dementia)

Parkinson's disease
Huntington's disease
Depression
Alcoholism

FAMILY PROCESSES, INTERRUPTED

Family Processes, Interrupted
Family Processes, Dysfunctional

DEFINITION

The state in which a normally supportive family experiences or is at risk to experience a stressor that challenges its previously effective functioning ability.

DEFINING CHARACTERISTICS

Major (Must Be Present, One or More)

Family system cannot or does not:
Adapt constructively to crisis
Communicate openly and effectively among family members

Minor (May Be Present)

Family system cannot or does not:
Meet physical needs of all its members
Meet emotional needs of all its members
Meet spiritual needs of all its members
Express or accept a wide range of feelings
Seek or accept help appropriately

RELATED FACTORS

Any factor can contribute to *Interrupted Family Processes*. Some common factors are listed below.

Treatment-Related

Related to:

Disruption of family routines owing to time-consuming
treatments (e.g., home dialysis)

Physical changes owing to treatments of ill family member

Emotional changes in all family members owing to treatments of
ill family member

Financial burden of treatments for ill family member

Hospitalization of ill family member

Situational (Personal, Environmental)

Related to loss of family member:

Death	Incarceration
Going away to school	Desertion
Separation	Hospitalization
Divorce	

Related to gain of family member (e.g., birth, adoption, marriage, elderly relative)

Related to losses associated with:

Poverty	Change in family roles
Disaster	Working mother
Relocation	Retirement
Economic crisis	Birth of child with defect

Related to conflict (moral, goal, cultural)

Related to breach of trust among members

Related to social deviance by family member (e.g., crime)

NOC

Family Coping, Family Environment: Internal, Family
Normalization: Parenting

Goals

The family members will maintain a functional system of mutual
support for each other.

Indicators

- Frequently verbalize feelings to professional nurse and each
  other.
- Identify appropriate external resources available.

NIC

Family Involvement Promotion, Coping Enhancement, Family Integrity Promotion, Family Therapy, Counseling, Referral

Generic Interventions

Assist the family with appraisal of the situation.

What is at stake? Encourage the family to have a realistic perspective by providing accurate information and answers to questions.

- What are the choices? Assist the family to reorganize roles at home and set priorities to maintain family integrity and reduce stress.
- Where is help available? Direct the family to community agencies, home health care organizations, and sources of financial assistance as needed (see *Impaired Home Maintenance* for additional interventions).

Create a private and supportive hospital environment for the family.

Acknowledge strengths to the family when appropriate:

- "I can tell you are a very close family."
- "You know just how to get your mother to eat."
- "Your brother means a great deal to you."

Involve family members in care of ill member when possible (feeding, bathing, dressing, ambulating).

Involve family members in patient care conferences when appropriate.

Encourage family to acquire substitutes to care for the ill person to provide the family with time away.

Encourage verbalization of guilt, anger, blame, hostility, and subsequent recognition of feelings in family members.

Aid family members to change their expectations of the ill member in a realistic manner.

Provide the family with anticipatory guidance as illness continues:

Inform parents of the effects of prolonged hospitalization on children (appropriate to developmental age).

Prepare family members for signs of depression, anxiety, and dependency, which are a natural part of the illness experience.

Enlist help of other professionals when problems extend beyond realm of nursing (e.g., social worker, clinical psychologist, nurse therapist, clinical specialist, psychiatrist, child care specialist).

▶ Family Processes, Dysfunctional

Related to destructive family response patterns to alcohol abuse

DEFINITION

The state in which the psychosocial, spiritual, economic, and physiologic functions of the family unit are chronically disorganized, which leads to conflict, denial of problems, resistance to change, ineffective problem-solving and a series of self-perpetuating crises.

■■■■ AUTHOR'S NOTE

Dysfunctional Family Processes can be utilized with any family that is not functioning effectively for all members. Examples of related factors can be family member addictions (alcohol, gambling, shopping, drugs or a chronic health problem, e.g., mental health. Alcoholism is a family disease. The focus of the intervention section represents the consequences of the disturbed family dynamics related to alcohol abuse by a family member.

DEFINING CHARACTERISTICS
(LINDEMAN ET AL., 1994)

Major (80% to 100%)

Behaviors

DEFINING CHARACTERISTICS

Major

Deteriorated family relationships	Inconsistent parenting	Disturbed family dynamics
Closed communication systems	Family denial	Marital problems
Ineffective spouse communication	Intimacy dysfunction	Disruption of family roles

Minor

Cannot express or accept wide range of feelings
Inability to get or receive help appropriately
Orientation toward tension relief rather than goal achievement

Ineffective decision making
Contradictory, paradoxical communication
Triangulating family relationship
Inability to meet spiritual needs of members
Reduced ability to relate to one another for mutual growth and
    maturation
Inability to meet security needs of members
Does not demonstrate respect for individuality of its members

RELATED FACTORS

*Related to impaired ability to fulfill role responsibilities
secondary to:*
Any acute or chronic illness

Situational (Personal, Environmental)

*Related to impaired ability to constructively manage stressors
secondary to:*
Substance abuse, alcoholism
Negative role modeling
History of ineffective relationship with own parents
History of abusive relationship with parents
Related to unrealistic expectations of child by parent
Related to unrealistic expectations of parent by child
Related to unmet psychosocial needs of child by parent
Related to unmet psychosocial needs of parent by child
Dysfunctional Family Processes related to destructive family
    response patterns to alcohol abuse
Dysfunctional Family Processes related to destructive family
    responses to alcohol abuse

NOC

Family Coping, Family Functioning, Substance Abuse
Consequences

Goals

The family will acknowledge the alcoholism in the family.
The family will set short- and long-term goals.

Indicators

- Relate the effects of alcoholism on the family unit and individu-
  als.
- Identify destructive response patterns.
- Describe resources available for individual and family therapy.

NIC

Coping Enhancement, Referral, Family Process Maintenance, Substance Abuse Treatment, Family Integrity Promotion, Limit-Setting Support Group

Generic Interventions

Establish a Trusting Relationship.

Be consistent; keep promises.
Be accepting and noncritical.
Do not pass judgment on what is revealed.
Focus on family member responses.

Allow the Family as Individuals and as a Group to Share Their Pent-Up Feelings.

Emphasize that Family Members Are Not Responsible for the Person's Drinking.

Explore the Family's Beliefs About Their Situation and Their Goals.

Discuss characteristics of alcoholism. Review a screening test that outlines characteristics of alcoholism (e.g., the Michigan Alcoholism Screening Test).
Discuss causes, and correct misinformation.
Assist to establish short- and long-term goals.

Discuss Ineffective Methods Families Use:

Hiding alcohol or car keys
Anger, silence, threats, crying
Making excuses for work, family, or friends
Bailing the person out of jail

Assist Family Members to Gain Insight into the Effects of Their Attempts to Control the Drinking.

Does not stop drinking
Increases family anger
Removes the responsibility for drinking from the person
Prevents the person from suffering the consequences of his or her drinking behavior

Emphasize that Helping the Alcoholic Means First Helping Themselves.

Focus on changing their response.
Allow the person to be responsible for his or her drinking behavior.

Describe activities that will improve their life as individuals and as a family.

Initiate one stress-management technique (e.g., aerobic exercises, assertiveness course, walking, meditation, relaxation breathing).

Plan time as a family together outside the home (e.g., museum, zoo, picnic). If the alcoholic person is included, the person must contract not to drink during the activity and agree on a consequence if he or she does.

Discuss with the Family that, During Recovery, Their Usual Family Dynamics Will Be Dramatically Changed.

Discuss the Possibility of Relapse and the Contributing Factors.

If Additional Family or Individual Nursing Diagnoses Exist, Refer to Child Abuse or Domestic Violence Under Disabled Family Coping.

Initiate Health Teaching Regarding Community Resources and Referrals as Indicated.

Al-Anon
Alcoholics Anonymous
Family therapy
Individual therapy
Self-help groups (e.g., adult children of alcoholics)

FATIGUE

DEFINITION

The self-recognized state in which an individual experiences an overwhelming sustained sense of exhaustion and decreased capacity for physical and mental work that is not relieved by rest.

AUTHOR'S NOTE

Fatigue is different from tiredness. Tiredness is a transient, temporary state from lack of sleep, improper nutrition, sedentary lifestyle, or a temporary increase in work or social

(continued)

■■■■ **AUTHOR'S NOTE** *(Continued)*
responsibilities. Fatigue is a pervasive, subjective, drained
feeling that cannot be eliminated. Persons with fatigue are
taught energy-conservation techniques. *Activity Intolerance* is
different from *Fatigue* in that the person with *Activity Intolerance* will be assisted to increase endurance to progress and
increase activity. The person with chronic fatigue will not
return to the previous level of functioning.

DEFINING CHARACTERISTICS (VOITH ET AL., 1987)

Major (80% to 100%)

Verbalization of an unremitting and overwhelming lack of
energy
Inability to maintain usual routines
Verbalization of distress

Minor (50% to 79%)

Perceived need for additional energy to accomplish routine tasks
Increase in physical complaints
Emotionally labile or irritable
Impaired ability to concentrate
Decreased performance
Lethargic or listless
Sleep disturbances

RELATED FACTORS

Many factors can cause fatigue. It may be useful to combine
related factors, such as related to muscle weakness, build-up of
waste products, inflammatory process, and infections secondary
to AIDS.

Pathophysiologic

Related to:
Acute infections (e.g., mononucleosis, hepatitis, viruses)
Chronic infections (Epstein-Barr)
Pregnancy

Related to inadequate tissue oxygenation secondary to:
Congestive heart failure
Chronic obstructive lung disease
Anemia
Peripheral vascular disease

Related to biochemical changes secondary to:

Endocrine/metabolic disorders

Diabetes mellitus	Pituitary disorders
Hypothyroidism	Addison's disease

Chronic diseases (e.g., renal failure, cirrhosis, Lyme disease)

Related to muscle wasting secondary to:

Myasthenia gravis	Parkinson's disease
Multiple sclerosis	AIDS
Amyotrophic lateral sclerosis	

Related to hypermetabolic state, competition between body and tumor for nutrients, anemia, and stressors associated with cancer

Related to nutritional deficits or changes in nutrient metabolism secondary to:

Nausea	Side effects of medications
Vomiting	Gastric surgery
Diarrhea	Diabetes mellitus

Related to chronic inflammatory process secondary to:

AIDS	Cirrhosis
Arthritis	Inflammatory bowel disease
Lupus erythematosus	Renal failure
Hepatitis	

Treatment-Related

Related to biochemical changes secondary to:

Chemotherapy

Radiation therapy

Side effects of (specify)

Related to surgical damage to tissue and anesthesia

Related to increased energy expenditure secondary to, for example, amputation, gait disorder, use of walker, crutches

Situational (Personal, Environmental)

Related to prolonged decreased activity and deconditioning secondary to:

Anxiety	Social isolation
Fever	Nausea/vomiting
Diarrhea	Depression
Pain	Obesity

Related to excessive role demands

Related to overwhelming emotional demands

Related to extreme stress

Related to sleep disturbance

Maturational

Child/Adolescent

Related to hypermetabolic state secondary to:
Mononucleosis   Fever

Related to chronic insufficient nutrients secondary to:
Obesity   Excessive dieting
Eating disorders

Related to effects of newborn care on sleep patterns and need for continuous attention

Related to hypermetabolic state during first trimester

NOC

Activity Tolerance, Endurance, Energy Conservation

Goals

The person will participate in activities that stimulate and balance physical, cognitive, affective, and social domains.

Indicators
- Discuss the causes of fatigue.
- Share feelings regarding the effects of fatigue on his or her life.
- Establish priorities for daily and weekly activities.

NIC

Mutual Goal Setting, Energy Management

Generic Interventions

Explain the causes of the person's fatigue.

Allow expression of feelings regarding the effects of fatigue on the person's life.

Assist the individual to identify strengths, abilities, interests.

Instruct the individual to record fatigue levels each hour during a 24-hour period (select a usual day).

Ask individual to rate fatigue 0 to 10 using the Rhoten (1982) fatigue scale (0 = not tired, peppy; 10 = total exhaustion).

Record the activities at the time of each rating.

Together, analyze the 24-hour fatigue levels:
- Times of peak energy
- Times of exhaustion
- Activities associated with increasing fatigue

Assist the individual to identify what tasks can be delegated.

Plan the important tasks during periods of high energy.

Assist the individual to identify priorities and eliminate nonessential activities.

Teach energy conservation techniques:
- Place work items within easy reach.
- Reduce trips up and down stairs.
- Distribute difficult tasks throughout the week.
- Rest before difficult tasks, and stop before fatigue ensues.
- Install grab rails.
- Eat small meals (five times daily).
- Request drivers instead of driving.
- Delegate or barter for household chores.

Explain the psychological and physiological benefits of exercise, and discuss what is realistic.

Provide significant others with opportunities to discuss their feelings in private.

Explain the effects of conflict and stress on energy levels.

Assist to learn effective coping skills (e.g., sharing, assertiveness, relaxation techniques).

Refer to community services (Meals on Wheels, housekeeper).

🎎 Maternal Interventions

Explain the reason for fatigue in first and third trimesters:
- Increased basal metabolic rate
- Changes in hormonal levels
- Anemia
- Increased cardiac output (third trimester)

Emphasize the need for naps and 8 hours of sleep.

Discuss the importance of exercise (e.g., walking).

Advise to avoid overexertion.

For postpartum women, discuss factors that increase fatigue (Gardner & Campbell, 1991):
- Labor more than 30 hours, difficult labor, or reports of high labor pain
- Hemoglobin <10 g/dL or postpartum hemorrhage
- Preexisting chronic disease
- Episiotomy, tear, or cesarean section
- Sleeping difficulties
- Ill neonate or a congenital anomaly
- Nonsupportive partner
- Dependent children at home
- Child care problems
- Unrealistic expectations

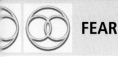

Geriatric Interventions

Consider if chronic fatigue is the consequence of late-life depression.

Refer individual suspected of depression for evaluation.

FEAR

DEFINITION

The state in which an individual or group experiences a feeling of physiologic or emotional disruption related to an identifiable source that is perceived as dangerous.

■■■■ **AUTHOR'S NOTE**
See *Anxiety.*

DEFINING CHARACTERISTICS

Major (Must Be Present, One or More)

Feelings of dread, fright, apprehension, alarm

Behaviors of avoidance; narrowing of focus on danger; and deficits in attention, performance, control, and self-assurance

Minor (May Be Present)

Verbal Reports of Panic, Obsessions

Behavioral acts of:

Crying	Dysfunctional immobility
Aggression	Compulsive mannerisms
Escape	Increased questioning/
Hypervigilance	verbalization

Visceral-Somatic Activity

Musculoskeletal

Trembling	Fatigue/weakness of limbs
Muscle tightness	

Cardiovascular

Palpitations	Increased blood pressure
Rapid pulse	

Respiratory

Shortness of breath

Increased rate

Gastrointestinal

Anorexia

Diarrhea/urge to defecate

Nausea/vomiting

Dry mouth/throat

Genitourinary

Urinary frequency/urgency

Skin

Flush/pallor

Paresthesia

Sweating

Central Nervous System/Perceptual

Syncope

Absentmindedness

Insomnia

Nightmares

Lack of concentration

Dilated pupils

Irritability

RELATED FACTORS

Fear can occur as a response to a variety of health problems, situations, or conflicts. Some common sources are indicated below.

Pathophysiologic

Related to perceived immediate and long-term effects of:

Loss of body part

Cognitive impairment

Loss of body function

Long-term disability

Disabling illness

Terminal disease

Sensory impairment

Treatment-Related

Related to loss of control and unpredictable outcome secondary to:

Hospitalization

Surgery and its outcome

Anesthesia

Invasive procedures

Radiation

Situational (Personal, Environmental)

Related to loss of control and unpredictable outcome secondary to:

Pain

Divorce

New environment

Success

New persons

Failure

Lack of knowledge

Language barrier

Change or loss of significant other
Related to potential loss of income

Maturational

Preschool

Related to:

Separation from parents, peers
Being alone
Strangers, animals, snakes
Bodily harm

Age-related fears (dark,
  strangers, ghosts, monsters)

School Age (6 to 12 years)

Related to:

Being lost
Bad dreams
Being in trouble (12 years)

Weapons (8 years)
Thunder, lightning
  (6 to 8 years)

Adolescent

Related to uncertainty of:

Appearance
Peer support

Scholastic success

Related to vulnerability to violence
Related to separation from support system

Adult

Related to uncertainty of:

Marriage
Pregnancy
Parenthood

Job security
Effects of aging

Older Adult

Related to:

Anticipated dependence
Prolonged suffering
Vulnerability to crime
Financial insecurity
Abandonment

NOC

Anxiety Level, Fear Level

Goals

The adult will relate an increase in psychological and physiologic comfort.

Indicators

- Show decreases in visceral response (pulse, respirations).
- Differentiate real from imagined situations.
- Describe effective and ineffective coping patterns.
- Identify his or her own coping responses.

The child will exhibit or relate an increase in psychological and physiologic comfort.

- Discuss fears.
- Exhibit less crying.

NIC

Anxiety Reduction, Coping Enhancement, Presence, Counseling, Relaxation Therapy

Generic Interventions

Orient to environment using simple explanations.

Speak slowly and calmly.

Allow personal space.

Use simple, direct statements (avoid detail).

Encourage expression of feelings (helplessness, anger).

Encourage responses that reflect reality. Discuss which aspects can be changed and which cannot.

Provide an emotionally nonthreatening atmosphere. Set up a consistent daily schedule.

When intensity of feelings has decreased, bring behavioral cues into the person's awareness.

Teach relaxation techniques:

- Slow, rhythmic breathing
- Progressive relaxation of muscle groups
- Self-coaching
- Thought-stopping
- Guided imagery

👥 Pediatric Interventions

Accept the child's fear and provide an explanation, if possible, or some form of control; share with the child that these fears are okay:

- Fear of imaginary animals, intruders ("I don't see a lion in your room, but I will leave the light on for you, and if you need me again, please call.")
- Fear of parent being late (Establish a contingency plan, e.g., "If you come home from school and Mommy is not here, go to Mrs. S. next door.")

- Fear of vanishing down a toilet or bathtub drain. Wait until the child is out of the tub before releasing drain. Wait until the child is off the toilet before flushing. Leave toys in bathtub, and demonstrate how they do not go down the drain.
- Fear of dark. Give child a night light.

Fear of dogs, cats:

- Allow child to watch a child and a dog playing from a distance.
- Do not force child to touch the animal.

Discuss with parents the normalcy of fears in children; explain the necessity of acceptance and the negative outcomes of punishment or of forcing the child to overcome the fear.

Provide the child with opportunity to observe how other children cope successfully with feared object.

Maternal Interventions

Explore fears and emotional responses to pregnancy (Reeder et al., 1997).

First trimester

- Uncertainty about future role as mother
- Uncertainty about timing of pregnancy

Third trimester

- Fears about own well-being and "performance" during labor
- Fears about well-being of the fetus

FLUID VOLUME, DEFICIENT

Fluid volume, deficient
Risk for Deficient Fluid Volume

DEFINITION

The state in which an individual who is not NPO experiences or is at risk of experiencing dehydration.

AUTHOR'S NOTE

This diagnosis represents situations in which nurses can prescribe definitive treatment to prevent fluid depletion or to reduce or eliminate related factors, such as insufficient oral intake. Situations that represent hypovolemia caused by hemorrhage or NPO status should be considered collaborative problems, not nursing diagnoses. Nurses monitor to detect these situations and collaborate with doctors for treatment. These situations can be labeled *Risk for Complication of Bleeding* or *Risk for Complication of Hypovolemia*.

DEFINING CHARACTERISTICS

Major (Must Be Present, One or More)

Insufficient oral fluid intake
Negative balance of intake and output
Weight loss
Dry skin/mucous membranes

Minor (May Be Present)

Increased serum sodium
Decreased urine output or excessive urine output
Concentrated urine or urinary frequency
Thirst, nausea, or anorexia

RELATED FACTORS

Pathophysiologic

Related to excessive urinary output
Uncontrolled diabetes
Diabetes insipidus (inadequate antidiuretic hormone)
Related to increased capillary permeability and evaporative loss from burn wound
Related to losses secondary to:
Fever or increased metabolic rate
Abnormal drainage (e.g., wound, excessive menses)
Peritonitis
Diarrhea

Situational (Personal, Environmental)

Related to vomiting/nausea
Related to decreased motivation to drink liquids secondary to depression or fatigue

Related to fad diets/fasting
Related to high-solute tube feedings
Related to difficulty swallowing or feeding self secondary to
oral pain or fatigue
Related to extreme heat/sun, dryness
Related to excessive loss through indwelling catheters or drains
Related to insufficient fluids for exercise effort or weather
conditions
Related to excessive use of laxatives, enemas, diuretics, or
alcohol

Maturational

Infant/Child
Related to increased vulnerability secondary to decreased fluid
reserve and decreased ability to concentrate urine

Older Adult
Related to increased vulnerability secondary to decreased fluid
reserve and decreased sensation of thirst

NOC

Electrolyte and Acid-Base Balance, Fluid Balance,
Hydration

Goals

The person will maintain a urine specific gravity within a normal
range.

Indicators
- Increase intake of fluids to a specified amount according to age
  and metabolic needs.
- Identify risk factors for fluid deficit, and relate the need for in-
  creased fluid intake as indicated.
- Demonstrate no signs and symptoms of dehydration.

NIC

Fluid/Electrolyte Management, Fluid Monitoring

Generic Interventions

Assess likes and dislikes; provide favorite fluids within dietary
  restrictions.
Plan an intake goal for every 8 hours (e.g., 1000 mL during day,
  800 mL during evening, 300 mL at night).

Assess the person's understanding of the reasons for maintaining adequate hydration and methods for reaching goal of fluid intake.

Have the person maintain a written record (log) of fluid intake, urinary output, and daily weight (if necessary).

Monitor intake; ensure at least 1500 mL of oral fluids is taken every 24 hours.unless contraindicated.

Monitor output; ensure an output of at least 5 mL/Kg. per hour. Monitor for a decrease in urine specific gravity.

Weigh daily in same type of clothing at same time. A 2% to 4% weight loss indicates mild dehydration; a 5% to 9% weight loss indicates moderate dehydration.

Monitor levels of serum electrolytes, blood urea nitrogen, urine and serum osmolality, creatinine, hematocrit, and hemoglobin.

Teach that coffee, tea, and grapefruit juice are diuretics and can contribute to fluid loss.

Consider the additional fluid losses associated with vomiting, diarrhea, fever, tubes, drains.

For wound drainage:

- Keep careful records of the amount and type of drainage.
- Weigh dressings, if necessary, to estimate fluid loss.
- Cover wounds to minimize fluid loss.

Pediatric Interventions

Monitor weight, body temperature, moisture in oral cavity, wet diapers, and urine volume and concentration.

Offer:

- Appealing forms of fluids (popsicles, frozen juice bars, snow cones, water, milk, Jell-O with vegetable coloring added; let child help make it)
  - Unusual containers (colorful cups, straws)
  - A game or activity (have child take a drink when it is child's turn in a game)

Geriatric Interventions

Teach to drink 8 to 10 glasses of fluid daily, not including caffeine drinks unless contraindicated (e.g., renal or cardiac insufficiency).

Advise at least four glasses of water: caution on caffeine and sugar drinks.

Explain not to rely on thirst as an indicator of a need for fluids.

Teach to monitor hydration by color of urine.

Evaluate if person is restricting intake to avoid incontinence.

▶ Risk for Deficient Fluid Volume

DEFINITION

A state in which an individual is at risk for decreased intravascular, interstitial, and/or intracellular fluid. This refers to dehydration, water loss alone without change of sodium.

DEFINING CHARACTERISTICS

Deviations affecting access to fluids
Deviations affecting intake of fluids
Deviations affecting absorption of fluids
Excessive losses through normal routes, e.g., diarrhea
Extremes of age
Extremes of weight
Factors influencing fluid needs, e.g., hypermetabolic state
Loss of fluid through abnormal routes, e.g., tubes
Knowledge deficiency
Medication, e.g., diuretics

AUTHOR'S NOTE

If the individual is NPO, refer to the collaborative problem *Risk for Complications of Hypovolemia*. If the person can drink, refer to *Deficient Fluid Volume* for interventions.

NOC

Refer to *Deficient Fluid Volume*.

Goals

The individual will demonstrate continued hydrated state with a urine output >5 mL/kg/hour.

FLUID VOLUME, EXCESS

DEFINITION

The state in which an individual experiences or is at risk of experiencing intracellular or interstitial fluid overload.

■■■ **AUTHOR'S NOTE**
This diagnosis represents situations in which nurses can
prescribe definitive treatment to reduce or eliminate factors
that contribute to edema or can teach preventive actions.
Situations that represent vascular fluid overload should be
considered collaborative problems, not nursing diagnoses.
They can be labeled *Risk for Complications of Congestive Heart
Failure* or *Risk for Complications of Hypervolemia*.

DEFINING CHARACTERISTICS

Major (Must Be Present, One or More)

Edema (peripheral, sacral)
Taut, shiny skin

Minor (May Be Present)

Intake greater than output
Shortness of breath
Weight gain

RELATED FACTORS

Pathophysiologic

*Related to compromised regulatory mechanisms secondary to
acute or chronic renal failure*

*Related to portal hypertension, lower plasma colloidal osmotic
pressure, and sodium retention secondary to liver disease,
cirrhosis, cancer, or ascites*

Related to impaired venous return secondary to:
Varicose veins
Peripheral vascular disease
Thrombus
Chronic phlebitis
Immobility

Treatment-Related

*Related to sodium and water retention secondary to
corticosteroid therapy*

Situational (Personal, Environmental)

Related to excessive sodium intake/fluid intake
Related to low protein intake (e.g., fad diets, malnutrition)

Related to dependent venous pooling/venostasis secondary to immobility, tight cast or bandage, or standing or sitting for long periods
Related to venous compression by pregnant uterus
Related to inadequate lymphatic drainage secondary to mastectomy

Maturational

Older Adult

Related to impaired venous return secondary to increased peripheral resistance and decreased efficiency of valves

NOC

Electrolyte Balance, Hydration

Goals

The person will exhibit decreased edema (specify site).

Indicators
- Relate causative factors.
- Relate methods of preventing edema.

NIC

Electrolyte Management, Fluid Management, Fluid Monitoring, Skin Surveillance

Generic Interventions

For Edema:

Monitor skin for signs of pressure ulcers.
Gently wash between skin folds, and dry carefully.
Avoid tape when possible.
Change position at least every 2 hours.

Assess for Evidence of Dependent Venous Pooling or Venostasis

Keep Edematous Extremity Elevated Above the Level of the Heart Whenever Possible (Unless Contraindicated by Heart Failure)

Assess Dietary Intake and Habits that May Contribute to Fluid Retention (e.g., Salt Intake)

Teach the person to:
- Read labels for sodium content.
- Avoid convenience foods, canned foods, and frozen foods.
- Cook without salt, to use spices to add flavor (lemon, basil, tarragon, mint).
- Use vinegar in place of salt for flavor (e.g., 2 to 3 teaspoons of vinegar to 4 to 6 quarts, according to taste).

Instruct the Person to Avoid Panty Girdles/Garters, Knee-Highs, and Leg Crossing and to Practice Keeping Legs Elevated When Possible

For inadequate lymphatic drainage in arm:
- Keep extremity elevated on pillows.
- Take blood pressures in unaffected arm.
- Do not give injections or start intravenous fluids in affected arm.
- Protect affected arm from injury.
- Teach the person to avoid using strong detergents, carrying heavy bags, holding a cigarette, injuring cuticles or hangnails, reaching into a hot oven, wearing jewelry or a wristwatch, or using Ace bandages.
- Caution the person to see a physician if the arm becomes red, swollen, or unusually hard.

Protect Edematous Skin from Injury

🚹 Maternal Interventions

Explain the cause of fluid retention (e.g., increased estrogen production, posture that affects blood flow and renal function).

Explain the importance of lying on side at night and during the day (several times).

Teach women to:
- Elevate feet often.
- Drink at least 2000 mL of fluids (three to four servings).
- Eat enough protein and avoid highly salted foods.

Assess for early signs of pregnancy-induced hypertension:
- Weight gain of over 2 lb in 1 week
- Finger edema

FLUID VOLUME, RISK FOR IMBALANCED

DEFINITION (NANDA)

At risk to experience a decrease, increase, or rapid shift from one to the other of intravascular, interstitial, and/or intracellular fluid.

■■■ **AUTHOR'S NOTE**

This diagnosis can represent a multitude of clinical conditions, such as edema, hemorrhage, dehydration, and compartment syndrome. If the nurse is monitoring an individual for *Imbalanced Fluid Volume*, labeling the specific imbalance as a collaborative problem, such as *Risk for Complications of Hypovolemia*, *Compartment Syndrome*, *Increased Intracranial Pressure*, *Gastrointestinal Bleeding*, or *Postpartum Bleeding*, would clinically be more useful. For example, most intra-operative clients are monitored for hypovolemia; if the procedure is neurosurgery, cranial pressure would also be monitored. If the procedure is orthopedic, compartment syndrome would be addressed. Refer to Section 3 for specific collaborative problems and interventions.

RISK FACTORS (NANDA)

Need to be developed (NANDA, 2001)

GASTROINTESTINAL MOTILITY, DYSFUNCTIONAL

DEFINITION

The state in which a individual is experiencing increased, decreased, ineffective or lack of peristaltic activity within the gastrointestinal system.

DEFINING CHARACTERISTICS

Absence of flatus
Abdominal cramping
Abdominal distention
Abdominal pain
Accelerated gastric emptying
Bile-colored gastric residual
Change in bowel sounds (e.g., absent, hypoactive, hyperactive)
Diarrhea
Dry stool, difficulty passing stools
Hard stools
Increased gastric residual
Nausea
Regurgitation
Vomiting

RELATED FACTORS

Aging
Anxiety
Enteral feedings
Food intolerance (e.g., gluten lactose)
Immobility
Ingestion of contaminates (e.g., food, water)
Malnutrition
Pharmaceutical agents (e.g., narcotics/opiates, antibiotics,
    laxatives, anesthesia)
Prematurity
Sedentary lifestyle
Surgery

AUTHOR'S NOTE
This new NANDA-I diagnosis is too broad for clinical usefulness for it can represent a collaborative problem as:

- *Risk for Complications of Gastrointestinal Dysfunction*
- *Risk for Complications of Paralytic Ileus*
- *Risk for Complications for GI Bleeding*

Or it can represent a nursing diagnosis such as:

- Diarrhea
- Constipation
- Sedentary Lifestyle
- Risk for Imbalanced Fluid Volume
- Imbalanced Nutrition
- Disuse Syndrome

Interventions/Goals

The nurse should examine the assessment data to determine the focus.

- To monitor for physiological complications that require nursing and medical interventions as Risk for Complications of Paralytic Illeus or GI Bleeding (collaborative problem). Refer to Section 3.
- To prevent or treat a physiological dysfunction as constipation, diarrhea, fluid imbalance, compromised nutrition, or complications of immobility as Risk for Imbalanced Nutrition, Deficient Fluid Volume, Diarrhea, Disuse Syndrome, or Risk for Constipation (nursing diagnoses) Refer to Section 1.

▶ Risk for Complications of Dysfunctional Gastrointestinal Motility

DEFINITION (NANDA)

At risk for increased, decreased, ineffective or lack of peristaltic activity within the gastrointestinal system.

RISK FACTORS (NANDA)

Abdominal Surgery
Aging
Anxiety
Change in food
Change in water
Decreased gastrointestinal circulation
Diabetes mellitus
Food intolerance (gluten, lactose)
Gastroesophageal reflux disease (GERD)
Immobility
Infection (e.g., bacterial, parasitic, viral)
Pharmaceutical agents (e.g., antibiotics, laxatives, narcotics/
    opiates, proton pump inhibitors)
Prematurity
Sedentary lifestyle
Stress
Unsanitary food

■■■■ **AUTHOR'S NOTE**
Refer to author's note for Dysfunctional Gastrointestinal
Motility.

Interventions/Goals

Refer to Section 3 under Risk for Complications of Gastrointestinal Dysfunctions.

GASTROINTESTINAL TISSUE PERFUSION, RISK FOR INEFFECTIVE

DEFINITION (NANDA)

At risk for decrease in gastrointestinal circulation.

RISK FACTORS (NANDA)

Abdominal aortic aneurysm
Abdominal compartment syndrome
Abnormal partial thromboplastin time

Abnormal prothrombin time
Acute gastrointestinal bleed
Acute gastrointestinal hemorrhage
Age >60 years
Anemia
Coagulopathies (e.g., sickle cell anemia)
Diabetes mellitus
Disseminated intravascular coagulation
Female gender
Gastric paresis (e.g., diabetes mellitus)
Gastrointestinal disease (e.g., duodenal or gastric ulcer, ischemic colitis, ischemic pancreatitis)
Hemodynamic instability
Liver dysfunction
Myocardial infarction
Poor left ventricular performance
Renal failure
Stroke
Treatment-related side effects (e.g., cardiopulmonary bypass, medications, anesthesia, gastric surgery)
Vascular disease (e.g., peripheral vascular disease, aortoiliac occlusive disease)

▓▓▓■ AUTHOR'S NOTE

This diagnosis is too general for clinical use because it represents a variety of physiological complications related to GI perfusion. These complications are collaborative problems and should be separated to more specific complications as:

- Risk for Complications of GI Bleeding
- Risk for Complications of Paralytic Ileus
- Risk for Complications of Hypovolemia/Shock

Interventions/Goals

Refer to Section 3 for interventions/rationale and goals for Risk for Complications of GI Bleeding or Paralytic Ileus or Hypovolemia/Shock.

GLUCOSE, RISK FOR UNSTABLE BLOOD

DEFINITION (NANDA)

The state in which an individual is at risk for variations of blood glucose/sugar levels from the normal range.

RISK FACTORS (NANDA)

Deficient knowledge of diabetes management
Developmental level
Dietary intake
Inadequate blood glucose monitoring
Lack of acceptance of the diagnosis
Lack of adherence to diabetes management
Lack of diabetes management
Medication management
Mental health status
Physical activity status
Pregnancy, rapid growth periods
Stress
Weight gain, weight loss

■■■ AUTHOR'S NOTE

This NANDA diagnosis represents multiple issues in the management of a client with diabetes mellitus. If the focus is to monitor blood glucose level, especially for a hospitalized person, use the collaborative problem *Risk for Complications of Hypo/Hyperglycemia*. If the problem is related to knowledge deficit, use *Risk-Prone Health Behavior*. If the problem is multiple factors, use *Ineffective Self-Health Management*.

GRIEVING

Grieving
Grieving, Anticipatory*
Grieving, Complicated
Grieving, Risk for Complicated

DEFINITION

A state in which an individual or family experiences a natural human response involving psychosocial and physiologic reactions to an actual or perceived loss (person, object, function, status, relationship).

DEFINING CHARACTERISTICS

Major (Must Be Present)

The person reports an actual, anticipated or perceived loss
    (person, object, function, status, relationship) with varied
    responses, e.g.,

Denial	Delusions
Guilt	Phobias

---

*This diagnosis is no longer on the NANDA list. It has been retained by the author for its usefulness.

Anger
Despair
Feelings of worthlessness
Suicidal thoughts
Crying
Sorrow

Anergia
Inability to concentrate
Visual, auditory, and tactile
hallucinations about the
object or person
Longing/searching behaviors

RELATED FACTORS

Many situations can contribute to feelings of loss. Some common situations are listed below.

Pathophysiologic

Related to loss of function or independence secondary to:
Neurologic
Cardiovascular
Sensory
Musculoskeletal

Digestive
Renal
Trauma

Treatment-Related

Related to losses associated with, for example, long-term dialysis, surgery (mastectomy, colostomy, hysterectomy)

Situational (Personal, Environmental)

Related to negative effects and losses (e.g., chronic pain, terminal illness, death)
Related to losses in lifestyle associated with:
Childbirth
Marriage
Separation
Divorce

Child leaving home
(e.g., college or marriage)
Retirement

Related to loss of normalcy secondary to, for example, handicap, scars, illness

Maturational

Related to losses attributed to aging, friends, occupation, function, home
Related to loss of hopes, dreams
Related to anticipated loss of (specify)

NOC

Coping, Family Coping, Grief Resolution, Psychosocial
Adjustment: Lifechange

Goals

The individual will express his or her grief.

Indicators
- Describe the meaning of the death or loss to him or her.
- Share his or her grief with significant others (children, spouses).

NIC

Family Support, Grief Work Facilitation, Coping Enhancement, Anticipatory Guidance, Emotional Support

Generic Interventions

Promote a Trusting Relationship

- Never try to lessen the loss, e.g., " she didn't suffer long" " you can have another baby"
- Provide privacy, but be careful not to isolate the person or family inadvertently

Support the Person and the Family's Grief Reactions

Explain Grief Reactions

Shock and disbelief
Developing awareness
Restitution
Somatic manifestations

Assess for Experiences with Loss

Recognize and Reinforce the Strengths of Each Family Member

Encourage the Family Members to Evaluate Their Feelings and Support One Another

Allow Each Member Privacy to Share Grief

Provide a presence of simply "being " with the bereaved

Promote Physical Well-Being: Nutrition, Sleep-Rest, Exercise

Promote Grief Work with Each Response

Denial
Explain the use of denial by one family member to the other members.
Do not push the client to move past denial without emotional readiness.

Isolation
Reinforce the person's self-worth by allowing privacy.
Encourage client/family to increase social activities gradually
(e.g., support groups, church groups).

Depression
Identify the level of depression, and develop the approach
accordingly.
Use empathic sharing; acknowledge grief ("It must be very
difficult").

Anger
Explain to family that anger is an attempt to control one's
environment more closely because of inability to control loss.
Encourage verbalization of the anger.

Guilt
Encourage the client to identify positive contributions/aspects of
the relationship.
Avoid arguing and participating in the person's system of
"shoulds" and "should nots."

Fear
Focus on the present, and maintain a safe and secure
environment.

Rejection
Explain this response to family members.

Hysteria
Reduce environmental stresses (e.g., limit personnel).
Provide the person with a safe, private area to display grief.
Determine whether family has special requests regarding viewing
the deceased (Vanezis & McGee, 1999):
- Respect their requests.
- Prepare them for any body changes.
- Remove all equipment; change soiled linen.
- Support their request (e.g., holding, washing, touching, kiss-
ing).

Identify Factors that Can Impede Successful Completion of the Mourning Process (Varcorolis, 2007):

High dependence on deceased
Unresolved conflicts
Age of deceased
Inadequate support system

Number of previous losses
Physical and psychological health of person grieving

**Teach the Person and the Family Signs of
Resolution. Refer to Complicated Grieving**

Identify Agencies that May Be Helpful

👥 Pediatric Interventions

Encourage parents and staff to be truthful, and offer explanations
that can be understood.

Encourage parents or significant others to nurture children
during the grieving process.

Explore with the child his or her concept of death in the context
of maturational level.

Correct misconceptions about death, illness, and rituals
(funerals).

Prepare the child for grief responses of others.

If the child plans to attend the funeral or visit the funeral home,
a thorough explanation of the setting, rituals, and expected
behaviors of mourners is necessary beforehand. (The family
can plan the visit of the child to be short and to occur before
the other mourners arrive.)

Allow child to share fears.

Allow child to remain with significant others while they grieve
at home.

Provide accurate explanations for sibling illness or death.

👥 Maternal Interventions

**Assist Parents of a Deceased Infant (Newborn,
Stillbirth, Miscarriage) with Grief Work (Mina, 1985)**

Use baby's name when discussing loss.

Allow parents to share their hopes and dreams.

Provide access to hospital chaplain or own religious leader.

Encourage parents to see and hold their infant to validate the
reality of the loss.

Prepare a memory packet (wrapped in clean baby blanket)
(photograph, identification bracelet, footprints with birth
certificate, lock of hair, crib card, fetal monitor strip, infant's
blanket).

Encourage parents to share the experience with siblings at home
(refer to pertinent literature for consumers).

Provide for follow-up support and referral services after
discharge (e.g., social service, support group).

Assist Others to Comfort Grieving Parents

Stress the importance of openly acknowledging the death.
If the baby or fetus was named, use the name in discussions.
Send sympathy cards.

▶ Grieving, Anticipatory

DEFINITION

The state in which an individual or group experiences reactions in response to an expected significant loss.

DEFINING CHARACTERISTICS

Major (Must Be Present)

Expressed distress at potential loss

Minor (May Be Present)

Denial
Guilt
Anger patterns
Sorrow
Change in eating habits

Change in sleep patterns
Change in social patterns
Change in communication
Decreased libido

RELATED FACTORS

See *Grieving*.

NOC
Refer to *Grieving*

Goals

The person will express his or her grief.

Indicators
• Participate in decision-making for the future.
• Share his or her concerns with significant others.

NIC
Refer to *Grieving*

Generic Interventions

Encourage the person to share concerns, fears, effects on
   lifestyle.

Promote the integrity of the person and family by
acknowledging strengths and normalcy of reactions.
Prepare the person and family for grief reactions.
Promote family cohesiveness.
Provide for the concept of hope by:
- Supplying accurate information
- Resisting the temptation to give false hope
- Discussing concerns willingly

Promote grief work with each response.

Denial

Initially support and then strive to increase the development of
awareness (when individual indicates readiness for awareness).

Isolation

Listen and spend designated time consistently with the person
and family.
Offer the person and family opportunity to explore their
emotions.

Depression

Begin with simple problem-solving, and move toward
acceptance.
Enhance self-worth through positive reinforcement.

Anger

Allow crying to release this energy.
Encourage concerned support from significant others and
professional support.

Guilt

Allow crying.
Promote more direct expression of feelings.
Explore methods to resolve guilt.

Fear

Help the person and family recognize the feeling.
Explore the person's and family's attitudes about loss, death, etc.
Explore the person's and family's methods of coping.

Rejection

Allow verbal expression of this feeling state to diminish the
emotional strain.
Recognize that expression of anger may create a rejection of self
to significant others.

Caution against the use of sedatives and tranquilizers, which may prevent or delay emotional expressions of loss.

Teach signs of pathologic responses and referrals needed.

Discuss options available during terminal stage:
- Home care
- Institution
- Hospice

Discuss benefits of home care of terminal family member (Vickers & McGee, 2000):
- Unlimited access to the person
- Keeps family together
- More opportunities for support and assistance from extended family and friends
- Dying person is less isolated

Discuss the problems of home care and fears:
- 24-hour responsibility
- Unprepared for experience
- Feelings of inadequacy
- Lack of family cohesiveness

Encourage continuing usual schedule or activities (work and play).

▶ Grieving, Complicated

DEFINITION

The state in which an individual or group experiences prolonged unresolved grief and manifests in functional impairment.

AUTHOR'S NOTE

How one responds to loss is highly individual. Responses to acute loss should not be labeled dysfunctional, regardless of the severity. *Complicated Grieving* is characterized by its sustained or prolonged detrimental response in the grieving person. The validation of *Complicated Grieving* cannot occur until several months or 1 to 2 years after the death. Careful assessment with the grieving person can help to determine if the grieving process is being integrated into his or her life or if it is damaging his or her life. In many clinical settings, the diagnosis of *Risk for Complicated Grieving* for individuals at risk for unsuccessful reintegration after a loss may be more useful.

DEFINING CHARACTERISTICS

Major (Must Be Present, One or More)

Unsuccessful adaptation to loss
Prolonged denial, depression
Delayed emotional reaction
Inability to assume normal patterns of living
Grief avoidance
Yearning

Minor (May Be Present)

Social isolation or withdrawal
Failure to develop new relationships/interests
Failure to restructure life after loss
Rumination
Self-blame
Verbalizes persistent painful memories

RELATED FACTORS

Situational (Personal, Environmental)

Related to:
- Unavailable (or lack of) support system
- Negation of the loss by others
- History of a difficult relationship with the lost person or object
- Multiple past or present losses
- History of ineffective coping strategies
- Unexpected death
- Expectations to "be strong"
- History of unresolved losses
- Thwarted grieving response secondary to role, work responsibilities

NOC
See *Grieving*

Goals

The individual will verbalize intent to seek professional assistance.

Indicators
- Acknowledge the loss.
- Acknowledge an unresolved grief process.

NIC
See also *Grieving*, Referral, Support Group

Generic Interventions

Teach the normal tasks of mourning (Worden, 2002), and help the person recognize at which task he or she is:
- Acknowledging the loss
- Experiencing the pain
- Adjusting to the loss
- Reinvesting and goal-setting

Encourage person to share perceptions of the situation.
- Review relationship with the lost concept, person.
- Empathically point out misrepresentations.
- Discuss the appropriateness of guilt, anger, or sorrow.
- Encourage expressions of anger or rage.

If denial persists, see *Ineffective Denial*.

Help identify activities that have been ignored or abandoned since loss. Encourage the selection of one to resume.

Encourage participation in large motor activities (e.g., brisk walks, exercise bicycle).

Emphasize past successful coping.

Discuss community resources available for sharing experiences with others.

Refer for counseling if indicated.

▶ Risk for Complicated Grieving

DEFINITION

Risk for Complicated Grieving: The state in which an individual is at risk for a disorder that occurs after the death of a significant other or a significant loss, e.g., divorce, in which the experience or distress accompanying bereavement fails to follow normative expectations and manifests in functional impairment.

RISK FACTORS

Death of significant other

Lack of support

Significant loss or losses, e.g., divorce, termination, natural disaster, war

Goals

Refer to *Grieving*

Interventions

Identify clients at high risk for complicated grieving response:
Length of relationship: more than 55 years, less than 5 years

Medical issues: pending treatments, surgeries, history of acute or
   chronic illness
Significant mental health issues of deceased or grieving person
Substance abuse
Suicide in family history, potential for suicide
Family conflicts
Refer also to Complicated Grieving

GROWTH AND DEVELOPMENT, DELAYED

Growth and Development, Delayed
Development, Risk for Delayed
Growth, Risk for Disproportionate
Adult Failure to Thrive

DEFINITION

The state in which an individual has or is at risk for an impaired
ability to perform tasks of his or her age group or impaired growth.

AUTHOR'S NOTE
The focus of this diagnosis will be children and adolescents.
When an adult has not accomplished a developmental task,
the nurse should assess for the altered functioning that has
resulted from the failure to meet a developmental task, for
example, *Impaired Social Interaction* or *Ineffective Coping*.

DEFINING CHARACTERISTICS

Major (Must Be Present, One or More)

Inability to perform or difficulty performing skills or behaviors
   typical of age group, for example, motor, personal/social,
   language/cognition *and/or*
Altered physical growth: Weight lagging behind height by two
   standard deviations; pattern of height and weight percentiles
   indicating a drop in pattern

Minor (May Be Present)

Inability to perform self-care or self-control activities
   appropriate for age

Flat affect, listlessness, decreased responses, slow social responses, limited signs of satisfaction to caregiver, limited eye contact, difficulty feeding, decreased appetite, lethargic, irritable, negative mood, regression in self-toileting, regression in self-feeding

Infants: watchfulness, interrupted sleep pattern

RELATED FACTORS

Pathophysiologic

Related to compromised physical ability and dependence secondary to:

Congenital heart defects

Cerebral damage

Congenital defects

Malabsorption syndrome

Gastroesophageal reflux

Congenital anomalies of extremities

Muscular dystrophy

Acute illness

Prolonged pain

Repeated acute illness, chronic illness

Inadequate caloric or nutritional intake

Congestive heart failure

Cerebral palsy

Cystic fibrosis

Treatment-Related

Related to separation from significant others, school; or inadequate sensory stimulation secondary to:

Prolonged, painful treatments

Repeated or prolonged hospitalization

Traction or casts

Prolonged bed rest

Isolation due to disease processes

Confinement for ongoing treatment

Situational (Personal, Environmental)

Related to:

Parental stressor secondary to lack of knowledge

Change in usual environment

Separation from significant others (parents, primary caregiver)

School-related stressors

Loss of significant other

Loss of control over environment (established rituals, activities, established hours of contact with family)

Related to inadequate, inappropriate parental support (neglect, abuse)

Related to inadequate sensory stimulation (neglect, isolation)

Maturational

Infant–Toddler: Birth to 3 Years

Related to limited opportunities to meet social, play, or educational needs secondary to:
Separation from parents/significant others
Restriction of activity secondary to (specify)
Inadequate parental support
Inability to trust significant other
Inability to communicate (deafness)
Multiple caregivers

Preschool Age: 4 to 6 Years

Related to limited opportunities to meet social, play, or educational needs secondary to:
Loss of ability to communicate
Lack of stimulation
Lack of significant other
Related to loss of significant other (death, divorce)
Related to loss of peer group
Related to removal from home environment

School Age: 6 to 11 Years
Related to loss of significant other
Related to loss of peer group
Related to strange environment

Adolescent: 12 to 18 Years
Related to loss of independence and autonomy secondary to (specify)
Related to disruption of peer relationships
Related to disruption in body image
Related to loss of significant other

NOC
Child Development (Specify Age)

Goals

The child/adolescent will continue to demonstrate appropriate behavior.

Indicators (specify for age)
- Self-care
- Social skills

- Language
- Cognitive skills
- Motor skills

NIC

Development Enhancement, Parenting Promotion, Infant/Child Care

Generic Interventions

Teach parents the age-related developmental tasks (Table II.1).
Carefully assess child's level of development in all areas of functioning by using specific assessment tools (e.g., Brazelton Assessment Table, Denver Developmental Screening Tool).
Provide opportunities for an ill child to meet age-related developmental tasks.

Birth to 1 Year

Provide increased stimulation using variety of colored toys in crib (e.g., mobiles, musical toys, stuffed toys of varied textures, frequent periods of holding and speaking to infant).
Hold while feeding; feed slowly and in relaxed environment.
Provide periods of rest prior to feeding.
Observe mother and child during interaction, especially during feeding.
Investigate crying promptly and consistently.
Assign consistent caregiver.
Encourage parental visits/calls and involvement in care if possible.
Provide buccal experience if infant desires (i.e., thumb, pacifier).
Allow hands and feet to be free if possible.

1 to 3½ Years

Assign consistent caregiver.
Encourage self-care activities (i.e., self-feeding, self-dressing, bathing).
Reinforce word development by repeating words child uses, naming objects by saying words, and speaking to child often.
Provide frequent periods of play with peers present and with a variety of toys (puzzles, books with pictures, manipulative toys, trucks, cars, blocks, bright colors).
Explain all procedures as you do them.
Provide safe area where the child can locomote; use walker, provide creeping area, and hold hand while taking steps.
Encourage parental visits/calls and involvement in care if possible.

TABLE II.1 AGE-RELATED DEVELOPMENTAL TASKS/NEEDS

Developmental Tasks/Needs

Birth to 1 Year	1–3½ Years	3½–5 Years	5–11 Years	11–15 Years
Personal/Social	**Personal/Social**	**Personal/Social**	**Personal/Social**	**Personal/Social**
Learns to trust and anticipate satisfaction	Establishes self-control, decision-making, self-independence (autonomy)	Attempts to establish self as like parents but independent	Learns to include values and skills of school, neighborhood, peers	Family values continue to be significant influence
Sends cues to mother/ caregiver	Extremely curious, prefers to do things independently	Explores environment on own initiative	Peer relationships important	Peer group values have increasing significance
Begins understanding self as separate from others (body image)	Demonstrates independence through negativism	Boasts, brags, has feelings of indestructibility	Focuses more on reality, less on fantasy	Early adolescence: outgoing and enthusiastic
Motor	Very egocentric: believes he or she controls the world	Family is primary group	Family is main base of security and identity	Emotions are extreme, mood swings, introspection
Responds to sound	Learns about words through senses	Peers increasingly important	Sensitive to reactions of others	Sexual identity fully mature
Social smile	**Motor**	Assumes sex roles	Seeks approval, recognition	Wants privacy/ independence
Reaches for objects	Begins to walk and run well	Aggressive	Enthusiastic, noisy, imaginative, desires to explore	Develops interests not shared with family
Begins to sit, creep, pull up, and stand with support	Drinks from cup, feeds self	**Motor**	Likes to complete a task	Concern with physical self
Attempts to walk	Develops fine motor control	Locomotion skills increase, and coordinates easier		
	Climbs			

Language/Cognition
Learns to signal wants/needs with sounds, crying
Begins to vocalize with meaning (two-syllable words: dada, mama)
Comprehends some verbal/nonverbal messages (no, yes, bye-bye)
Learns about words through senses
Fears
Loud noises
Falling

Begins self-toileting
Language/Cognition
Has poor time sense
Increasingly verbal (4–5-word sentences by age 3½)
Talks to self/others
Misconceptions about cause/effect
Fears
Loss/separation from parents
Darkness
Machines/equipment
Intrusive procedures
Unknown
Inanimate, unfamiliar objects

Rides tricycle/bicycle
Throws ball, but has difficulty catching
Language/Cognition
Egocentric
Language skills flourish
Generates many questions: how, why, what?
Simple problem-solving; uses fantasy to understand, problem-solve
Fears
Mutilation
Castration

Enjoys helping
Motor
Moves constantly
Physical play prevalent (sports, swimming, skating, etc.)
Language/Cognition
Organized, stable thought
Concepts more complicated
Focuses on concrete understanding
Fears
Rejections, failure
Immobility
Mutilation
Death

Explores adult roles
Motor
Well developed
Rapid physical growth
Secondary sex characteristics
Language/Cognition
Plans for future career
Able to abstract solutions and problem-solve in future tense
Fears
Mutilation
Disruption in body image
Rejection from peers

Provide comfort measures after painful procedures.

3½ to 5 Years

Encourage self-care: self-grooming, self-dressing, mouth care, hair care.

Provide frequent playtime with others and with variety of toys (e.g., models, musical toys, dolls, puppets, books, mini-slide, wagon, tricycle).

Read stories aloud.

Ask for verbal responses and requests.

Say words for equipment, objects, and people, and ask the child to repeat.

Allow time for individual play and exploration of play environment.

Encourage parental visits/calls and involvement in care if possible.

Monitor television, and use television as means to help child understand time ("After *Sesame Street*, your mother will come.")

5 to 11 Years

Talk with child about care provided.

Request input from child (e.g., diet, clothes, routine).

Allow child to dress in clothes instead of pajamas.

Provide periods of interaction with other children on unit.

Provide craft project that can be completed each day or week.

Continue schoolwork at intervals each day.

Praise positive behaviors.

Read stories, and provide variety of independent games, puzzles, books, video games, painting, or other activity.

Introduce the child by name to persons on unit.

Encourage visits and telephone calls from parents, siblings, and peers.

11 to 15 Years

Speak frequently with the child about feelings, ideas, concerns about condition or care.

Provide opportunity for interaction with others of the same age on unit.

Identify interest or hobby that can be supported on unit in some manner, and support it daily.

Allow hospital routine to be altered to suit child's schedule.

Allow the child to dress in own clothes if possible.

Involve child in decisions about care.

Provide opportunity for involvement in variety of activities (e.g., reading, video games, movies, board games, art, trips outside or to other areas).

Encourage visits and telephone calls from parents, siblings, and peers.

Refer to community programs specific to contributing factors (e.g., social services, family services, counseling).

▶ Development, Risk for Delayed

DEFINITION

The state in which an individual is at risk for an impaired ability to perform tasks of his or her age group.

RISK FACTORS

Refer to *Delayed Growth and Development*.

Generic Interventions and Goals

Refer to *Delayed Growth and Development*.

▶ Growth, Risk for Disproportionate

DEFINITION

The state in which an individual is at risk for impaired growth.

RISK FACTORS

Refer to *Delayed Growth and Development*.

Goals

The child/adolescent will continue to demonstrate age-appropriate growth.

Indicators
- Height
- Weight
- Head circumference

Generic Interventions

Refer to *Delayed Growth and Development*.

▶ Adult Failure to Thrive

DEFINITION

The state in which an individual experiences insidious and progressive physical and psychosocial deterioration characterized by limited coping and diminished resilience.

DEFINING CHARACTERISTICS

Major

Declining physical functioning   Weight loss
Declining cognitive functioning   Social withdrawal
Depression   Self-care deficit
Loneliness   Apathy
Giving-up   Anorexia
Denial of symptoms

RELATED FACTORS

The cause of failure to thrive in adults, usually the elderly, is unknown. Researchers have identified some factors that may contribute to this condition.

Situational (Personal, Environmental)

Related to diminished coping abilities
Related to limited ability to adapt to effects of aging
Related to loss of social skills and the resultant social isolation
Related to loss of social relatedness
Related to increasing dependency and feelings of helplessness

NOC

Psychological Adjustment: Life Change, Will to Live, Physical Aging

Goals

The person will participate to increase functioning.

Indicators

• Increase social relatedness.
• Maintain or increase self-care activities.

NIC

Coping Enhancement, Hope Instillment, Spiritual Support, Social Enhancement

Generic Interventions

Consult with therapist to evaluate for depression and medication therapy as indicated.

Evaluate pattern of socialization (refer to *Risk for Loneliness*).

Provide opportunities to increase social relatedness:

- Music therapy
- Recreation therapy
- Reminiscence therapy

Engage in useful, meaningful conversations about likes, dislikes, interests, hobbies and work history

Speak as one adult to another, use average volume, good eye contact

Encourage to be as independent as possible

Maintain standards of empathic, respectful care.

Attempt to obtain information that will provide useful and meaningful topics for conversations (likes, dislikes; interests, hobbies; work history). Interview early in the day.

Encourage significant others and caregivers to speak slowly with a low voice pitch and at an average volume (unless hearing deficits are present), as one adult to another, with eye contact, and as if expecting person to understand.

Provide respect and promote sharing:

- Pay attention to what the person is saying.
- Pick out meaningful comments and continue talking.

Call the person by name and introduce yourself each time contact is made; use touch if welcomed.

Engage in useful and meaningful adult conversations:

- Likes, dislikes
- Interests, work history

RISK-PRONE HEALTH BEHAVIORS

DEFINITION

State in which a person has an inability to modify lifestyle/behaviors in a manner consistent with a change in health status.

DEFINING CHARACTERISTICS

Major (Must Be Present, One or More)

Minimizes health status change

Failure to take action that prevents health problems

RELATED FACTORS

Situational (Personal, Environmental)

Related to:
- Low self-efficacy
- Negative attitude toward health care
- Multiple stressors
- Inadequate social support
- Inadequate resources
- Inadequate finances
- Multiple responsibilities

Related to impaired ability to understand secondary to:
- Low literacy
- Language barriers

AUTHOR'S NOTE

This new nursing diagnosis replaces the NANDA diagnosis *Impaired Adjustment*. *Risk-Prone Health Behaviors* has some commonalities with *Ineffective Health Maintenance* and *Noncompliance*. This author recommends that *Ineffective Health Maintenance* be used to describe a person with an unhealthy lifestyle that puts him or her at risk for a chronic health problem or disease. *Noncompliance* describes a person who wants to comply, but factors are present that deter adherence. *Risk-Prone Health Behaviors* describes a person with a health problem who is not participating in management of the health problem because of lack of motivation or comprehension or personal barriers.

NOC

Adherence Behavior, Symptom Control, Treatment Behavior: Illness/Injury

Goals

The person will verbalize intent to modify one behavior to manage health problem indicators:

- Describe the health problem.
- Describe the relationship of present practices/behavior to decreased health.
- Engage in goal setting.

NIC

Interventions, Health Education, Mutual Goal Setting, Self-Responsibility, Teaching: Disease Process, Decision-Making Support

Generic Interventions

If low literacy is suspected, start with what the person is most stressed about.

Speak simply.

Repeat and ask the person to repeat.

Use pictures.

Use appropriate examples.

Demonstrate and ask for a return demonstration.

Use videotapes and audiotapes.

Engage in collaborative decision making (Bodenheimer, MacGregor, & Shariffi, 2005).

List some choices for improving the person's health, e.g., for diabetes:

Exercise	Healthy eating
Medication	Blood glucose monitoring
Client-defined choice	

- Ask if there is one activity on the list they would like to focus on.
- Provide information as directed by the client.
  - Ask: What do you want to know about _____?
  - Provide information the person wants to know.
  - Ask the person if he or she understood.
  - Ask if there are other questions.
- Ask the person to repeat the goal, behavior, or activity.
- Assess readiness to change.
- Determine how important the person thinks the behavior change is, e.g., How important is it to you to increase your activity? Rate from 0 to 10
  - 0–not important   10–important
- Determine how confident the person is to make the change, e.g., How confident are you that you can get more exercise? Rate from 0 to 10.
- Determine if the person is ready for change.
- If the importance level is 7 or above, assess confidence level. If the importance level is low, provide more information regarding the risks of not changing behavior.
- If the level of confidence is 4 or less, ask the person why is not a 1.

- Ask the person what is needed to change the low score to an 8.
- Collaboratively set a goal and an action plan that is realistic, e.g.,
  How often each week could you walk around the block two times?
- Ask person if you can call him or her in 2 weeks to find how they are doing. Gradually extend the time to monthly calls.

HEALTH MAINTENANCE, INEFFECTIVE

DEFINITION

The state in which an individual or group experiences or is at risk of experiencing a disruption in health because of an unhealthy lifestyle or lack of knowledge about managing a condition.

■■■■ AUTHOR'S NOTE
Ineffective Health Maintenance can describe persons who desire to change an unhealthy lifestyle (obesity, tobacco use). *Ineffective Self-Health Management* can be used for those who need teaching for self-management of a disease or condition.

DEFINING CHARACTERISTICS (IN THE ABSENCE OF DISEASE)

Major (Must Be Present, One or More)

Reports or demonstrates an unhealthy practice or lifestyle, e.g.:

Reckless driving   Inadequate oral hygiene
Substance abuse   Inadequate hygiene
Excessive sun exposure   Overeating
Sedentary lifestyle   High-fat diet

Minor (May Be Present)

Reports or Demonstrates:

Skin and Nails
Malodorous   Sunburn

Skin lesions (pustules, rashes, dry or scaly skin)

Unusual color, pallor
Unexplained scars

Respiratory System

Frequent infections
Chronic cough

Dyspnea with exertion

Oral Cavity

Frequent sores (on tongue, buccal mucosa)
Loss of teeth at early age
Lesions associated with lack of oral care or substance abuse (leukoplakia, fistulas)

Gastrointestinal System and Nutrition

Obesity
Anorexia
Cachexia

Chronic anemia
Chronic bowel irregularity
Chronic dyspepsia

Musculoskeletal System

Frequent muscle strain, backaches, neck pain
Diminished flexibility and muscle strength

Genitourinary System

Frequent sexually-transmitted infections
Frequent use of potentially unhealthful over-the-counter products (e.g., chemical douches, perfumed vaginal products, nasal sprays)

Constitutional

Chronic fatigue, headaches, apathy

Psychoemotional

Emotional fragility
Frequent feelings of being overwhelmed

RELATED FACTORS

A variety of factors can produce altered health maintenance. Some common causes are listed below.

Situational (Personal, Environmental)

Related to:

Lack of motivation
Lack of education or readiness
Lack of access to adequate health care services
Inadequate health teaching
Impaired ability to understand secondary to (specify)

Maturational

Child

Related to lack of education of age-related factors. Examples include:

Sexuality and sexual
  development
Safety hazards

Substance abuse
Poor nutrition
Inactivity

Adolescent

Same as children
Cycle, automobile safety practices
Substance abuse (alcohol, other drugs, tobacco)

Adult

Related to lack of education of age-related factors. Examples include:

Parenthood
Sexual function

Safety practices

Older Adult

Related to lack of education of age-related factors. Examples include:

Effects of aging
Sensory deficits
See Table II.2 for age-related conditions.

NOC

Health-Promoting Behavior, Health-Seeking Behaviors, Knowledge: Health Promotion, Knowledge: Health Resources, Participation: Health Care Decisions, Risk Detection, Treatment

Goals

The individual or caregiver will verbalize an intent to engage or engage in health maintenance behaviors.

Indicator

Identify barriers to health maintenance.

NIC

Health Education, Self-Responsibility Facilitation, Health Screening, Risk Identification, Family Involvement Promotion

TABLE II.2 PRIMARY AND SECONDARY PREVENTION FOR AGE-RELATED CONDITIONS

Developmental Level	Primary Prevention	Secondary Prevention
Infancy (0–1 y)	Parent education	Complete physical examination every 2–3 mo
	Infant safety	Screening at birth
	Nutrition	Congenital hip dysplasia
	Breastfeeding	Phenylketonuria (PKU)
	Sensory stimulation	Sickle cell disease
	Infant massage and touch	Cystic fibrosis
	Visual stimulation	Vision (startle reflex)
	Activity	Hearing (response to and localization of sounds)
	Colors	Tuberculin test at 12 mo
	Auditory stimulation	Developmental assessments
	Verbal	Screen and intervene for high risk
	Music	Low birth weight
	Immunizations	Maternal substance abuse during pregnancy
	DTap, hepatitis B	Alcohol: fetal alcohol syndrome
	H. influenzae	Cigarettes: sudden infant death syndrome (SIDS)
	Pneumococcal	Drugs: addicted neonate
	Oral hygiene	Maternal infections during pregnancy
	Teething biscuits	
	Fluoride	
	Avoid sugared food and drink	

(continued)

TABLE II.2 PRIMARY AND SECONDARY PREVENTION FOR AGE-RELATED CONDITIONS (Continued)

Developmental Level	Primary Prevention	Secondary Prevention
Preschool (1–5 y)	Parent education Teething Discipline Nutrition Accident prevention Normal growth and development Child education Dental self-care Dressing Bathing with assistance Feeding self-care Immunizations DTap IPV MMR HIB Influenza (for high risk) Varicella (unless had disease) Hepatitis A (high risk) Pneumococcal Hepatitis B (if not completed as infant)	Complete physical examination between 2 and 3 y and pre-school (urinalysis, CBC) Tuberculin test at 3 y Developmental assessments (annual) Speech development Hearing Vision Screen and intervene Lead poisoning Developmental lag Neglect or abuse Strabismus Hemoglobin or hematocrit Vision, hearing deficit Strong family history of arteriosclerotic disease (e.g., MI, CVA, peripheral vascular disease), diabetes, hypertension, gout, or hyperlipidemia—fasting serum cholesterol at age 2 years, then every 3–5 years if normal.

Dental/oral hygiene
Fluoride treatments
Fluoridated water
Dietary counsel

		Complete physical examination
School age (6–11 y)	Health education of child	Tuberculin test every 3 y (at ages 6 and 9)
	Food pyramid	Developmental measurements
	Accident prevention	Language
	Outdoor safety (e.g., helmets)	Vision: Snellen charts at school
	Substance abuse counsel	6–8 y, use "E" chart
	Anticipatory guidance for physical	Over 8 y, use alphabet chart
	changes at puberty	Hearing: audiogram
	Immunizations	
	Tetanus at 11–12 y	
	DTap Boosters between	
	OPV 4 and 6 y	
	MMR	
	Varicella (at age 11–12 if no history of	
	infection)	
	Pneumococcal (high risk)	
	Gardasil (girls age 11–26, one time	
	series of three injections)	
	Professional dental hygiene every 6–12 mo	
	Continue fluoridation	
	Complete physical examination (yearly)	

(continued)

TABLE II.2 PRIMARY AND SECONDARY PREVENTION FOR AGE-RELATED CONDITIONS (Continued)

Developmental Level	Primary Prevention	Secondary Prevention
Adolescence (12–19 y)	Health education Proper nutrition and healthful diets Sex education (abstinence, family planning, sexually transmitted diseases) Safe driving skills Adult challenges Seeking employment and career choices Dating and marriage Confrontation with substance abuse Safety in athletics, water Skin care, sunscreens Professional dental hygiene every 6–12 mo Immunization Hepatitis B series, Hepatitis A series (if needed) Gardasil (females age 11–26, one time series of three injections)	Complete physical examination (yearly) Blood pressure Cholesterol profile Tuberculin test at 12 y, and yearly if high risk, RPR, CBC, urinalysis, urine for chlamydia and gonorrhea (male) Female: breast self-examination, monthly Male: testicular self-examination monthly Female, if sexually active: Pap test and pelvic examination three years after intial sexual activity, then yearly (chlamydia and cervical gonorrhea cultures with pelvic examination) earlier if problems are encountered. Screening and interventions if high risk: Depression Suicide Substance abuse Pregnancy Family history of alcoholism or domestic violence HIV infection

	Health education	

Young adult (20–39 y)	Weight management with good nutrition as basal metabolic rate changes
	Lifestyle counseling
	  Stress management skills
	Injury prevention
	"Safe sex"
	Parenting skills
	Substance abuse
	Environmental health choices
	Professional dental hygiene every 6–12 mo
	
	Immunization
	  Tetanus at 20 y and every 10 y
	  Female: rubella, if zero negative for antibodies
	  Hepatitis B series if needed
	  Gardasil (females age 11–26, one time series of three injections)
		Sexually transmitted infections
		Complete physical examination at about 20 y, then every 5–6 y
		Female: breast self-examination monthly
		Gynecologic exam—same as adolescent 12–19 if high risk otherwise every 2 years beginning at age 21 sexually active or not
		Male: testicular self-examination monthly
		All females: baseline mammography at age 40 then every 1–2 y unless positive family history for breast cancer, screening should begin 5 years earlier than the age of relative with onset of breast cancer
		Parents-to-be: high-risk screening for Down syndrome, Tay-Sachs disease
		Pregnant female: screen for sexually transmitted diseases, rubella titer, Rh factor
		Annual screening and interventions if high risk
		Female with previous breast cancer: annual mammography at 35 y and after
		Female with mother or sister who has had breast cancer, same as above
		Family history of colorectal cancer or high risk: annual stool guaiac, digital rectal examination, and sigmoidoscopy or colonoscopy
		PPD if exposed to tuberculosis
		Glaucoma screening at 35 years along with routine physical exams
		Cholesterol profile every 5 years if normal
		Cholesterol profile every 1–2 years if borderline

(continued)

TABLE II.2 PRIMARY AND SECONDARY PREVENTION FOR AGE-RELATED CONDITIONS (Continued)

Developmental Level	Primary Prevention	Secondary Prevention
Middle-aged adult (40–59 y)	Health education: continue with young adult, perimenopausal Midlife changes, male and female counseling "Empty-nest syndrome" Anticipatory guidance for retirement Grandparenting Professional dental hygiene every 6–12 mo Immunizations Tetanus every 10 years Influenza—annual if high risk (i.e., major chronic disease [COPD, CAD, DM]) Pneumococcal—single dose if high risk (COPD, Immune compromised, DM)	Complete physical examination every 5–6 y with complete laboratory evaluation (serum/urine tests, x-ray, ECG) Dexascan screening for osteoporosis once then as needed if high risk e.g., chronic steroid use, surgical menopause. Female: breast self-examination monthly, Pap test every 1–3 y Male: testicular self-examination monthly All females: mammography every 1–2 y 50 years and over unless positive family history for breast cancer Eye examination every 1–2 y Pregnant female: perinatal screening by amniocentesis if desired Colonoscopy at 50 and 51 y, then every 10 y if negative or more frequent as advised Stool guaiac test annually at 50 y and thereafter Screening and intervention if high risk Oral cancer: screen more often if substance abuser, smoker Skin cancer PSA yearly after age 40 for blacks, Hispanics and after 50 for others

Old adult (60–74 y)	Health education: continue with previous counseling	Complete physical examination every 2 y with laboratory assessments
	Home safety	Blood pressure annually
	Retirement	Female: breast self-examination monthly
	Loss of spouse	Male: testicular self-examination monthly
	Special health needs	Female: annual mammogram, Pap test every 1–3 y, depending on risk
	Nutritional changes	Dexascan when post menopausal with frequency determined by baseline findings
	Changes in hearing or vision	Annual stool guaiac test
	Professional dental/oral hygiene every 6–12 mo	Colonoscopy frequency per recommendation of primary
	Immunizations	Complete eye examination yearly
	Tetanus every 10 y	Podiatric evaluation with foot care PRN
	Influenza—annual if high risk	Screen for high risk
	Pneumococcal (one time only)	Depression
	Zosterix (herpes zoster vaccine) one time only	Suicide
		Alcohol/drug abuse
		Elder abuse

(continued)

229

TABLE II.2 PRIMARY AND SECONDARY PREVENTION FOR AGE-RELATED CONDITIONS (Continued)

Developmental Level	Primary Prevention	Secondary Prevention

Old-aged adult (75 y and over)	Health education: continue counsel
	Anticipatory guidance
	  Dying and death
	  Loss of spouse
	  Increasing dependency on others
	Professional dental/oral hygiene every 6–12 mo
	Immunizations
	  Tetanus every 10 y
	  Influenza—annual
	  Pneumococcal—if not already received
		Complete physical examination annually
		Female: mammogram every 1–2 y
		Colonoscopy, frequency per recommendation of primary
		Complete eye examination yearly
		Podiatrist PRN

(Source: U.S. Department of Health and Human Services [2008]. *Clinician's handbook of preventive services: Putting prevention into practice*. Washington, DC: U.S. Government Printing Office.)

Generic Interventions

Assess Knowledge of Primary Prevention:

Safety—accident prevention (e.g., car, machinery, outdoor safety, occupational)

Healthful diet (e.g., "basic four," low fat and salt, high complex carbohydrate, sufficient intake of vitamins, minerals, 2 to 3 quarts of water daily)

Weight control

Avoidance of substance abuse (alcohol, drugs, tobacco)

Avoidance of sexually transmitted diseases

Dental/oral hygiene (daily, dentist)

Immunizations

Regular exercise pattern

Stress management

Lifestyle counseling (e.g., safe sex, family planning, parenting skills, financial planning)

Teach Importance of Secondary Prevention (Refer to Table II.2)

Determine Knowledge Needed to Manage Condition:

Causes

Treatments

Medications

Diet

Activity

Risk factors

Signs/symptoms of complications

Restrictions

Follow-up care

Assess If Needed At-Home Resources Are Available

Caregiver

Finances

Equipment

Determine If Referrals Are Indicated (e.g., Social Services, Housekeeping, Home Health).

HEALTH-SEEKING BEHAVIORS

DEFINITION

The state in which an individual in stable health actively seeks ways to alter personal health habits and/or the environment to move toward a higher level of wellness.*

DEFINING CHARACTERISTICS

Major (Must Be Present)

Expressed or observed desire to seek information for health promotion

Minor (May Be Present)

Expressed or observed desire for increased control of health
Expression of concern about current environmental conditions on health status
Stated or observed unfamiliarity with community wellness resources
Demonstrated or observed lack of knowledge of health-promotion behaviors

---

*Stable health is defined as a condition in which the client's well-being is maximized; signs and symptoms of disease, if present, are controlled; and disabilities follow a predictable, non-acute course.

RELATED FACTORS

Situational (Personal, Environmental)

Related to anticipated role changes; for example, marriage, parenthood, "empty nest syndrome," retirement

Related to lack of knowledge of:
Preventive behavior (disease)
Screening practices for age and risk
Optimal nutrition and weight control
Regular exercise program
Constructive stress management
Supportive social networks

Maturational

See Table II.2.

NOC

Adherence Behavior, Health Behaviors, Health Promoting Behaviors, Well-Being

Goals

The person will agree with self-responsibility for wellness (physical, dental, safety, nutritional, family).

Indicators

- Describe screening that is appropriate for age and risk factors.
- Perform self-screening for cancer.
- Participate in a regular physical exercise program.
- State an intent to use positive coping mechanisms and constructive stress management.
- Eat a balanced diet to maintain or achieve a BMI <26.

NIC

Health Education, Risk Identification, Values Clarification, Behavior Modification, Coping Enhancement, Knowledge: Health Resources

Generic Interventions

Determine the Person's or Family's Knowledge or Perception of:

Life cycle challenges (e.g., marriage, parenting, aging, finances).

Need to maintain responsible relationships with health care providers.

Ability to attain a higher level of health through anticipatory planning for life cycle events (e.g., financial planning).

Need to provide and nurture reciprocity in social support.

Determine the Person's or Family's Past Patterns of Health Care

Expectations

Interactions with health care system or providers

Influences of family, cultural group, peer group, mass media

Provide Specific Information Concerning Age-Related Health Promotion (Refer to Table II.2)

Discuss Client's Food Choices, and Assist as He or She Identifies New Goals for Health Promotion

Assist in the selection of foods to sustain life and facilitate body functioning.

Provide information, when needed, about developmental considerations for dependents.

Discuss the risk of excess use of:

Salt	Snack foods
Fried foods	Processed meats
Fats	Soda, fruit drinks

Discuss the Benefits of a Regular Exercise Program

Discuss the Elements of Constructive Stress Management:

Assertiveness training

Problem solving

Relaxation techniques

Discuss Strategies for Developing Positive Social Networks

Promote Self-Actualization in the Client Who Is Seeking to Promote Health

Demonstrate an interested but nonjudgmental attitude.

View the client–nurse relationship as collaborative; the client remains in control of choices, actions, and evaluations.

Facilitate adoption of new behaviors rather than defining them.

Listen, reflect, and converse to clarify the client's current behavior patterns and desired goals.

Enhance the client's strengths, empower with choices and self-control, and always demonstrate respect for those choices.

HOME MAINTENANCE, IMPAIRED

DEFINITION

The state in which an individual or family experiences or is at risk to experience difficulty in maintaining a safe, hygienic, growth-producing home environment.

■■■■ **AUTHOR'S NOTE**
This diagnosis can describe situations in which the individual or family needs specific support or instruction to manage home care of a family member or activities of daily living.

DEFINING CHARACTERISTICS

Major (Must Be Present, One or More)

Expressions or observations of:
- Difficulty in maintaining home hygiene
- Difficulty in maintaining a safe home
- Inability to keep up home
- Lack of sufficient finances

Minor (May Be Present)

Repeated infections
Accumulated wastes
Overcrowding

Unwashed cooking and
  eating equipment
Offensive odors
Infestations

RELATED FACTORS

Pathophysiologic

Related to compromised functional ability secondary to chronic debilitating disease

Diabetes mellitus
Chronic obstructive
  pulmonary disease
Congestive heart failure
Cancer

Arthritis
Multiple sclerosis
Muscular dystrophy
Parkinson's disease
Cerebrovascular accident

Situational (Personal, Environmental)

Related to change in functional ability of (specify family member) secondary to:

Injury (fractured limb, spinal cord injury)

Surgery (amputation, ostomy)
Impaired mental status (memory lapses, depression, severe
anxiety, panic)
Substance abuse (alcohol, other drugs)
Related to unavailable support system
Related to loss of family member
Related to lack of knowledge
Related to insufficient finances

Maturational

Infant
*Related to multiple care requirements secondary to high-risk
newborn*

Older Adult

*Related to multiple care requirements secondary to family
member with deficits (cognitive, motor, sensory)*

NOC
Family Functioning, Safe Home Environment

Goals

The person or caregiver will demonstrate the ability to perform
skills necessary for the care of the home.

Indicators
• Identify factors that restrict self-care and home management.
• Express satisfaction with home situation.

NIC
Home Maintenance Assistance, Environmental
Management: Safety, Environmental Management

Generic Interventions

Determine with the person and family the information needed to
be taught and learned.
Determine the type of equipment needed, considering
availability, cost, and durability.
Determine the type of assistance needed (e.g., meals, housework,
transportation), and assist the individual to obtain them.
Discuss the implications of caring for a chronically ill family
member (refer to *Caregiver Role Strain*):

- Amount of time
- Effects on other role responsibilities (spouse, children, job)
- Physical requirements (lifting)

Arrange for a home visit.

Allow the caregiver opportunities to share problems and feelings.

Refer to community agencies as indicated (e.g., nursing, social service, meals).

HOPELESSNESS

DEFINITION

A sustained subjective emotional state in which an individual sees no alternatives or personal choices available to solve problems or to achieve what is desired and cannot mobilize energy on own behalf to establish goals.

AUTHOR'S NOTE

Hopelessness differs from *Powerlessness* in that a hopeless person sees no solution to the problem or way to achieve what is desired, even if he or she has control of his or her life. A powerless person may see an alternative or answer to the problem yet be unable to do anything about it because of perceived lack of control and resources.

DEFINING CHARACTERISTICS

Major (Must Be Present, One or More)

Expresses profound, overwhelming, sustained apathy in response to situations perceived as impossible

Physiologic

Slowed responses to stimuli

Lack of energy

Increased sleep

Emotional

The hopeless person often has difficulty experiencing feelings but may feel:

- Unable to seek good fortune, luck, or God's favor
- Lack of meaning or purpose in life
- "Empty" or "drained"
- A sense of loss and deprivation
- Helpless
- Incompetent
- Entrapped
- Demoralized
- Negative recent and future perspective

Person exhibits:

- Passiveness, lack of involvement in care
- Decreased verbalization
- Decreased affect
- Lack of ambition, initiative, and interest
- "Giving up–given up" complex
- Inability to accomplish anything
- Slowed thought processes
- Lack of responsibility for own decisions and life
- Isolating behavior

Cognitive

Decreased problem-solving and decision-making capabilities
Deals with past and future, not here and now
Decreased flexibility in thought processes
Rigidity (e.g., "all or none" thinking)
Lacks imagination and wishing capabilities
Unable to identify and/or accomplish desired objectives and goals
Unable to plan, organize, or make decisions
Unable to recognize sources of hope
Suicidal thoughts

Minor (May Be Present)

Physiologic
Anorexia
Weight loss

Emotional
Person feels:

- "A lump in the throat"
- Discouraged with self and others
- "At the end of my rope"
- Tense
- Overwhelmed (feels he or she just "can't")
- Loss of gratification from roles and relationships
- Vulnerable

Person exhibits:
- Poor eye contact—turns away from speaker; shrugs in response to speaker
- Decreased motivation
- Sighing
- Regression
- Resignation
- Depression

Cognitive

Decreased ability to integrate information received
Loss of time perception for past, present, and future
Decreased ability to recall the past
Inability to communicate effectively
Distorted thought perceptions and associations
Unreasonable judgment

RELATED FACTORS

Pathophysiologic

Any chronic and/or terminal illness can cause or contribute to hopelessness (e.g., heart disease, kidney disease, cancer, AIDS).

Related to impaired ability to cope secondary to (e.g.):

Failing or deteriorating physiologic condition
New and unexpected signs or symptoms of previous disease process
Prolonged pain, discomfort, weakness
Impaired functional abilities (walking, elimination, eating)

Treatment-Related

Related to:

Prolonged treatments (e.g., chemotherapy, radiation) that cause discomfort (pain, nausea, vomiting)
Treatments that alter body image (e.g., surgery, chemotherapy)
Prolonged diagnostic studies
Prolonged dependence on equipment for life support (e.g., dialysis, ventilator)
Prolonged dependence on equipment for monitoring bodily functions (telemetry)

Situational (Personal, Environmental)

Related to:

Prolonged activity restriction (e.g., fractures, spinal cord injury)
Prolonged isolation (e.g., infectious diseases, reverse isolation for suppressed immune system)

Abandonment of or separation from significant others (parents, spouse, children, others)

Inability to achieve goals that one values in life (marriage, education, children)

Inability to participate in activities one desires (walking, sports)

Loss of something or someone valued (spouse, children, friend, financial resources)

Prolonged caretaking responsibilities (spouse, child, parent)

Exposure to long-term physiologic or psychological stress

Loss of belief in transcendent values/God

Ongoing, repetitive losses related to AIDS (individual, community)

Repetitive natural disasters (hurricanes, floods)

Prolonged exposure to violence/war

Maturational

Child

Related to:

Loss of caregivers

Loss of trust in significant other (parents, sibling)

Rejection or abandonment by caregivers

Loss of autonomy related to illness (e.g., fracture)

Loss of bodily functions

Inability to achieve developmental tasks (trust, autonomy, initiative, industry)

Rejection by family

Adolescent

Related to:

Loss of significant other (peer, family)

Loss of bodily functions

Change in body image

Inability to achieve developmental task (role identity)

Adult

Related to:

Impaired bodily functions, loss of body part

Impaired relationships (separation, divorce)

Loss of job, career

Loss of significant others (death of children, spouse)

Inability to achieve developmental tasks (intimacy, commitment, productivity)

Older Adult

Related to:

Sensory deficits

Motor deficits

Cognitive deficits
Loss of independence
Loss of significant others, things
Inability to achieve developmental tasks (integrity)

NOC

Decision-Making, Depression Control, Hope, Quality of Life

Goals

Short-Term

The person will express feelings of optimism about the present.

Indicators

- Share suffering openly and constructively with others.
- Reminisce and review life positively.
- Consider own values and the meaning of life.
- Express confidence in a desired outcome and goals.
- Express confidence in self and others.
- Practice energy conservation.
- Develops, improves and maintains positive relationships with others
- Participates in a significant role
- Expresses spiritual beliefs

Long-Term

The person will express positive expectations about the future, expressing purpose and meaning in life.

Indicators

Demonstrate an increase in energy level, as evidenced by activities (e.g., self-care, exercise, hobbies).

Demonstrate initiative, self-direction, and autonomy in decision-making and problem-solving.

Makes positive statements about the future similar to the following:

- "I am looking forward to . . ."
- "There are more good times ahead."
- "I expect to succeed in . . ."
- "I expect to get more out of the good things in life."
- "I have faith in the future."

Develop, improve, and maintain positive relationships with others.

Participate in a significant role.

Express spiritual beliefs.
Redefine the future and set realistic goals.
Exhibit peace and comfort with situation.

NIC

Hope Instillation, Values Clarification, Decision-Making Support, Spiritual Support, Support System Enhancement

Generic Interventions

Convey empathy to promote verbalization of doubts, fears, and concerns.

Determine risk for suicide (refer to *Risk for Suicide*).

Encourage verbalization of why and how hope is significant in client's life.

Encourage expressions of how hope is uncertain and areas in which hope has failed.

Teach how to deal with the hopeless aspects by separating them from the hopeful aspects.

Assess and mobilize the person's internal resources (autonomy, independence, rationality, cognitive thinking, flexibility, spirituality).

Assist with identification of sources of hope (e.g., relationships, faith, things to accomplish).

Create an environment in which spiritual expression is encouraged.

Assist with development of realistic short- and long-term goals (progress from simple to more complex; may use a "goals poster" to indicate type and time for achieving specific goals).

Teach how to anticipate pleasurable experiences (e.g., walking, reading favorite book, writing letter).

Assess and mobilize person's external resources (significant others, health care team, support groups, God or higher powers).

Help person to recognize that he or she is loved, cared about, and important in the lives of others regardless of failing health.

Encourage sharing of concerns with others who have had a similar problem or disease and have had positive experiences from coping effectively with it.

Assess belief support system (values, religious activities, relationship with God, meaning and purpose of prayer; refer to *Spiritual Distress*).

Allow time and opportunities to reflect on the meaning of suffering, death, and dying.
Initiate referrals as indicated (e.g., counseling, spiritual leader).

👫 Pediatric Interventions (Adolescent)

Provide truthful explanations.
Engage in activities.
If appropriate, discuss knowledge of survivors.
Focus on future.
Discuss topics interesting to the child.
Use humor if appropriate.

INFANT BEHAVIOR, DISORGANIZED

Infant Behavior, Disorganized
Infant Behavior, Risk for Disorganized

DEFINITION

The state in which the neonate has an alteration in integration and modulation of the physiologic and behavioral systems of adaptation (autonomic, motor, state, organizational, self-regulatory, and attention-interactional).

■■■ AUTHOR'S NOTE

This diagnosis describes an infant who has difficulty regulating and adapting to external stimuli. This difficulty is the result of immature neurobehavioral development and increased environmental stimuli associated with neonatal units. When an infant is overstimulated or stressed, she or he uses energy to adapt, which depletes the supply of energy needed for physiologic growth. The goal of nursing care is to assist the infant with energy conservation by reducing environmental stimuli, allowing the infant sufficient time to adapt to handling, and providing sensory input when appropriate to the infant's physiologic and neurobehavioral status.

DEFINING CHARACTERISTICS (VANDENBERG, 1990; HOCKENBERRY & WILSON, 2009)

Autonomic System

Cardiac
Increased rate

Respiration
Pauses, tachypnea, gasping

Color changes
Paling around nostrils, perioral duskiness, mottled, cyanotic, gray, flushed, ruddy

Visceral
Hiccups, gagging, grunting, spitting up
Straining as if actually producing a bowel movement

Motor
Seizures

Sneezing

Tremor/startling

Yawning

Twitching

Sighing

Coughing

Motor System

Fluctuating Tone
Flaccidity of:
    Trunk   Face
    Extremities
Hypertonicity:
    Leg extensions   Arching
    Salutes   Finger splays
    Airplaning   Tongue extensions
    Sitting on air   Fisting
Hyperflexions:
    Trunk   Fetal tuck
    Extremities

Frantic Diffuse Activity

State System (Range)

Difficulty maintaining state control
Difficulty in transitions from one state to another
Sleeping:
    Twitches   Whimpers
    Sounds   Grimacing
    Jerky moves   Fussy in sleep
    Irregular respirations

Awake:

Eye-floating	Panicked, worried, or dull look
Glassy-eyed	Weak cry
Strained, fussy	Irritability
Staring	Abrupt state changes
Gaze aversion	

Attention-Interaction System

Attempts at engaging behaviors elicit stress

Impaired ability to orient, attend, engage in reciprocal social interactions

Difficult to console

Self-Regulatory System

Limited or absent use of self-regulatory behaviors to maintain or regain control:

- Postural changes
- Foot, leg bracing
- Sucking fists
- Finger folding
- Hand to mouth

Stressed with more than one mode of stimuli

RELATED FACTORS

Pathophysiologic

Related to immature or impaired central nervous system secondary to:

Prematurity

Prenatal exposure to drugs

Congenital anomalies

Hypoglycemia

Infection

Hyperbilirubinemia

Decreased oxygen saturation

Related to nutritional deficits secondary to: reflux emesis, colic, swallowing problems, or feeding intolerances

Related to excess stimulation secondary to: pain, hunger, oral hypersensitivity, or temperature variation

Treatment-Related

Related to excess stimulation secondary to, for example, invasive procedures, chest physical therapy, restraints, lights (e.g., bililights), tubes, tape, medication administration, movement, feeding, noise (e.g., prolonged, alarms)

Related to inability to see caregivers secondary to eye patches

Situational (Personal, Environmental)

Related to multiple caregivers
Related to imbalance of task touch and consoling touch
*Related to decreased ability to self-regulate secondary to
sudden movement, noise, fatigue, or insufficient sleep*

NOC

Neurological Status, Preterm Infant Organization, Sleep,
Comfort Level

Goal

The infant will demonstrate increased signs of stability.

Indicators

- Smooth, stable respirations; pink, stable color; consistent tone, improved posture; calm; focused alertness; well-modulated sleep; responsive to auditory, visual, and social stimuli
- Self-regulatory skills such as sucking, hand to mouth, hand holding, position changes

The parent(s)/caregiver(s) will describe techniques to reduce environmental stress in agency and/or at home.

- Describe situations that stress the infant.
- Describe signs/symptoms of stress in the infant.

NIC

Environmental Management, Neurological Monitoring,
Sleep Enhancement, Newborn Care, Parent Education:
Newborn, Positioning

Generic Interventions

Assess for Causative/Contributing Factors:

Pain
Fatigue
Disorganized sleep-wake pattern
Feeding problems
Excessive stimulation—personal, environmental

Reduce or Eliminate Contributing Factors If Possible

Pain

Determine the baseline behavioral manifestations of the infant
and document.

Observe for responses different from baseline that have been associated with neonatal pain responses

Facial responses (open mouth, brow bulge, grimace, chin quiver, nasolabial furrow, taut tongue)

Motor responses (flinch, muscle rigidity, clenched hands, withdrawal)

If unsure whether behavior indicates pain but pain is suspected, consult with physician for an analgesic trial. Evaluate the infant's response.

Aggressively manage obvious pain stimuli (e.g., postsurgical, lack of feeding, painful procedures, hyperglycemia; Acute Pain Management Guideline Panel, 1992).

- Consult with physician for an analgesic.
- Provide analgesic before painful procedures.
- Consider topical analgesia for frequent painful procedures (e.g., heelstick, venipuncture).

When administering analgesics (Acute Pain Management Guideline Panel, 1992):

- Reduce initial dose, and monitor respiratory response cautiously.
- Determine optimal dose and interval.
- Monitor when pain breaks through.
- Determine if the infant appears comfortable after the dose.

When indicated, wean infant from the drug slowly over a period of days. Assess response to withdrawal. Consult with physician to manage withdrawal symptoms if indicated.

Fatigue/Disorganized Sleep-Wake Patterns

Evaluate the need for and, if needed, the frequency of each intervention.

Organize care plan for every-4-hour interventions.

Feeding Problems

Reduce the stress of feeding:

- Initiate contact slowly.
- Touch the infant's back lightly.
- Swaddle the infant with hands crossing midline.
- When this is tolerated, pick the infant up, facing out toward room to eliminate visual stimulation.
- Prevent auditory stimulation (e.g., do not talk).
- Give bottle; provide jaw support if needed.

After the infant is settled, use soothing techniques, hand holding, vertical rocking.

Allow the infant's behavioral cues to set the pace and tone of the interaction.

Position to facilitate feeding.

Provide Comfort Measures When Infant Is in a Nonarousal State

Tactile stimulation (e.g., kangaroo care, massage)
Music, intrauterine sounds; play music, and evaluate response
Swaddling, rocking

Reduce Environmental Stimuli

Noise

Do not tap on incubator.
Place a folded blanket on top of incubator if it is the only work surface available.
Slowly open and close portholes.
Pad incubator doors to reduce banging.
Remove water from ventilator tubing.
Speak softly at the bedside and only when necessary.
Slowly drop the head of the mattress.
Position the infant's bed away from sources of noise (e.g., telephone, intercom, unit equipment).
Evaluate the effectiveness of a quiet hour each shift. Collect data before and after to evaluate effects on staff, infants, and parents

Lights

Use full-spectrum light instead of white light at bedside.
Cover cribs, incubators, and radiant warmers completely during sleep periods; partially during awake times.
Shade the infant's eyes with a blanket tent or cutout box.
Avoid usual stimuli on cribs (e.g., toys)

Position the Infant in Postures that Permit Flexion, and Minimize Flailing, Arching, and Squirming

Avoid oversized diapers
Use prone-lying positions

Reduce the Stress Associated with Handling

When moving or lifting the infant, contain the infant with your hands by wrapping or placing rolled blankets around his or her body.
Maintain containment during procedures and caregiving activities.
Handle slowly and gently.
Initiate all interactions and treatments with one sense stimulus at a time (e.g., touch), and then slowly progress to visual, auditory, movement.

Assess for cues for readiness, impending disorganization, or stability; respond to cues.

Allow infant to be protected and undisturbed for 2- to 3-hour intervals.

Use suctioning or postural drainage as needed instead of routinely.

Reduce Disorganized Neurobehavior During Transport (Transfer)

Have a plan for transport with assigned roles for each team member.

Establish behavior cues of stress for this infant with primary nurse before transport.

Swaddle the infant or place in a nest made of blankets.

Ensure the transport equipment is ready (e.g., ventilator). Warm the mattress or use sheepskin.

Carefully and smoothly move the infant. Avoid talking if possible.

If stress behaviors manifest, stop and allow the infant to return to a stable state.

Reposition every 2–3 hours or sooner if infant behavior suggests discomfort.

Enhance Parent Participation

Encourage parents to share their feelings, fears, and expectations. Gently correct misconceptions.

Teach the behavioral cues and signs of stress in their infant.

Assist parents to interact with their infant as appropriate to status and maturity.

Initiate Health Teaching and Referrals as Indicated

Teach caregivers to continually observe the changing capabilities to determine the appropriate positioning and bedding options

Provide parents with teaching related to

Health Concerns
Feeding, hygiene
Safety, temperature
Illness, infection
Growth, development

State Modulation
Appropriate stimulation
Sleep-wake patterns

Parent–Infant Interaction
Behavior cues
Signs of stress

Infant's Environment
Animate, inanimate stimulation
Role of father and siblings
Playing with infant

Parental Coping and Support
Refer for follow-up home visits.

▶ Infant Behavior, Risk for Disorganized

DEFINITION

The state in which the neonate is at risk for an alteration in integration and modulation of the physiologic and behavioral systems of adaptation (autonomic, motor, state, organizational, self-regulatory, and attentional-interactional).

RISK FACTORS

Refer to Related Factors.

Related Factors

Refer to *Disorganized Infant Behavior*.

Interventions

Refer to *Disorganized Infant Behavior*.

INFECTION, RISK FOR

Infection, Risk for
Infection Transmission, Risk for

DEFINITION

The state in which an individual is at risk to be invaded by an opportunistic or pathogenic agent (virus, fungus, bacterium, protozoan, or other parasite) from endogenous or exogenous sources.

■■■■ **AUTHOR'S NOTE**
Risk for Infection describes a situation when host defenses are
compromised, making the host more susceptible to environmental pathogens. Nursing interventions focus on minimiz-
ing introduction of organisms or increasing resistance to
infection (e.g., improving nutritional status).

RISK FACTORS

Presence of risk factors (see Related Factors)

RELATED FACTORS

A variety of health problems and situations can create favorable
conditions that encourage the development of infections. Some
common factors are listed below.

Pathophysiologic

Related to compromised host defenses secondary to:

Cancer   AIDS
Renal failure   Hepatic disorders
Hematologic disorders   Respiratory disorders
Diabetes mellitus   Immunosuppression
Alcoholism   Altered or insufficient
Immunodeficiency   leukocytes
Periodontal disease   Altered integumentary system
Arthritis

Related to compromised circulation secondary to:

Lymphedema
Obesity
Peripheral vascular disease

Treatment-Related

Related to a site for organism invasion secondary to:

Surgery   Presence of invasive lines
Dialysis   Intubation
Total parenteral nutrition   Enteral feedings

Related to compromised host defenses secondary to:

Radiation therapy
Organ transplant
Medication therapy (specify; e.g., chemotherapy,
    immunosuppressants)

Situational (Personal, Environmental)

Related to compromised host defenses secondary to:

Prolonged immobility

Stress

Increased length of hospital stay

Smoking

Malnutrition

History of infections

Related to a site for organism invasion secondary to:

Trauma (accidental, intentional)

Postpartum period

Bites (animal, insect, human)

Thermal injuries

Warm, moist, dark environment (skin folds, casts)

Related to contact with contagious agents (nosocomial or community-acquired)

Maturational

Newborn

Related to increased vulnerability of infant secondary to:

Lack of maternal antibodies (dependent on maternal exposure)

Lack of normal flora

Open wounds (umbilical, circumcision)

Immature immune system

Infant/Child

Related to increased vulnerability secondary to lack of immunization

Older Adult

Related to increased vulnerability of elderly secondary to: debilitated condition, decreased immune response, or multiple chronic diseases

NOC

Infection Severity, Immune Status

Goals

The person will report risk factors associated with infection and precautions needed.

Indicators

- Demonstrate meticulous hand washing technique by the time of discharge.
- Describe methods of transmission of infection.
- Describe the influence of nutrition on prevention of infection.

Infection Control, Wound Care, Incision Site Care, Health Education

Generic Interventions

Identify Individuals at Risk for Nosocomial Infections

Assess for factors that Increase the Risk of Infection
- Infection (preoperatively)
- Abdominal or thoracic surgery
- Surgery longer than 2 hours
- Genitourinary procedure
- Instrumentation (ventilator, suction, catheters, nebulizers, tracheostomy, invasive monitoring)
- Anesthesia
- Age younger than 1 year or older than 65 years
- Obesity
- Underlying disease conditions (chronic obstructive pulmonary disease, diabetes, cardiovascular, blood dyscrasias)
- Substance abuse
- Medications (steroids, chemotherapy, antibiotic therapy)
- Nutritional status (intake less than minimum daily requirements)
- Smoker

Reduce the Entry of Organisms into Individuals

Meticulous hand washing
Aseptic technique
Isolation measures
No unnecessary diagnostic or therapeutic procedures
Reduction of airborne microorganisms

Protect the Immune-Deficient Individual from Infection

Instruct individual to ask all visitors and personnel to wash their hands before approaching him or her.
Limit visitors when appropriate.
Restrict invasive devices (intravenous line, laboratory specimens) to those that are necessary.
Teach individual and family members signs and symptoms of infection.

Reduce Individual's Susceptibility to Infection

Encourage and maintain caloric and protein intake in diet (see *Imbalanced Nutrition*).

Monitor use or overuse of antimicrobial therapy.
Administer prescribed antimicrobial therapy within 15 minutes of scheduled time.
Minimize length of stay in hospital.

Observe for Clinical Manifestations of Infection (e.g., Fever, Cloudy Urine, Purulent Drainage)

Instruct Individual and Family Regarding the Causes, Risks, and Communicability of the Infection

Report Communicable Diseases As Appropriate to Public Health Department

👫 Pediatric Interventions

Monitor for signs of infection (e.g., lethargy, feeding difficulties, vomiting, temperature instability, subtle color changes).
Provide umbilical cord care. Teach cord care and signs of infection (e.g., increased redness, purulent drainage).
Teach signs of infection of circumcised area (e.g., bleeding, increased redness, or unusual swelling).

👫 Maternal Interventions

Explain the increased vulnerability to infection during pregnancy.
Teach how to prevent urinary tract infections during pregnancy:
• Drink at least eight 8-oz glasses of water.
• Void frequently.
• Void before and after intercourse (Reeder et al., 1997).
Teach how to prevent infection postpartum:
• Wipe from front to back.
• Clean perineal area after voiding or defecating (e.g., sitz bath, squirt bottle).
• Change perineal pads after each voiding.
• Teach proper breast care.
Identify risk factors for postpartum infections:
• Anemia
• Poor nutrition
• Lack of prenatal care
• Obesity
• Intercourse after membrane rupture
• Immunosuppression
• Prolonged labor
• Prolonged membrane rupture
• Intrauterine fetal monitoring (in high-risk mothers)
• Bleeding

Instruct on signs and symptoms of infection (e.g., fever, purulent drainage), and report promptly.

Ⓒ Geriatric Considerations

Explain that the usual signs of infection may not be present (e.g., fever, chills).

Assess for anorexia, weakness, change in mental status, or hypothermia.

Monitor skin and urinary system for signs of fungal, viral, or mycobacterial pathogens.

▶ Infection Transmission, Risk for*

DEFINITION

Risk for Infection Transmission: The state in which an individual is at risk for transferring an opportunistic or pathogenic agent to others.

Risk Factors

Presence of risk factors (see Related Factors)

Related Factors

Pathophysiologic

Related to:

Colonization with highly antibiotic-resistant organism
Airborne transmission exposure
Contact transmission exposure (direct, indirect, contact droplet)

Treatment-Related

Related to contaminated wound
Related to devices with contaminated drainage (urinary and chest tubes, suction equipment, endotracheal tubes)

Situational (Personal, Environmental)

Related to:

Disaster with hazardous infectious material
Unsanitary living conditions (sewage, personal hygiene)
Areas considered high risk for vector-borne diseases (malaria, rabies, bubonic plague, natural disasters)

---

*This diagnosis is not currently on the NANDA list, but has been included for clarity or usefulness.

Areas considered high risk for vehicle-borne diseases (hepatitis
    A, shigella, *Salmonella*)
Lack of knowledge of sources or prevention of infection
Intravenous drug use
Multiple sexual partners
Unprotected sexual intercourse
Natural disaster (e.g., flood, hurricane)

Maturational

Newborn

*Related to birth outside a hospital setting in an uncontrolled
environment*
*Related to exposure during prenatal or perinatal period to
communicable disease via mother*

NOC
Infection Severity, Risk Control, Risk Detection

Goals

The person will describe the mode of transmission of disease by
the time of discharge.

Indicators
• Relate the need to be isolated until noninfectious.
• Demonstrate meticulous hand washing during hospitalization.

NIC
Teaching: Disease Process, Infection Protection

Generic Interventions

Identify susceptible host individuals based on focus assessment
    for risk factors and history of exposure.
Identify the mode of transmission based on infecting agent:
• Airborne
• Contact
    • Direct
    • Indirect
    • Contact droplet
• Vehicle-borne (e.g., food, water, blood, body fluids)
• Vector-borne (insects, animals)
Initiate appropriate isolation precautions. Consult with infection
    control practitioner.

Secure appropriate room assignment, depending on the type of
   infection and hygienic practices of the infected person.
Adhere to the Universal Infection Precautions.
In the case of acute exposure to HIV (e.g., sexual assault,
   needlestick, break in barrier with an HIV-infected person),
   immediately refer to health care facility (e.g., emergency
   room, occupational health) to evaluate the immediate
   initiation of postexposure prophylaxis with antiviral therapy
   (CDC, 2008).
Refer to infection control practitioner for follow-up with the
   health department concerning family exposure and cause of
   exposure, and assist in appropriate isolation of the client.
Teach client regarding the chain of infection and patient
   responsibility in the hospital and at home.

INJURY, RISK FOR

Injury, Risk for
Aspiration, Risk for
Falls, Risk for
Poisoning, Risk for
Suffocation, Risk for
Trauma, Risk for

DEFINITION

The state in which an individual is at risk for harm because of a
perceptual or physiologic deficit, a lack of awareness of hazards,
or maturational age.

■■■■ AUTHOR'S NOTE

This diagnosis has five subcategories: *Risk for Aspiration,
Falls, Poisoning, Suffocation,* and *Trauma*. Should the nurse
choose to isolate interventions only for prevention of poisoning, then the diagnosis *Risk for Poisoning* would be useful.

RISK FACTORS

Presence of risk factors (see Related Factors for specific factors)

RELATED FACTORS

Pathophysiologic

Related to altered cerebral function secondary to, for example, tissue hypoxia, vertigo, syncope

Related to altered mobility secondary to:

Unsteady gait

Amputation

Arthritis

Cerebrovascular accident

Parkinsonism

Loss of limb

Related to impaired sensory function (e.g., vision, hearing, thermal/touch, smell)

Related to fatigue

Related to orthostatic hypotension

Related to vestibular disorders

Related to carotid sinus syncope

Related to lack of awareness of environmental hazards secondary to, for example, confusion, hypoglycemia, depression, electrolyte imbalances

Related to tonic-clonic movements secondary to seizures

Treatment-Related

Related to effects of (specify) on mobility or sensorium:

Medications

Sedatives

Vasodilators

Antihypertensives

Hypoglycemics

Diuretics

Phenothiazines

Psychotropics

Related to casts/crutches, canes, walkers

Situational (Personal, Environmental)

Related to decrease in or loss of short-term memory

Related to faulty judgment secondary to, for example, dehydration (e.g., summer), stress, alcohol

Related to prolonged bed rest

Related to vasovagal reflex

Related to household hazards (specify):

Unsafe walkways

Unsafe toys

Inadequate lighting

Bathrooms (tubs, low toilets)

Stairs

Slippery floors

Faulty electric wires

Improperly stored poisons

Related to automotive hazards

Related to fire hazards

Related to unfamiliar setting (hospital, nursing home)
Related to improper footwear
Related to inattentive caregiver
Related to improper use of aids (crutches, canes, walkers, wheelchairs)
Related to history of accidents

Maturational

Infant/Child
Related to lack of awareness of hazards

Older Adult

Related to faulty judgment secondary to:
Sensory deficits
Medication
Cognitive deficits

NOC

Risk Control, Safety Status: Falls Occurrence, Safety Behavior: Home Physical Environment, Safety Behavior: Personal

Goals

The person will relate fewer injuries and less fear of injury.

Indicators
- Identify factors that increase the risk for injury.
- Relate an intent to use safety measures to prevent injury (e.g., remove throw rugs or anchor them).
- Relate an intent to practice selected prevention measures (e.g., wear sunglasses to reduce glare).
- Increase daily activity, if feasible.

NIC

Fall Prevention, Environmental Management: Safety, Health Education, Surveillance: Safety, Risk Identification

Generic Interventions

Orient each new admission to surroundings, explain the call system, and assess the person's ability to use it.
Closely supervise the person during the first few nights to assess safety.

Use night light.

Encourage the person to request assistance during the night.

Keep bed at lowest level during the night.

Teach proper use of crutches, canes, walkers, prosthesis.

Instruct the person to wear shoes that fit properly and that have nonskid soles.

Assess for the presence of side effects of drugs that may cause vertigo.

Teach the person to:

- Eliminate throw rugs, litter, and highly polished floors.
- Provide nonslip surfaces in bathtub or shower by applying commercially available traction tapes.
- Provide handgrips in bathroom.
- Provide railings in hallways and on stairs.
- Remove protruding objects (e.g., coat hooks, shelves, light fixtures) from stairway walls.

Institute safety precautions for confused persons (Schoenfelder, 2000).

- Observe frequently.
- Ask roommate, if capable, to alert nurses of a problem.
- Use low bed, with side rails up.
- Use mattress on floor.
- Place bedside table or commode chair in front of patient when sitting in a chair.
- Consider an alarm system.
- Place person in room near traffic (e.g., nurses' station).
- Provide a distraction: music, companion, simple craft, pet therapy.

🚼 Pediatric Interventions

Teach parents to expect frequent changes in infants' and children's ability and to take precautions (e.g., infant who suddenly rolls over for the first time might be on a changing table unattended).

Discuss with parents the necessity of constant monitoring of small children.

Provide parents with information to assist them in selecting a babysitter.

Determine previous experiences and knowledge of emergency measures.

Observe the interaction of the sitter with the child.

Teach parents to expect children to mimic them and to teach their children what they can do with or without supervision (seat belts, helmets, safe driving).

Explain and expect compliance with certain rules (depending on age) concerning:
- Streets
- Playground equipment
- Water (pools, bathtubs)
- Bicycles
- Fire
- Animals
- Strangers

Instruct how to "child-proof" the home.

Explain why children should not ride in front (air bags).

Refer to local fire department for assistance in staging home fire drills.

Encourage parents to learn basic life-saving skills (CPR, Heimlich maneuver).

Teach children how to dial 911.

Teach parents to assist their children in handling peer pressure that involves risk-taking behavior.

🅖 Geriatric Interventions

Assess for orthostatic hypotension. Compare brachial blood pressure (supine, standing).

Discuss physiology of orthostatic hypotension with client.

Teach techniques to reduce orthostatic hypotension.
- Change positions slowly.
- Move from lying to an upright position in stages.
- During day, rest in a recliner rather than in bed.
- Avoid prolonged standing.

Teach to avoid dehydration and vasodilation (e.g., hot tubs).

Teach exercises to increase strength and flexibility.

Perform ankle-strengthening exercises daily (Schoenfelder, 2000).
- Stand behind a straight chair, with feet slightly apart.
- Slowly raise both heels until body weight is on balls of feet; hold for count of 3 (e.g., "1 Mississippi, 2 Mississippi, 3 Mississippi").
- Do 5 to 10 repetitions; increase repetitions as strength increases.

Walk at least two or three times a week.
- Use ankle exercises as a warm-up before walking.
- Begin walking with someone at side if needed for 10 minutes.
- Increase time and speed according to capabilities.

▶ Aspiration, Risk for

DEFINITION

The state in which a person is at risk for entry of secretions, solids, or fluids into the tracheobronchial passages.

RISK FACTORS

Presence of favorable conditions for aspiration (see Related Factors).

RELATED FACTORS

Pathophysiologic

Related to reduced level of consciousness secondary to:

Anesthesia	Coma
Head injury	Presenile dementia
Cerebrovascular accident	Seizures

Related to depressed cough and gag reflexes

Related to increased intragastric pressure secondary to:

Lithotomy position	Obesity
Enlarged uterus	Ascites

Related to impaired swallowing or decreased laryngeal and glottic reflexes secondary to:

Achalasia	Catatonia
Scleroderma	Myasthenia gravis
Esophageal strictures	Guillain-Barré syndrome
Cerebrovascular accident	Multiple sclerosis
Parkinson's disease	Muscular dystrophy
Debilitating conditions	

Related to tracheoesophageal fistula

Related to impaired protective reflexes secondary to:

Facial/oral/neck surgery or trauma
Paraplegia or hemiplegia
Treatment-Related

Related to depressed laryngeal and glottic reflexes secondary to:

Presence of tracheostomy/endotracheal tube
Sedation
Tube feedings

Related to impaired ability to cough secondary to:

Wired jaw
Imposed prone position

Situational (Personal, Environmental)
Related to inability/impaired ability to elevate upper body
Related to eating when intoxicated

Maturational
Premature
Related to impaired sucking/swallowing reflexes

Neonate
Related to decreased muscle tone of inferior esophageal sphincter

Older Adult
Related to poor dentition

NOC
Aspiration Control

Goals
The person will not experience aspiration.

Indicators
- Relate measures to prevent aspiration.
- Name foods or fluids that are high risk for aspiration.

NIC
Aspirations: Precautions, Airway Management, Positioning, Airway Suctioning

Generic Interventions
Reduce the Risk of Aspiration
For individuals with decreased strength, decreased sensorium, or autonomic disorders:
- Maintain a side-lying position if not contraindicated by injury.
- Assess for position of the tongue, ensuring that it has not dropped backward, occluding the airway.
- Keep the head of the bed elevated if not contraindicated.
- Clear secretions from mouth and throat with a tissue or gentle suction.
- Reassess frequently for presence of obstructive material in mouth and throat.

For persons with tracheostomies or endotracheal tubes:
- Inflate cuff (during continuous mechanical ventilation, during and after eating, during and 1 hour after tube feeding, during intermittent positive-pressure breathing treatments).
- Suction every 1 to 2 hours and as needed.

For persons with gastrointestinal tubes and feedings:
- Verify that feeding tube has not moved upward since insertion.
- Aspirate for residual contents before each feeding for tubes positioned gastrically.
- Elevate head of bed for 30 to 45 minutes during feeding period and 1 hour after to prevent reflux by reverse gravity.
- Administer feeding if residual contents are less than 150 mL (intermittent), *or*
- Administer feeding if residual is not greater than 150 mL at 10% to 20% of hourly rate (continuous).
- Regulate gastric feedings using an intermittent schedule, allowing periods of stomach emptying between feeding intervals.

Ensure emergency management of obstructions is known.

👥 Pediatric Interventions

Position infant in side-lying position or supine, not prone.
Teach parents:
- Not to prop bottle
- To keep small objects (e.g., coins) out of reach
- To remove all plastic bags
- To inspect toys for removable parts or long strings

Teach what foods to avoid for young children (e.g., fruits with pits, nuts, gum, whole grapes, hot dogs, popcorn kernels).
Teach emergency management of airway obstruction:
- Back blows and chest thrusts (infants)
- Heimlich maneuver (children)

▶ Falls, Risk for

DEFINITION

The state in which an individual has increased susceptibility to falling.

RISK FACTORS

Presence of risk factors (see Related Factors under *Risk for Injury*).

■■■■ **AUTHOR'S NOTE**

This nursing diagnosis can be used to specify an individual at risk for falls. If the person is at risk for various types of injuries (e.g., as a cognitively impaired person), the broader diagnosis *Risk for Injury* is more useful.

Goals

The person will relate fewer falls and less fear of falling.

Indicators

- Identify factors that increase the risk for injury.
- Relate an intent to use safety measures to prevent injury (e.g., remove throw rugs or anchor them).
- Relate an intent to practice selected prevention measures (e.g., wear sunglasses to reduce glare).
- Increase daily activity, if feasible.

Generic Interventions

Refer to *Risk for Injury*.

❱ Poisoning, Risk for

DEFINITION

The state in which an individual is at risk of accidental exposure to or ingestion of drugs or dangerous substances.

Risk Factors

Presence of risk factors (see Related Factors under *Risk for Injury*).

❱ Suffocation, Risk for

DEFINITION

The state in which an individual is at risk for smothering and asphyxiation.

RISK FACTORS

Presence of risk factors (see Related Factors under *Risk for Injury*)

▶ Trauma, Risk for

DEFINITION

The state in which an individual is at risk of accidental tissue injury (e.g., wound, burns, fracture).

RISK FACTORS

Presence of risk factors (see Related Factors under *Risk for Injury*)

INJURY, RISK FOR PERIOPERATIVE POSITIONING

DEFINITION

The state in which an individual is at risk for harm as a result of positioning requirements for surgery and loss of usual protective responses secondary to anesthesia.

AUTHOR'S NOTE

This diagnosis focuses on identifying the vulnerability for tissue, nerve, and joint injury resulting from required positions for surgery. The addition of the term "perioperative positioning" to the *Risk for Injury* diagnosis adds etiology to the label.

If a client has no preexisting risk factors that make him or her more vulnerable to injury, this diagnosis could be used with no related factors because they are evident. If related factors are desired, the statement could read, for example, *Risk for Perioperative Positioning Injury related to position requirements for surgery and loss of usual sensory protective measures secondary to anesthesia*. When a client has preexisting risk factors, the statement should include them: for example, *Risk for Perioperative Positioning Injury related to compromised tissue perfusion secondary to peripheral arterial disease*.

RISK FACTORS

Presence of risk factors (see Related Factors).

RELATED FACTORS
Pathophysiologic

Related to increased vulnerability secondary to:

Chronic disease	Radiation therapy
Renal, hepatic dysfunction	Cancer
Osteoporosis	Infection
Compromised immune system	Thin body frame

Related to compromised tissue perfusion secondary to:

Diabetes mellitus	Cardiovascular disease
Peripheral vascular disease	Anemia
Hypothermia	History of thrombosis
Ascites	Dehydration
Edema	

Related to vulnerability of stoma during positioning
Related to preexisting contractures or physical impairments secondary to: for example, rheumatoid arthritis, polio

Treatment-Related

Related to position requirements and loss of usual sensory protective responses secondary to anesthesia*
Related to surgical procedures of 2 hours or longer
Related to vulnerability of implants or prostheses (e.g., pacemakers) during positioning

Situational (Personal, Environmental)

Related to compromised circulation secondary to:

Obesity	Pregnancy
Tobacco use	

Maturational

Related to increased vulnerability to tissue injury secondary to decreased circulatory volume (infant, elder)

NOC

Circulation Status, Neurological Status, Tissue Perfusion: Peripheral

Goals

The person will have no neuromuscular damage or injury related to the surgical position.

Indicators
- Padding is used as indicated for procedure.
- Limbs are secured when at risk.
- Limbs are flexed when indicated.

NIC

Positioning: Intraoperative, Surveillance, Pressure Management

Generic Interventions

Determine if client has preexisting risk factors (refer to Risk Factors). Communicate findings to the surgical team.

Prior to positioning, assess and document the following:
- Range-of-motion ability
- Physical abnormalities
- External/internal prostheses or implants
- Neurovascular status
- Circulatory status

Move the person from the stretcher to the operating room bed according to protocol. Lift; do not pull or drag. Do not leave unattended.

Discuss the surgical position desired with the surgeon. Advise if any preexisting factors exist. Determine if the position will be arranged before or after anesthesia.

Always ask the anesthesiologist's or nurse anesthetist's permission before moving or repositioning an anesthetized person.

Reduce vulnerability to tissue injury:
- Align neck and spine at all times.
- Gently manipulate joints. Do not abduct more than 90 degrees.
- Do not let limbs extend off the operating room bed. Reposition slowly and gently.
- Use a draw sheet above the elbows to tuck in arms at side, or abduct arm on an arm board with padding.

Protect eyes and ears from pressure. Ensure that ears are not bent. Use eye shields if needed.

Depending on the surgical position, pad areas vulnerable to injury. Refer to unit protocols.

If feasible, ask client if he or she feels pain, burning, pressure, or any discomforts after positioning.

Continually assess that team members are not leaning on the client, especially on the limbs.

Ensure that the head is lifted slightly every 30 minutes.

When repositioning or returning the person to a supine position after certain surgical positions (e.g., Trendelenburg, lithotomy, reverse Trendelenburg, jack-knife, lateral), slowly change position to prevent severe hypotension.

Assess client's skin condition when surgery is completed, and document findings. Inform postanesthesia nurses whether preexisting risk factors are present that increase vulnerability postoperatively.

DEFICIENT KNOWLEDGE

DEFINITION

The state in which an individual or group experiences a deficiency in cognitive knowledge or psychomotor skills concerning the condition or treatment plan.

AUTHOR'S NOTE

Deficient Knowledge does not represent a human response, alteration, or pattern of dysfunction; rather, it is an etiologic or contributing factor (Jenny, 1987). Lack of knowledge can contribute to a variety of responses (e.g., anxiety, self-care deficits). All nursing diagnoses have related client/family teaching as a part of nursing interventions (e.g., *Impaired Bowel Elimination, Impaired Verbal Communication*). When the teaching relates directly to a specific nursing diagnosis, incorporate the teaching into the plan. When specific teaching is indicated before a procedure, the diagnosis *Anxiety related to unfamiliar environment or procedure* can be used. When information is given to assist a person or family with self-care at home, the diagnosis *Ineffective Therapeutic Regimen Management* may be indicated.

DEFINING CHARACTERISTICS

Major (Must Be Present, One or More)

Verbalizes a deficiency in knowledge or skill or requests information

Expresses an inaccurate perception of health status

Does not correctly perform a desired or prescribed health behavior

Minor (May Be Present)

Lack of integration of treatment plan into daily activities
Exhibits or expresses psychological alteration (e.g., anxiety, depression) resulting from misinformation or lack of information

LATEX ALLERGY RESPONSE

Latex Allergy Response
Latex Allergy Response, Risk for

DEFINITION

The state in which an individual experiences an immunoglobulin E–mediated allergic response to latex.

DEFINING CHARACTERISTICS

Major

Positive skin test to natural rubber latex (NRL) extract

Minor

Allergic conjunctivitis   Rhinitis
Urticaria   Asthma

RELATED FACTORS

Biopathophysiologic

Related to hypersensitivity response to the protein component of NRL

NOC

Immune Hypersensitivity Control

Goals

The person will report no exposure to latex.

Indicators
- Describe products of NRL.
- Describe strategies to avoid exposure.

NIC
Allergy Management, Latex Precautions, Environmental Risk Protection

Generic Interventions

Explain the importance of completely avoiding direct contact with all NRL products.

Advise that a person with a history of mild skin reaction to latex is at risk for anaphylaxis.

Instruct the patient to wear a medical alert bracelet stating "Latex Allergy" and to carry autoinjectable epinephrine.

Instruct to warn all health care providers (e.g., dental, medical, surgical) of the allergy.

Use nonlatex alternative supplies:
- Clear disposable amber bags
- Silicone baby nipples
- 2 × 2 gauze pads with silk tape in place of adhesive bandages
- Clear plastic or Silastic catheters
- Vinyl or Neoprene gloves
- Silk or plastic tape, not plastic or adhesive

Protect from exposure to latex:
- Cover skin with cloth before applying blood pressure cuff.
- Do not allow rubber stethoscope tubing to touch person.
- Do not inject through rubber parts (e.g., heparin locks); use syringe and stopcock.
- Change needles after each puncture of rubber stopper.
- Cover rubber parts with tape.

Teach what products are commonly made of latex

Health Care Equipment:
- NRL gloves, powdered or unpowdered, including those labeled "hypoallergenic"
- Blood pressure cuffs, stethoscopes, tourniquets
- Electrode pads
- Airways, endotracheal tubes
- Syringe plunges, bulb syringes
- Masks for anesthesia
- Rubber aprons
- Catheters, wound drains

- Injection ports
- Tops of multidose vials
- Adhesive tape
- Ostomy pouches
- Wheelchair cushions
- Briefs with elastic
- Pads for crutches

Office/Household Products:

- Erasers, rubber bands, dishwashing gloves, balloons
- Condoms, diaphragms
- Baby bottle nipples, pacifiers, hot water bottles
- Rubber balls and toys
- Racquet handles, cycle grips
- Tires
- Carpeting
- Shoe soles
- Elastic in underwear
- Rubber cement

▶ Latex Allergy Response, Risk for

DEFINITION

The state in which an individual is at risk for experiencing an immunoglobulin E–mediated allergic response to latex.

RISK FACTORS

Biopathophysiologic

Related to history of atopic eczema, asthma
Related to history of allergic rhinitis

Treatment-Related

Related to frequent urinary catheterizations
Related to frequent rectal disimpaction
Related to frequent surgical procedures

Situational (Personal, Environmental)

*Related to history of allergy to banana, kiwi, avocado, tomato,
raw potato, peach, chestnuts, mango, papaya, passion fruit*
History of allergy to gloves, condoms, etc.
Frequent occupational exposure to natural rubber latex, such as:

Health care workers	Housekeepers
Food handlers	Greenhouse workers' products
Workers making NRL	

Goals

Refer to *Latex Allergy Response*.

Generic Interventions

Refer to *Latex Allergy Response*.

LIVER FUNCTION, RISK FOR IMPAIRED

DEFINITION

A state in which an individual is at risk for liver dysfunction.

DEFINING CHARACTERISTICS

Hepatotoxic medications, e.g., statins, acetaminophen
HIV coinfection
Substance abuse, e.g., alcohol, cocaine
Viral infections, e.g., hepatitis A, B, and C, Epstein-Barr

AUTHOR'S NOTE

This new NANDA diagnosis is the same focus as the collaborative problem *Risk for Complications of Liver Dysfunction*. Students should consult with their instructor for which terminology should be used.

RISK FOR LONELINESS

DEFINITION

The state in which an individual is at risk for experiencing discomfort associated with a desire or need for contact with others.

AUTHOR'S NOTE
Risk for Loneliness was added to the NANDA list in 1994.
Social Isolation is also on the NANDA list. *Social Isolation* is a
conceptually incorrect diagnosis because it does not represent a response but instead is the cause. *Loneliness* and *Risk
for Loneliness* better describe the negative state of aloneness.

Loneliness is a subjective state that exists whenever a person says it does and is perceived as imposed by others. Loneliness is *not* the result of voluntary solitude that is necessary
for personal renewal, nor is it the creative aloneness of the
artist or the initial aloneness one may experience as a result
of seeking individualism and independence (e.g., moving to a
new city, going away to college).

RISK FACTORS
See Related Factors.

RELATED FACTORS
Pathophysiologic
Related to fear of rejection secondary to:
Obesity
Cancer (disfiguring surgery of head or neck, superstitions of
   others)
Physical handicaps (paraplegia, amputation, arthritis, hemiplegia)
Emotional handicaps (extreme anxiety, depression, paranoia,
   phobias)
Incontinence (embarrassment, odor)
Communicable diseases (AIDS, hepatitis)
Psychiatric illness (schizophrenia, bipolar affective disorder,
   personality disorders)
Related to difficulty accessing social events secondary to:
Debilitating diseases
Physical disabilities

Treatment-Related
Related to therapeutic isolation

Situational (Personal, Environmental)
Related to insufficient planning for retirement
Related to death of a significant other
Related to divorce

Related to disfiguring appearance

Related to fear of rejection secondary to: for example, obesity, extreme poverty, hospitalization or terminal illness (dying process), or unemployment

Related to moving to another culture (e.g., unfamiliar language)

Related to history of unsatisfying social experiences secondary to: drug abuse, alcohol abuse, immature behavior, unacceptable social behavior, or delusional thinking

Related to loss of usual means of transportation

Related to change in usual residence secondary to long-term care or relocation

Maturational

Child

Related to protective isolation or a communicable disease

Older Adult

Related to loss of usual social contacts secondary to retirement, relocation, death of (specify), or loss of driving ability

NOC

Loneliness, Social Development

Goals

The person will report decreased feelings of loneliness.

Indicators
• Identify the reasons for feelings of isolation.
• Discuss ways of increasing meaningful relationships.

NIC

Socialization Enhancement, Spiritual Support, Behavior Modification: Social Skills, Presence, Anticipatory Guidance

Generic Interventions

The nursing interventions for a variety of contributing factors that might be associated with a diagnosis of *Risk for Loneliness* are very similar.

Identify Causative and Contributing Factors

Reduce or Eliminate Causative and Contributing Factors

Promote Social Interaction

Support the individual who has experienced a loss as he or she works through grief (see *Grieving*).

Validate the normalcy of grieving.

Encourage the person to talk about feelings of loneliness and the reasons they exist.

Mobilize the person's support system of neighbors and friends.

Discuss the importance of quality socialization rather than a great number of interactions.

Refer to social skills teaching (see *Social Interaction, Impaired*).

Offer feedback on how the person presents himself or herself to others (see *Social Interaction, Impaired*).

Decrease Barriers to Social Contact

Determine available transportation in the community (public, church-related, volunteer).

Determine if person must be taught how to use alternate transportation (e.g., drive a car).

Identify activities that help keep people busy, especially during times of high risk of loneliness (see *Deficient Diversional Activity*).

Assist with the development of alternate means of communication for persons with compromised sensory ability (e.g., amplifier on phone; see *Impaired Communication*).

Assist with the management of aesthetic problems (e.g., consult enterostomal therapist if odor is a problem).

Assist the person in locating stores that sell clothing especially made for those who have had disfiguring surgery (e.g., mastectomy).

Refer to *Impaired Urinary Elimination* for specific interventions to control incontinence.

For Individuals with Poor or Offensive Social Skills:

Engage in one-to-one social dialogue. Explain the difference between casual and meaningful conversation.

Discuss the characteristics of meaningful conversation:

- Initiating interactions
- Being spontaneous
- Being alert
- Showing interest
- Giving and receiving compliments
- Showing interest in others, in activities
- Requesting help when needed

- Using increased eye contact
- Using appropriate speech tone and nonverbal behavior

Allow person opportunities to observe others engaged in meaningful conversation.

Observe the person socializing, and discuss the interactions after. Offer praise. Gently discuss alternative approaches. Role-play skills.

Initiate Referrals as Indicated:

Community-based groups that contact the socially isolated

Self-help groups for clients isolated due to specific medical problems (Reach to Recovery, United Ostomy Association)

Wheelchair groups

Psychiatric consumer rights associations

Ⓒ Geriatric Interventions

Discuss the Anticipated Effects of Retirement on the Person's Life. Assist with Planning (Stanley & Beare, 2000)

Plan to ensure adequate income.

Decrease time at work the last 2 to 3 years (e.g., shorter days, longer vacations).

Cultivate friends outside of work.

Develop routines at home to replace work structure.

Rely on others rather than spouse for leisure activities.

Cultivate leisure activities that are realistic (energy, cost).

Prepare self for ambivalent feelings and short-term negative impact on self-esteem.

Identify Strategies to Expand the World of the Isolated:

Senior centers and church groups

Foster grandparent program

Day care centers for the elderly

Retirement communities

House sharing, group homes

College classes open to older persons

Pets

Telephone contact

Psychiatric day hospital or activity program

Identify Community Sources for Socialization

Refer to Transportation Services If Needed

RISK FOR DISTURBED MATERNAL/FETAL DYAD

DEFINITION

The state in which a pregnant woman is at risk for disruption of the symbiotic maternal/fetal dyad as a result of comorbid or pregnancy–related conditions.

RISK FACTORS

Complications of pregnancy (e.g., premature rupture of membranes, placenta previa or abruption, late prenatal care, multiple gestations)

Compromised Oxygen transport (e.g., anemia, cardiac disease, asthma, hypertension, seizures, premature labor, hemorrhage)

Impaired glucose metabolism (e.g., diabetes, steroid use)

Physical abuse

Substance abuse (e.g., tobacco, alcohol, drugs)

Treatment-related side effects (e.g., medications, surgery, chemotherapy)

■■■■ AUTHOR'S NOTE

This new NANDA-I nursing diagnosis represents numerous situations or factors that can compromise the pregnant woman and/or the fetus. The primary responsibility of nursing is to monitor the status of the mother, fetus, and pregnancy and to collaborate with medicine for monitoring (e.g., electronic fetal, Doppler, laboratory tests) and treatments.

For example, if a pregnant woman is using cocaine, the collaborative problem *Risk for Complications of Maternal-Fetal Dyad secondary to cocaine use* would be valid because cocaine contributes to preterm labor and fetal complications.

In another situation, such as placenta previa, *Risk for Complications of Prenatal Bleeding* would be valid. In addition, some nursing diagnoses may be valid as *Ineffective Denial, Disabled Family Coping*.

INTERVENTIONS/GOALS

Refer to Section 3 under Risk for Complications of Maternal/Infant Dyad, for interventions for this generic Collaborative problem or for more specific collaborative problems such as:

- Risk for Complications of Non-Assuring Fetal Status
- Risk for Prenatal Bleeding
- Risk for Complications of Postpartum Bleeding

MOBILITY, IMPAIRED PHYSICAL

Mobility, Impaired Physical
Impaired Bed Mobility
Impaired Walking
Impaired Wheelchair Mobility
Impaired Transfer Ability

DEFINITION

The state in which an individual experiences or is at risk of experiencing limitation of physical movement but is not immobile.

■■■ AUTHOR'S NOTE

Impaired Physical Mobility describes an individual with limited use of arm(s) or leg(s) or limited muscle strength. *Impaired Physical Mobility* should not be used to describe complete immobility; instead, *Disuse Syndrome* is more applicable. Limitation of physical movement can also be the etiology of other nursing diagnoses, such as *Self-Care Deficit* or *Risk for Injury*.

Nursing interventions for *Impaired Physical Mobility* focus on strengthening and restoring function and preventing deterioration.

DEFINING CHARACTERISTICS (LEVIN ET AL., 1989)

Major (80% to 100%)

Compromised ability to move purposefully within the environment (e.g., bed mobility, transfers, ambulation)

Range-of-motion (ROM) limitations

Minor (50% to 80%)

Imposed restriction of movement
Reluctance to move

RELATED FACTORS

Pathophysiologic

Related to decreased strength and endurance secondary to:

Neuromuscular impairment
Autoimmune alterations (e.g., multiple sclerosis, arthritis)
Nervous system diseases (e.g., parkinsonism, myasthenia gravis)
Muscular dystrophy
Partial or total paralysis (e.g., spinal cord injury, stroke)
Central nervous system tumor
Increased intracranial pressure
Sensory deficits

Musculoskeletal impairment
Fractures
Connective tissue disease (systemic lupus erythematosus)

Related to edema (increased synovial fluid)

Treatment-Related

Related to external devices (casts or splints, braces, intravenous tubing).
Related to insufficient strength and endurance for ambulation with (specify; e.g., prosthesis, crutches, walker)

Situational (Personal, Environmental)

Related to fatigue, decreased motivation, or pain

Maturational

Children
Related to abnormal gait secondary to:
Congenital skeletal deficiencies
Osteomyelitis
Congenital hip dysplasia
Legg-Calvé-Perthes disease

Older Adults
Related to decreased motor agility or muscle weakness

NOC

Ambulation: Walking, Joint Movement: Active, Mobility Level

Goals

The person will report an increase in strength and endurance of limbs.

Indicators

- Demonstrate the use of adaptive devices to increase mobility.
- Use safety measures to minimize potential for injury.
- Describe rationale for interventions.
- Demonstrate measures to increase mobility.

NIC

Exercise Therapy: Joint Mobility, Exercise Promotion: Strength Training, Exercise Therapy: Ambulation, Positioning, Teaching: Prescribed Activity: Exercise, Teaching: Assistance Device, Teaching: Safety

Generic Interventions

Refer to **Disuse Syndrome** for Interventions to Prevent the Complications of Immobility

Teach to Perform Active ROM Exercises on Unaffected Limbs at Least Four Times a Day

Perform passive ROM exercises on affected limbs:
- Perform slowly.
- Support the extremity above and below the joint.

Gradually progress from active ROM to functional activities.

Position in Alignment to Prevent Complications

Use a foot board.

Avoid prolonged periods of sitting or lying in the same position.

Change position of the shoulder joints every 2 to 4 hours.

Use a small pillow or no pillow when in Fowler's position.

Support the hand and wrist in natural alignment.

If the client is supine or prone, place a rolled towel or small pillow under the lumbar curvature or under the end of the rib cage.

Place a trochanter roll or sandbags alongside the hips and upper thighs.

If the client is in the lateral position, place pillow(s) to support the leg from groin to foot and a pillow to flex the shoulder and elbow slightly; if needed, support the lower foot in dorsal flexion with a sandbag.

Use hand and wrist splints.

Provide Progressive Mobilization.*

Assist slowly to sitting position.

Allow to dangle legs over the side of the bed for a few minutes before standing.

Limit the time to 15 minutes, three times a day, the first few times out of bed.

Increase time out of bed, as tolerated, by 15-minute increments.

Progress to ambulation, with or without assistive devices.

If client is unable to walk, assist out of bed to a wheelchair or chair.

Encourage ambulation for short, frequent walks (at least three times daily), with assistance if unsteady.

Increase lengths of walks progressively each day.

Observe and Teach the Use of:

Crutches
No pressure should be exerted on axilla; hand strength should be used.

Type of gait varies with diagnosis.

Measure crutches 2 to 3 inches below axilla and tips 6 inches away from feet.

Walkers
Use arm strength to support weakness in lower limbs.

Gait varies with individual's problems.

Wheelchairs
Practice transfers.

Practice maneuvering around barriers.

Prostheses
Stump wrapping before application of the prosthesis

Application of the prosthesis

Principles of stump care

Importance of cleaning the stump, keeping it dry, and applying the prosthesis only when the stump is dry

---

*This may require a primary care professional's order.

Slings

Assess for correct application; sling should be loose around neck
   and should support elbow and wrist above level of the heart.
Remove slings for ROM.

Ace Bandages

Observe for correct position.
Apply with even pressure, wrapping distally to proximally.
Observe for bunching.
Observe for signs of skin irritation (redness, ulceration) or
   tightness (compression).
Rewrap twice per day or as needed unless contraindicated (e.g.,
   if bandage is postoperative compression dressing, check
   physician's orders).

Teach Safety Precautions

Protect areas of decreased sensation from extremes of heat and
   cold.
Practice falling and how to recover from falls while transferring
   or ambulating.
For decreased perception of lower extremity (post-CVA
   "neglect"), instruct the individual to check where limb is
   placed when changing positions or going through doorways;
   check to make sure that both shoes are tied, that affected leg is
   dressed with trousers, and that pants are not dragging.
Instruct individuals who are confined to wheelchair to shift
   position and lift up buttocks every 15 minutes to relieve
   pressure; maneuver on curbs, ramps, inclines, and around
   obstacles; and lock wheelchair before transferring.

Encourage Use of Affected Arm When Possible

Encourage the person to use affected arm for self-care activities
   (e.g., feeding, dressing, brushing hair).
For post-CVA neglect of upper limb, see also *Unilateral Neglect.*
Instruct the person to use unaffected arm to exercise the affected
   arm.
Use appropriate adaptive equipment to enhance the use of arms:
   • Universal cuff for feeding in individuals who have poor con-
     trol in both arms, hands.
   • Large-handled or padded silverware to assist individuals with
     poor fine-motor skills.
   • Dishware with high edges to prevent food from slipping.
   • Suction-cup aids to hold dishes in place and prevent sliding
     of plate.
   • Use a warm bath to alleviate early morning stiffness and im-
     prove mobility.

Have Person Demonstrate:

Strengthening exercises
ROM exercises
Care of adaptive devices
Safety precautions

▶ Impaired Bed Mobility

DEFINITION

The state in which an individual experiences, or is at risk of experiencing, limitation of movement in bed.

AUTHOR'S NOTE

Impaired Bed Mobility is a clinically useful diagnosis when an individual is a candidate for rehabilitation to improve strength, range of motion, and movement. The nurse could consult with a physical therapist for a specific plan for the individual. This diagnosis would be inappropriate for an unconscious or terminally ill person.

DEFINING CHARACTERISTICS (NANDA)

Impaired ability to turn from side to side
Impaired ability to move from supine to sitting or from sitting to supine
Impaired ability to "scoot" or reposition self in bed
Impaired ability to move from supine to prone or from prone to supine
Impaired ability to move from supine to long sitting or from long sitting to supine

RELATED FACTORS

Refer to *Impaired Physical Mobility*.

Goals

Refer to *Impaired Physical Mobility*.

Generic Interventions

Refer to *Impaired Physical Mobility*.

▶ Impaired Walking

DEFINITION

The state in which an individual experiences or is at risk of experiencing limitation in walking.

DEFINING CHARACTERISTICS (NANDA)

Impaired ability to climb stairs
Impaired ability to walk required distances
Impaired ability to walk on an incline
Impaired ability to walk on uneven surfaces
Impaired ability to navigate curbs

RELATED FACTORS

Refer to *Impaired Physical Mobility*.

Goals

The person will increase walking distances (specify distance goal).

Indicators

• Demonstrate safe mobility.
• Use mobility aids correctly.

Generic Interventions

Explain that Safe Ambulation Is a Complete Movement Involving the Musculoskeletal, Neurologic, and Cardiovascular Systems and Cognitive Factors Such As Mentation and Orientation

If the Person Is Deconditioned, a Progressive Program of Exercise Is Needed; Consult with Physical Therapist for an Evaluation and Plan

Ascertain that Ambulatory Aids Are Being Used Correctly and Safely (e.g., Cane, Walker, Crutches).

Wears well-fitting, firm shoes
Can ambulate on inclines, uneven surfaces, and up and down stairs
Is aware of hazards (e.g., wet floors, throw rugs)

Provide Progressive Mobilization If Indicated:

Assist slowly to a sitting position.

Allow to dangle legs over the side of the bed for a few minutes before standing.

Limit the time to 15 minutes, three times a day, the first few times out of bed.

Increase time out of bed, as tolerated, by 15-minute increments.

Progress to ambulation, with or without assistive devices.

If client is unable to walk, assist out of bed to a wheelchair or chair.

Encourage ambulation for short, frequent walks (at least three times daily), with assistance if unsteady.

Increase lengths of walks progressively each day.

Evaluate Response to Ambulation. Refer to Activity Intolerance, If Needed

▶ Impaired Wheelchair Mobility

DEFINITION

The state in which an individual experiences or is at risk of experiencing difficulty with wheelchair mobility and safety.

DEFINING CHARACTERISTICS (NANDA)

Impaired ability to operate manual or power wheelchair on even or uneven surface

Impaired ability to operate manual or power wheelchair on an incline

Impaired ability to operate wheelchair on curbs

RELATED FACTORS

Refer to *Impaired Physical Mobility*.

Goals

The person will report satisfactory, safe wheelchair mobility.

Indicators
- Demonstrate safe use of wheelchair.
- Demonstrate safe transfer to wheelchair.

Generic Interventions

Determine Factors that Are Interfering with Proper Wheelchair Use

Knowledge
Strength
Mentation

Consult with Physical Therapist if Strengthening Exercises Are Indicated

Teach Transfer Techniques

Weight-bearing
Non–weight-bearing

Have Person Demonstrate Technique and Evaluate Effectiveness and Safety

▶ Impaired Transfer Ability

DEFINITION

The state in which an individual experiences or is at risk of experiencing difficulty with transfer to and from the wheelchair.

DEFINING CHARACTERISTICS (NANDA)

Impaired ability to transfer from bed to chair and from chair to bed

Impaired ability to transfer on or off a toilet or commode

Impaired ability to transfer in and out of tub or shower

Impaired ability to transfer between uneven levels

Impaired ability to transfer from chair to car or from car to chair

Impaired ability to transfer from chair to floor or from floor to chair

Impaired ability to transfer from standing to floor or from floor to standing

RELATED FACTORS

Refer to *Impaired Physical Mobility*.

NOC

Transfer Performance

Goals

The person will demonstrate transfer to and from wheelchair.

Indicators

- Identify when assistance is needed.
- Demonstrate ability to transfer in varied situations (e.g., toilet, bed, car, chair, uneven levels).

NIC

See also *Impaired Physical Mobility,* Positioning:
Wheelchair

Generic Interventions

Explain that safe ambulation is a complete movement involving
the musculoskeletal, neurologic, and cardiovascular systems
and cognitive factors such as mentation and orientation.

If the person is deconditioned, a progressive program of exercise
is needed; consult with physical therapist for an evaluation
and plan.

Explain that one should always transfer toward the unaffected
side.

Determine whether an assistive device is needed (e.g., walking
belt with handles, mechanical lift, transfer sheets).

Consult with physical therapist to determine how much
assistance is needed:
- Requires no assistance
- Requires only verbal cuing
- Support by clinician's hand if additional help is needed
- Requires physical assistance
- Needs mechanical device to execute transfer (e.g., lifts)

Advise that ability may fluctuate and to request assistance to
prevent injury.

MORAL DISTRESS

DEFINITION (NANDA)

The state in which an individual experiences psychological disequilibrium, physical discomforts, anxiety and/or anguish that
results when a person makes a moral decision but does not follow
through with the moral behavior.

AUTHOR'S NOTE
This NANDA I nursing diagnosis has application in all settings where nurses practice. The literature to support this

(continued)

■■■ **AUTHOR'S NOTE** *(Continued)*
diagnosis when submitted was focused primarily on moral distress in nursing. If moral distress occurs in a client or family, this author suggests a referral to a professional expert in this area, e.g., a counselor, therapist, or spiritual advisor.

This author will present *Moral Distress* as a Department of Nursing Standard of Practice. This standard would address prevention of moral distress with specific individual nurse, unit, and department interventions. Strategies for addressing moral distress for individual nurses, on units, in the department of nursing, and in the institution will be presented.

DEFINING CHARACTERISTICS

Major

Expresses anguish over difficulty acting on one's moral choice

Minor

Feelings of:
- Powerlessness
- Anxiety
- Guilt
- Fear
- Frustration
- Anger
- Avoidance

RELATED FACTORS

The following factors do not cause moral distress in every nurse. If the nurse does not support terminating ventilators on anyone, then she or he would not have moral distress if a terminally ill person was on a ventilator. *Moral Distress* results from a nurse not acting on his or her own moral beliefs and then suffering because of the inaction.

Situational (Personal, Environmental)

End-of-Life Decisions

Related to providing treatments which were perceived as futile for hopelessly ill persons, e.g., blood transfusions, chemotherapy, organ transplants, mechanical ventilation
Related to conflicting attitudes toward advance directives
Related to participation in life-saving actions when they only prolong dying

Treatment Decisions

Related to the client's/family's refusal of treatments deemed appropriate by the health care team

Related to inability of the family to make the decision to stop ventilator treatment on a hopelessly ill person

Related to a family's wishes to continue life support even though it is not in the best interest of the client

Related to performing a procedure that increases the person's suffering

Related to providing care that does not relieve the person's suffering.

Professional Conflicts

Related to insufficient resources for care, e.g., time, staff

Related to failure to be included in the decision-making process

Related to greater emphasis on technical skills and tasks than on relationships and caring

Cultural Conflicts

Related to decisions made for women by male family members

Related to cultural conflicts with the American health care system

NOC

Suffering Level, Social Support, Hope, Fear Control

Goal

The nurse will relate strategies to prevent or reduce moral distress.

Indicators

Share source(s) of moral distress with a colleague.

Identify two strategies to enhance decision-making with clients and family.

Identify two strategies to enhance discussion of the situation with the physician.

Identify institutional strategies to decrease moral distress in nurses.

NIC

Emotional Support, Decision-Making Support, Family Mobilization

Generic Interventions

Explore Moral Work and Action

Educate yourself about moral distress. Refer to articles on the reference list.

Share your stories of moral distress. Elicit stories from co-workers.

Read stories of moral action. Refer to Gordon's "Life Support: Three Nurses on the Front Lines" and Kritek's "Reflections on Healing: A Central Construct" on the reference list.

Investigate How Clinical Situations that Are Morally Problematic Are Managed in the Institution. If an Ethics Committee Exists, Determine Its Mission and Procedures.

Do Not Try to Avoid Moral Distress; It Is Inevitable and Can Build Moral Character When Moral Work Is Successful.

Dialogue with Unit Colleagues About the Situation that Causes You Moral Distress.

Initiate Discussions with Client and Family. Ask Questions to Explore What They Know. Elicit Their Feelings About the Situation. Explore Their End-of-Life Decisions.

Enlist a Colleague as a Coach or Engage as a Coach for a Coworker.

Begin to Address a Morally Unsatisfactory Clinical Situation with an Approach that Has a Low Risk. Evaluate the Risks Before Taking Action. Be Realistic.

Engage in Open Communication with Other Professional Colleagues Involved. Start Your Conversation with Your Concern, e.g., "I Am Not Comfortable with. . . . , The Family Is Asking/Questioning/Feeling. . . , Mr. . . . . Is Asking/Questioning/Feeling. . ."

Dialogue with Other Professionals, e.g., Chaplain, Manager, Social Worker, or Ethics Committee.

Actively Promote Advance Directives with Your Own Family, Friends, Colleagues, and Clients and Their Families Before Tragedy Occurs.

Incorporate Health Promotion and Stress Reduction in Your Lifestyle. Refer to **Stress Overload** and **Altered Health Maintenance**.

NEONATAL JAUNDICE

▶ (Refer to Risk for Complications of Hyperbilirubinemia in Section 3)

DEFINITION

The state in which there is a yellow orange tint of the neonate's skin and mucous membranes that occurs after 24 hours of life as a result of unconjugated bilirubin in the circulation.

DEFINING CHARACTERISTICS

Abnormal blood profile (hemolysis; total serum bilirubin >2mg/ dL: inherited disorder; total serum bilirubin in high risk range on age in hour-specific nomogram)

Abnormal skin bruising

Yellow-orange skin

Yellow sclera

RELATED FACTORS

Abnormal weight loss in breastfeeding newborn; 15% in term infant)

Feeding pattern not well established

Infant experiences difficulty making transition to extrauterine life

Neonate age 1-7 days

Stool (meconium) passage delayed

▄▄▄ AUTHOR'S NOTE

This new NANDA-I diagnosis is a collaborative problem which requires a laboratory test for diagnosis and treatment from medicine and nursing.

Interventions/Goals

Refer to Section 3 to Risk for Complications of Hyperbilirubine-mia for neonates at risk for or experiencing hyperbilirubinemia.

NONCOMPLIANCE

DEFINITION

The state in which an individual or group desires to comply, but factors are present that deter adherence to agreed-upon health-related advice given by health professionals.

AUTHOR'S NOTE

Noncompliance describes the individual who desires to comply, but the presence of certain factors prevents him or her from doing so. The nurse must attempt to reduce or eliminate these factors for the interventions to be successful. However, the nurse is cautioned against using the diagnosis of *Noncompliance* to describe an individual who has made an informed, autonomous decision not to participate. Behaviors may be acts of omission or commission and may be intentional or unintentional.

DEFINING CHARACTERISTICS

Major (Must Be Present)

Verbalization of difficulty with compliance or confusion about therapy *or*

Minor (May Be Present)

Missed appointments
Partially used or unused medications
Persistence of symptoms
Progression of disease process
Occurrence of undesired outcomes (postoperative morbidity, pregnancy, obesity, addiction, regression during rehabilitation)

RELATED FACTORS

Pathophysiologic

Related to impaired ability to perform tasks because of disability secondary to (e.g., poor memory, motor and sensory deficits)

Related to increasing number of disease-related symptoms despite adherence to advised regimen

Treatment-Related

Related to:
Side effects of therapy
Previous unsuccessful experiences with advised regimen
Impersonal aspects of referral process
Nontherapeutic environment
Cost of therapy
Complex unsupervised or prolonged therapy
Financial cost of therapy

Situational (Personal, Environmental)

Related to barriers to access secondary to:
Mobility problems
Financial issues
Lack of child care
Transportation problems
Inclement weather

Related to concurrent illness of family member
Related to nonsupportive family, peers, community
Related to barriers to care secondary to homelessness

Related to barriers to comprehension secondary to:

Cognitive deficits	Visual deficits
Hearing deficits	Poor memory
Anxiety	Fatigue
Decreased attention span	Motivation

Related to perception of seriousness and susceptibility

NOC

Adherence Behavior, Compliance Behavior, Symptom Control, Treatment Behavior: Illness/Dying

Goals

The person will report a desire to change or initiate change.

Indicators
- Describe reasons for suggested regimen.
- Identify barriers to adhering to regimen.

NIC

Health Education, Self-Modification Assistance, Self-Responsibility Facilitation, Coping Enhancement, Decision Making Support, Health System Guidance, Mutual Goal Setting, Teaching: Disease Process

Generic Interventions

Using Open-Ended Questions, Encourage Person to Talk about Experiences with Health Care (e.g., Hospitalizations, Family Deaths, Diagnostic Tests, Blood Tests, X-Ray Tests).

Ask Client Directly, "What Are Your Concerns About:

taking this drug?"
following this diet?"
having a blood test?"
going through the cystoscopy?"
having your gallbladder removed?"
using a diaphragm?"
paying for the operation?"

Explore the Person's Understanding of the Problem and His or Her Expectations of Treatment and of Outcomes. Determine If Beliefs are Realistic and Correct.

Assess Problematic Factors of Prescribed Therapy (e.g., Time, Cost, Complexity, Convenience, Adverse Effects).

Assess Person for Recent Changes in Lifestyle (Personal, Work, Family, Health, Financial).

Assist to Reduce Side Effects, If Possible.

For gastric irritation, suggest that drug be taken with milk or food; it may be advisable to eat yogurt (unless contraindicated).
For drowsiness, take medication at bedtime or late in afternoon; consult physician for dose reduction.

Discuss the Risks and Benefits of Adhering to the Prescribed Regimen.

Affirm Client's Right to Refuse All or Part of the Prescribed Regimen.

NUTRITION, IMBALANCED: LESS THAN BODY REQUIREMENTS

Nutrition, Imbalanced: Less Than Body Requirements
Impaired Dentition
Impaired Swallowing
Ineffective Infant Feeding Pattern

DEFINITION

The state in which an individual, who is not NPO, experiences or is at risk for inadequate intake or metabolism of nutrients for metabolic needs with or without weight loss.

> **AUTHOR'S NOTE**
> This diagnosis describes individuals who can ingest food but have an intake of less-than-adequate amounts. This diagnosis should not be used to describe individuals who are NPO or cannot ingest food. These situations should be described by the collaborative problems of *Risk for Complications of Electrolyte Imbalances* and *Risk for Complications of Negative Nitrogen Balance*. In addition, some nursing diagnoses that relate to an individual who is NPO are *Risk for Impaired Oral Mucous Membrane* and *Impaired Comfort*.

DEFINING CHARACTERISTICS

Major (Must Be Present, One or More)

One who is not NPO reports or has: inadequate food intake less than recommended daily allowance with or without weight loss *or*

Actual or potential metabolic needs in excess of intake

Minor (May Be Present)

Weight 10% to 20% or more below ideal for height and frame
Triceps skinfold, midarm circumference, and midarm muscle circumference less than 60% standard measurement

Muscle weakness and tenderness
Mental irritability or confusion
Decreased serum prealbumin
Decreased serum transferrin or iron-binding capacity
Sunken fontanelles in infants

RELATED FACTORS

Pathophysiologic

Related to increased caloric requirements and difficulty in ingesting sufficient calories secondary to:

Cancer	Chemical dependence
Trauma	Infection
GI complications	Burns (postacute phase)

Related to dysphagia secondary to:

CVA	Parkinson's disease
Amyotrophic lateral sclerosis	Neuromuscular disorders
Cerebral palsy	Muscular dystrophy
Cleft Lip/palate	Mobius syndrome

Related to decreased absorption of nutrients secondary to:

Crohn's disease	Cystic fibrosis
Lactose intolerance	Necrotizing enterocolitis

Related to decreased desire to eat secondary to altered level of consciousness

Related to self-induced vomiting, physical exercise in excess of caloric intake, or refusal to eat secondary to anorexia nervosa

Related to reluctance to eat for fear of poisoning secondary to paranoid behavior

Related to anorexia, excessive physical agitation secondary to bipolar disorder

Related to anorexia and diarrhea secondary to protozoal infection

Related to vomiting, anorexia, and impaired digestion secondary to pancreatitis

Related to anorexia, impaired protein and fat metabolism, and impaired storage of vitamins secondary to cirrhosis

Realted to anorexia, vomiting and impaired digestion secondary to GI malformation or necrotizing enterocolitis

Realyted to anorexia secondary to gastrointestinal reflux

Treatment-Related

Related to increased protein and vitamin requirements for wound healing and decreased intake secondary to: surgery, medications (cancer chemotherapy), surgical reconstruction of the mouth, wired jaw, or radiation therapy

Related to inadequate absorption as a side effect of (specify):

Colchicine   Neomycin
Pyrimethamine   Para-aminosalicylic acid
Antacid

Related to decreased oral intake, mouth discomfort, nausea, vomiting secondary to: radiation therapy, chemotherapy, or tonsillectomy

Situational (Personal, Environmental)

Related to decreased desire to eat secondary to: anorexia, depression, stress, social isolation, nausea and vomiting, or allergies

Related to inability to procure food (physical limitations, financial or transportation problems)

Related to inability to chew (damaged or missing teeth, ill-fitting dentures)

Related to diarrhea secondary to (specify)

Maturational

Infant/Child

Related to inadequate intake secondary to: lack of emotional/sensory stimulation or lack of knowledge of caregiver or inadequate production of breast milk

Related to malabsorption, dietary restrictions, and anorexia secondary to celiac disease, lactose intolerance, or cystic fibrosis

Related to sucking difficulties (infant) and dysphagia secondary to: cerebral palsy, cleft lip and palate, GI malformation, or Gastrointestuinal relux

Related to inadequate sucking, fatigue, and dyspnea secondary to:

Congenital heart disease   Prematurity
Viral syndrome   Hyperbilirubenemia
Respiratory distress syndrome   Developmental delay

Older Adult

Related to effects of declining metabolic rate, estrogen levels, and bone mineral density (women)

Related to degeneration of periodontal membrane with loose teeth

NOC

Nutritional Status, Symptom Control

Goals

The person will ingest daily nutritional requirements in accordance with his or her activity level and metabolic needs.

Indicators
- Relate importance of good nutrition.
- Identify deficiencies in daily intake.
- Relate methods to increase appetite.

NIC

Nutrition Management, Nutrition Monitoring, Nutrition Counseling

Generic Interventions

Determine daily caloric requirements that are realistic and adequate. Consult with dietitian.

Weigh daily; monitor laboratory results.

Explain the importance of adequate nutrition. Negotiate with client intake goals for each meal and snacks.

Teach client to use spices to help improve the taste and aroma of food (lemon juice, mint, cloves, basil, thyme, cinnamon, rosemary, bacon bits).

Encourage client to eat with others (meals served in dining room or group area or at local meeting place, such as community center, by church groups).

Plan care so that unpleasant or painful procedures do not take place before meals.

Provide pleasant, relaxed atmosphere for eating (no bedpans in sight; do not rush); try a "surprise" (e.g., flowers with meal).

Arrange plan of care to decrease or eliminate nauseating odors or procedures near mealtimes.

Teach or assist client to rest before meals.

Teach client to avoid cooking odors—frying foods, brewing coffee—if possible (take a walk; select foods that can be eaten cold).

Maintain good oral hygiene (brush teeth, rinse mouth) before and after ingestion of food.

Offer frequent small feedings (six per day plus snacks) to reduce the feeling of a distended stomach.

Arrange to have highest protein/calorie nutrients served at the time client feels most like eating (e.g., if chemotherapy is in early morning, serve in late afternoon).

Instruct person with decreased appetite to:
- Arrange to serve the highest protein/caloric foods when the person feels most like eating (e.g., with chemotherapy in early morning)
- Eat dry foods (toast, crackers) on arising.
- Try salty foods if permissible.
- Avoid overly sweet, rich, greasy, or fried foods.
- Try clear, cool beverages.
- Sip slowly through straw.
- Take whatever can be tolerated.
- Eat small portions low in fat, and eat more frequently.

Review high-calorie versus low calorie foods, avoid empty calorie foods (e.g., soda, bread)

Encourage family to bring in favorite foods

Try commercial supplements available in many forms (liquids, powder, pudding).

If person has an eating disorder
- Establish intake goals with client, physician, and nutritionist.
- Discuss the benefits of compliance and the consequences of nonadherence.
- If intake is refused, notify physician.
- Sit with person during meals. Limit meal times to 30 minutes.
- Observe for at least 1 hour after meals. Accompany to bathroom.
- Weigh on arising and after first voiding.
- Provide reinforcement for improvement, but do not focus discussions on food or eating.
- As person improves, explore issues of body image, weight gain, and control.

For a hyperactive person (Townsend, 1994):
- Provide high-protein, high-calorie finger foods and drinks.
- Offer frequent snacks. Avoid empty calories (e.g., soda).
- Walk or pace with person as finger foods are eaten.

Geriatric Interventions
Evaluate Ability to Process and Prepare Food

Finances
Transportation
Mobility
Manual dexterity

Explain Community Resources Available

Meals on Wheels
Senior centers
Supermarkets that deliver

For Women Older Than 50 Years, Advise to:

Increase calcium intake to 1200 mg/d (1500 mg/d if not taking
hormone replacement therapy).
Reduce calorie intake to 1700 to 1800.
Balance intake and exercise.
Include beta-carotene and vitamin C and E supplements daily.

▶ Impaired Dentition

DEFINITION

The state in which an individual experiences a disruption in tooth
development/eruption patterns or structural integrity of individual teeth.

AUTHOR'S NOTE

Impaired Dentition describes a multitude of problems with
teeth. It is unclear how this diagnosis would be used by
nurses or any health care professional. If the client has caries, abscesses, or misaligned or malformed teeth, the nurse
would refer him or her to a dental professional. If the tooth
problem is affecting comfort or nutrition, *Impaired Comfort*
or *Imbalanced Nutrition* would be the appropriate nursing
diagnosis.

DEFINING CHARACTERISTICS

Excessive plaque
Crown or root caries
Halitosis
Tooth enamel discoloration
Toothache
Loose teeth
Excessive calculus
Incomplete eruption for age (may be primary or permanent
teeth)
Malocclusion or tooth misalignment
Premature loss of primary teeth
Worn-down or abraded teeth

Tooth fracture(s)
Missing teeth or complete absence
Erosion of enamel
Asymmetric facial expression

▶ Impaired Swallowing

DEFINITION

The state in which an individual has abnormal functioning of the swallowing mechanisim associated with deficits in oral, pharyngeal or esophageal structure or function.

DEFINING CHARACTERISTICS

Major (Must Be Present)

Observed evidence of difficulty swallowing
and/*or*
Stasis of food in oral cavity
Choking
Coughing before a swallow
Coughing after fluid or food intake
Gagging

Minor (May Be Present)

Slurred speech   Regurgitation
Nasal-sounding voice   Vomiting
Drooling   Lack of chewing

RELATED FACTORS

Pathophysiologic

Related to decreased/absent gag reflex, mastication difficulties, or decreased sensations secondary to:

Cerebrovascular accident
Right or left hemispheric damage to the brain
Damage to the 5th, 7th, 9th, 10th, or 11th cranial nerves
Cerebral palsy   Parkinsonism
Muscular dystrophy   Myasthenia gravis
Amyotrophic lateral sclerosis   Guillain-Barré syndrome
    Poliomyelitis

Related to tracheoesophageal tumors, edema
Related to irritated oropharyngeal cavity
Related to decreased saliva

Treatment-Related

Related to surgical reconstruction of the mouth, throat, jaw, and/or nose

Related to mechanical obstruction secondary to tracheostomy tube

Related to esophagitis secondary to radiotherapy

Related to decreased consciousness secondary to anesthesia

Related to increased viscosity and diminished quantity of saliva (e.g., secondary to medications, radiation)

Situational (Personal, Environmental)

Related to fatigue

Related to limited awareness, distractibility

Maturational

Infant/Children

Related to decreased sensations or difficulty with mastication

Related to poor suck/swallow/breathe coordination

Refer to *Ineffective Infant Feeding Pattern*.

NOC

Aspiration Control, Swallowing Status

Goals

The person will report improved ability to swallow.

Indicators

- Describe causative factors when known.
- Describe rationale and procedures for treatment.

NIC

Aspiration Precautions, Swallowing Therapy, Surveillance, Referral, Positioning

Generic Interventions

Consult with a Speech Therapist for Evaluation and Recommended Plan of Care.

Alert all staff that impaired swallowing is present in the person (sign at bedside)

Reduce the Possibility of Aspiration.

Before beginning feeding, assess that person is adequately alert and responsive, is able to control mouth, has cough/gag reflex, and can swallow own saliva.

Have suction equipment available and functioning properly.

Position correctly:

- Sit upright (60 to 90 degrees) in chair or dangle feet at side of bed if possible (prop pillows if necessary).
- Assume position 10 to 15 minutes before eating, and maintain position for 10 to 15 minutes after finishing eating.
- Flex head forward on the midline about 45 degrees to keep esophagus patent.

Keep individual focused on task by giving directions until he or she has finished swallowing each mouthful.

Start with small amounts, and progress slowly as person learns to handle each step:

- Ice chips
- Part of eyedropper filled with water
- Use juice in place of water
- ¼, ½, 1 teaspoon semisolid
- Pureed food or commercial baby foods
- One-half cracker
- Soft diet/regular diet

Assist with Moving the Bolus of Food from the Anterior to the Posterior of Mouth.

Place Food in the Posterior Mouth Where Swallowing Can Be Ensured.

Prevent/Decrease Thick Secretions.

Progress to Ice Chips, Water, and Then Food When Danger of Aspiration is Decreased.

For Individuals with Impaired Cognition or Awareness:

Concentrate on solids rather than liquids, because liquids are generally less well tolerated.

Keep extraneous stimuli at minimum while eating (e.g., no television or radio, no verbal stimuli unless directed at task).

Have person concentrate on task of swallowing.

Have person sit up in chair with neck slightly flexed.

Instruct person to hold breath while swallowing.

Observe for swallowing and check mouth for emptying.

Avoid overloading mouth, because this decreases swallowing effectiveness.

Give solids and liquids separately.

Reinforce behaviors with simple one-word commands.

Feed Slowly, Making Certain Previous Bite Has Been Swallowed.

Consult with Speech Pathologist.

Teach Family Emergency Interventions for Obstruction (e.g., Heimlich Maneuver).

▶ Ineffective Infant Feeding Pattern

DEFINITION

A state in which an infant (birth to 9 months) demonstrates an impaired ability to suck or coordinate the suck-swallow response, resulting in inadequate oral nutrition for metabolic needs.

■■■■ **AUTHOR'S NOTE**

This diagnosis represents a specific type of nutritional problem of infants grouped under the more general diagnosis *Imbalanced Nutrition: Less Than Body Requirements*. The nursing role is to provide or assist caregivers to provide appropriate calories to gain weight. Specific feeding techniques and energy expenditure reduction are used to achieve oral feedings for all nutrition. Some infants with sucking or such swallow-response difficulties can meet nutritional needs unless additional factors that increase caloric needs are present (e.g., infection).

DEFINING CHARACTERISTICS

Major (Must Be Present, One or More)

Inability to initiate or sustain an effective suck; inability to coordinate sucking, swallowing, and breathing

Actual metabolic needs in excess of oral intake with weight loss or need for enteral feeding supplement

Minor (May Be Present)

Inconsistent oral intake (volume, time interval, duration)

Oral motor developmental delay

Tachypnea with increased respiratory effort

Regurgitation or vomiting after feeding

RELATED FACTORS

Pathophysiologic

Related to increased caloric need secondary to:

Body temperature instability	Wound healing
Growth needs	Infection
Tachypnea with increased respiratory effort	Major organ system disease or failure

Related to muscle weakness/hypotonia secondary to:

Malnutrition	Congenital defects
Prematurity	Major organ system disease or failure
Acute/chronic illness	Neurologic impairment/delay
Lethargy	

Treatment-Related

Related to hypermetabolic state and increased caloric needs secondary to:

Surgery	Painful procedures
Cold stress	Sepsis

Related to muscle weakness and lethargy secondary to sleep deprivation or medications (muscle relaxants, e.g., antiseizure medications, paralyzing agents in past, sedatives, narcotics)
Related to oral hypersensitivity
Related to previous prolonged NPO state

Situational (Personal, Environmental)

Related to inconsistent caregivers (feeders)
Related to lack of knowledge of or commitment of caregiver (feeder) to special feeding needs or regimen
Related to presence of noxious facial or absence of oral stimuli
Related to inadequate production of breast milk

NOC
Muscle Function, Nutritional Status, Swallowing Status

Goals

The infant will ingest adequate nutrition for growth appropriate to age and need.

Indicators
- The parent will demonstrate increasing skill.
- The parent will identify techniques that increase effective feeding.

NIC

Non-nutritive Swallowing, Swallowing Therapy, Aspiration Precautions, Bottle Feeding, Parent Education: Infant

👫 Pediatric Interventions

Assess the Infant's Feeding Pattern and Nutritional Needs.

Assess volume, duration, and effort during feeding; respiratory rate and effort; signs of fatigue.

Assess past caloric intake, weight gain, trends in intake and output, renal function, fluid retention.

Collaborate with Clinical Dietitian to Set Calorie, Volume, and Weight Gain Goals.

Collaborate with Parent(s) about Effective Techniques Used with This Infant.

Provide Specific Interventions to Promote Effective Oral Feeding.

Ensure a quiet, dim, calm environment

Eliminate painful procedures prior to feeding

Nutritive sucking for identified amount of time

Consistency in approach to feeding

Specific interventions for oral motor delays (position, equipment, jaw/mouth manipulation)

Control of adverse environmental stimuli and noxious stimuli to face and mouth

Choose nipple according to individual needs and successes

Position infant semi-upright

Use fingers to provide inward and forward support of cheeks during feeding

Do not:

Twist or turn nipple

Move nipple up and down in mouth

Move nipple in and out of mouth

Promote Sleep and Reduce Unnecessary Energy Expenditure.

If Needed, Plan for Enteral Feeding Includes Guidelines for Increasing Oral Feeding and

Decreasing Enteral Feeding as the Infant
Eats More Effectively by Mouth.

Establish Partnership with Parent(s)
in All Stages of Plan.

Provide Ongoing Information to Parent(s)
about Special Needs, and Assist Them in
Establishing Needed Resources (Equipment,
Nursing Care, Other Caregivers).

NUTRITION, IMBALANCED: MORE THAN BODY REQUIREMENTS

DEFINITION

The state in which an individual experiences or is at risk of experiencing weight gain related to an intake in excess of metabolic requirements.

AUTHOR'S NOTE

Obesity is a complex condition with sociocultural, psychological, and metabolic implications. This diagnosis, when used to describe obesity or overweight conditions, focuses on them as nutritional problems. The focus of treatment is behavioral modification and lifestyle changes. It is recommended that *Ineffective Health Maintenance related to intake in excess of metabolic requirements* be used in place of this diagnosis. In addition, *Ineffective Coping related to increased food consumption secondary to response to external stressors* may be used. When weight gain is the result of physiologic conditions (e.g., altered taste); pharmacologic interventions, such as corticosteroid therapy; or history of excessive weight gain during pregnancy, this diagnosis can be clinically useful.

DEFINING CHARACTERISTICS

Major (Must Be Present, One or More)

Overweight (weight 10% over ideal for height and frame) *or*
Obese (weight 20% or more over ideal for height and frame)
Triceps skinfold greater than 15 mm in men and 25 mm in
    women

Minor (May Be Present)

Reported undesirable eating patterns
Intake in excess of metabolic requirements
Sedentary activity patterns

RELATED FACTORS

Pathophysiologic

Related to altered satiety patterns secondary to (specify)
Related to decreased sense of taste and smell

Treatment-Related

Related to altered satiety secondary to:
Medications (corticosteroids, antihistamines)
Radiation (decreased sense of taste and smell)

Situational (Personal, Environmental)

Related to risk of gaining more than 25 to 30 lb when pregnant
Related to lack of basic nutritional knowledge
Related to sedentary activity patterns

Maturational

Adult/Older Adult
Related to decreased activity patterns and decreased metabolic
   needs

NOC

Nutritional Status, Weight Control

Goals

The person will describe why he or she is at risk for weight gain.

Indicators

- Describe reasons for increased intake with taste or olfactory deficits.
- Discuss nutritional needs during pregnancy.
- Discuss effects of exercise on weight control.

NIC

Nutrition Management, Weight Management, Teaching:
Individual, Behavioral Modification, Exercise Promotion

Generic Interventions

Increase Individual's Awareness of Amount/Type of Food Consumed.

Instruct person to keep a diet diary for 1 week:
- What, when, where, and why eaten
- Whether doing anything else (e.g., watching television, preparing dinner)
- Emotions just before eating
- Others present (spouse, children)

Review diet diary with individual to point out patterns (e.g., time, place, people, emotions, foods) that affect intake.

Review high- and low-calorie food items.

Assist Person to Set Realistic Goals (e.g., Decreasing Oral Intake by 500 Calories Will Result in a 1- to 2-Lb Loss Each Week).

Teach Behavior Modification Techniques.

Eat only at a specific spot at home (e.g., kitchen table).

Do not eat while doing other activities, such as reading or watching television; eat only when sitting.

Drink an 8-oz glass of water immediately before eating.

Use small plates (portions look bigger).

Prepare small portions, just enough for a meal, and discard leftovers.

Never eat from another person's plate.

Eat slowly, and chew thoroughly.

Put down utensils and wait 15 seconds between bites.

Eat low-calorie snacks that need to be chewed to satisfy oral need (carrots, celery, apples).

Decrease liquid calories; drink diet sodas or water.

Plan a Daily Walking Program, and Gradually Increase Rate and Length of Walk.

Start out at 5 to 10 blocks for 0.5 to 1 mile per day; increase 1 block or 0.1 mile per week.

Progress slowly.

Avoid straining or pushing too hard and becoming overly fatigued.

Stop immediately if any of the following signs occur:
- Tightness or pain in chest
- Severe breathlessness
- Lightheadedness
- Dizziness

- Loss of muscle control
- Nausea

Establish a regular time of day for physical activity; the goal is three to five times a week for a duration of 15 to 45 minutes and with a heart rate of 80% of stress test or gross calculation (170 beats/min for ages 20 to 29 years; decrease 10 beats/min for each additional decade of life; e.g., 160 beats/min for ages 30 to 39 years, 150 beats/min for ages 40 to 49 years).

Advise that intermittent physical activity that accumulates to 30 or more minutes daily is beneficial.

Suggest taking every opportunity to increase activity (e.g., walk down stairs instead of using elevator, park car farther from store).

Refer to Support Groups (e.g., Weight Watchers, Overeaters Anonymous, TOPS, Trim Clubs, the Diet Workshop, Inc.).

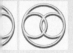

NUTRITION, IMBALANCED: POTENTIAL FOR MORE THAN BODY REQUIREMENTS

DEFINITION

The state in which an individual is at risk of experiencing an intake of nutrients that exceeds metabolic needs.

AUTHOR'S NOTE

This diagnosis is similar to *Risk for Imbalanced Nutrition: More Than Body Requirements*. It describes an individual who has a family history of obesity, who is demonstrating a pattern of higher weight, or who has had a history of excessive weight gain (e.g., previous pregnancy). Until clinical research differentiates this diagnosis from other accepted diagnoses, use *Ineffective Health Maintenance* (Actual or Risk) or *Risk for Imbalanced Nutrition: More Than Body Requirements* to direct teaching to assist families and individuals to identify unhealthy dietary patterns.

DEFINING CHARACTERISTICS

Reported or observed obesity in one or both parents
Rapid transition across growth percentiles in infants or children

Reported use of solid food as major food source before 5 months
   of age
Observed use of food as a reward or comfort measure
Reported or observed higher baseline weight at beginning of
   each pregnancy
Dysfunctional eating patterns

PARENTING, IMPAIRED

Parenting, Impaired
Parent-Infant-Child Attachment, Risk for Impaired
Parental Role Conflict

DEFINITION

The state in which one or more caregivers demonstrate real or
potential inability to provide a constructive environment that nurtures the growth and development of their child (children).

> **AUTHOR'S NOTE**
> A family's ability to function is at a high risk of develop-
> ing problems when the child or parent has a condition that
> increases the stress of the family unit. The term *parent* refers
> to any individual defined as the primary caregiver for a child.

DEFINING CHARACTERISTICS
Major (Must Be Present, One or More)

Inappropriate or non-nurturing parenting behaviors
Lack of parental attachment behavior

Minor (May Be Present)

Frequent verbalization of dissatisfaction or disappointment with
   infant or child
Verbalization of frustration of role
Verbalization of perceived or actual inadequacy
Diminished or inappropriate visual, tactile, or auditory
   stimulation of infant

Evidence of abuse or neglect of child
Growth and developmental delays in infant or child

RELATED FACTORS

Individuals or families who may be at risk for developing or experiencing parenting difficulties

Parent

Single
Adolescent
Abusive
Psychiatric disorder
Alcoholic

Addicted to drugs
Terminally ill
Acutely disabled
Accident victim

Child

Of unwanted pregnancy
With undesired
   characteristics
Mentally handicapped
Terminally ill

Of undesired gender
Physically handicapped
With hyperactive
   characteristics

Situational (Personal, Environmental)

Related to interruption of bonding process secondary to: illness (child, parent), incarceration, or relocation
Related to separation from nuclear family
Related to inconsistent caregivers or techniques
Related to lack of knowledge
Related to lack of available role model

Related to relationship problems (specify):
Marital discord
Separation
Live-in partner

Divorce
Stepparents
Relocation

Related to ineffective adaptation to stressors associated with illness, new baby, elder care, economic problems, or substance abuse

Maturational

Adolescent
Related to the conflict of meeting own needs over child's
Related to history of ineffective relationships with own parents
Related to parental history of abusive relationship with parents
Related to unrealistic expectations of child by parent
Related to unrealistic expectations of self by parent

Related to unrealistic expectations of parent by child
Related to unmet psychosocial needs of child by parent

NOC

Child Development (Specify), Family Coping, Family Environment: Internal, Family Functioning, Parent-Infant Attachment

Goals

The parent/primary caregiver will acknowledge a problem with parenting skills.

Indicators
- Provide a safe environment for child.
- Describe resources available for assistance with improvement of parenting skills.

NIC

Parenting Promotion, Developmental Enhancement, Anticipatory Guidance, Parent Education, Behavior Management

Generic Interventions

Encourage Parents to Share Parenting Difficulties and Usual or Recent Stressors.

If Abuse Is Suspected, Notify Appropriate Authorities (See Disabled Family Coping).

Provide Family with Information About:
Age-related developmental needs
Age-related problematic behavior

Observe Parents Interacting with Child.

Support strengths.
Role-model in uncomfortable or problematic areas.
Emphasize child's strengths or unique characteristics.

Allow Parents to Watch Nurse Care for Child.
Role-Model Comfort Measures and Sensory Stimulation (Verbal, Toys, Touch).

Encourage Parents to Participate in Care.

Explain All Procedures and the Associated Discomforts.

Encourage Parents to Be Present for Procedures When Possible and to Comfort Child.

Explore Parents' Expectations of Child; Differentiate Realistic from Unrealistic.

Assess Usual Discipline Methods for Appropriateness and Follow-Through.

Explore with Parents the Child's Problem Behavior (Herman-Staab, 1994):

Frequency, duration
Situational context (when, where, triggers)
Consequences of problem behavior (parental attention, discipline, inconsistencies in response)
Behavior desired by parents

Discuss Positive Parenting Techniques (Herman-Staab, 1994).

Convey to child that he or she is loved.
Catch child being good; use good eye contact.
Set aside "special time" when the parent guarantees a time with child without interruptions.
Ignore minor transgressions by having no physical contact, eye contact, or discussion about the behavior.
Practice active listening. Describe what child is saying, reflect back the child's feelings, and do not judge.
Use "I" statements when disapproving of behavior. Focus on the act, not the child, as undesirable.

Discuss Discipline Methods.

For small child—sit in chair 1 minute for each year of age (if child gets up, put back in chair, and reset timer).
For older child—deprive of favorite pastime (e.g., bicycle, television show).
Avoid hitting except for one hand slap for a small child for dangerous touching (e.g., stove, electric plug).
Do not threaten. Clarify punishment, and follow through with it.
Expect child to obey.
Parents should agree jointly and follow through with consistency.

Discuss Resources Available (e.g., Counseling, Community, Social Service, Parenting Classes).

**Initiate a Referral to Community
Nursing Service If Indicated.**

▶ Parent–Infant–Child Attachment, Risk for Impaired

DEFINITION

The state in which there is a risk for a disruption of a nurturing, protective, interactive process between a parent/primary caregiver and infant.

> **AUTHOR'S NOTE**
> This new diagnosis describes a parent or caregiver who is at risk for attachment difficulties with his or her infant. Barriers to attachment can be the environment, knowledge, anxiety, and health of the parent or infant. This diagnosis is appropriate as a risk or high-risk diagnosis. If the nurse diagnoses a problem in infant–parent attachment, the diagnosis *Risk for Impaired Parenting related to inadequate parent attachment* would be more useful so that the nurse could focus on improving attachment and preventing destructive parenting patterns.

RISK FACTORS

Refer to Related Factors.

RELATED FACTORS

Pathophysiologic

Related to interruption of bonding process secondary to:
Parental illness
Infant illness

Treatment-Related

Related to barriers to holding secondary to: bililights or intensive care monitoring

Situational (Personal, Environmental)

Related to unrealistic expectations (e.g., of child or self)
Related to unwanted pregnancy

Related to disappointment with infant (e.g., gender, appearance)

Related to ineffective adaptation to stressors associated with new baby and other responsibilities secondary to:

Health problems	Substance abuse
Mental illness	Relationship problems
Economic problems	

Related to history of ineffective relationship with own parents
Related to lack of knowledge or available role model for parental role
Related to physical disabilities of parent (e.g., blindness, paralysis, deafness)

Maturational

Adolescent
Related to difficulty delaying own gratification for the gratification of the infant

Goals

The parent will demonstrate increased attachment behaviors, such as holding infant close, smiling and talking to infant, and seeking eye contact with infant.

Indicators
• Be supported in his or her need to be involved in infant's care.
• Begin to verbalize positive feelings regarding infant.

Generic Interventions

Assess Causative or Contributing Factors.

Maternal
Unwanted pregnancy
Prolonged or difficult labor and delivery
Postpartum pain or fatigue
Lack of positive support system (mother, spouse, friends)
Lack of positive role model (mother, relative, neighbor)

Parental Inadequate Coping Patterns (one or both parents)
Alcoholic
Drug addict
Marital difficulties (separation, divorce, violence)
Change in lifestyle related to new role
Adolescent parent

Career change (e.g., working woman to mother)
Illness in family

Infant
Premature, defective, ill
Multiple birth

Eliminate or Reduce Contributing Factors if Possible.

Illness, Pain, Fatigue
Establish with mother what infant-care activities are feasible.
Provide mother with uninterrupted sleep periods of at least 2
    hours during the day and 4 hours during the night.
Provide relief for discomforts.

Lack of Experience or Lack of Positive Mothering Role Model
Explore with mother her feelings and attitudes concerning her
    own mother.
Assist her to identify someone who is a positive mother, and
    encourage her to seek that person's aid.
Outline the teaching program available to her during
    hospitalization.
Determine who will assist her at home initially.
Identify community programs and reference material that can
    increase her learning about child care after discharge.

Lack of Positive Support System
Identify parent's support system, and assess its strengths and
    weaknesses.
Assess the need for counseling.
  • Encourage the parents to express feelings about the experi-
    ence and about the future.
  • Be an active listener to the parents.
  • Observe the parents interacting with the infant.

Provide Opportunities for the Attachment Process.

Promote Attachment in the Immediate Postdelivery Phase.
Encourage mother to hold infant following birth (may need a
    short recovery period).
Provide skin-to-skin contact if desired; keep room warm (72° to
    76°F), or use a heat panel over the infant.
Provide mother with an opportunity to breastfeed if desired.
Delay the administration of silver nitrate to allow for eye
    contact.

Give family as much time as they need together, with minimum interruption from staff (the "sensitive period" lasts from 30 to 90 minutes).

Encourage father to hold infant.

Facilitate the Attachment Process During the Postpartum Phase.

Check mother regularly for signs of fatigue, especially if she had anesthesia.

Offer flexible rooming-in to the mother; establish with her the amount of care she will assume initially, and support her requests for assistance.

Discuss the future involvement of the father in the infant's care. (If desired, discuss opportunities for father to participate in his child's care at home.)

Provide Support to the Parents.

Listen to the mother's replay of her labor and delivery experience.

Allow for verbalization of feelings.

Indicate acceptance of feelings.

Point out the infant's strengths and individual characteristics to the parents.

Demonstrate the infant's responses to the parents.

Have a system of follow-up after discharge, especially for families considered at risk (e.g., phone call or a home visit by the community health nurse).

Assess the Need for Teaching.

Observe the parents interacting with the infant.

Support each parent's strengths.

Assist parents in areas in which they are uncomfortable (role-modeling).

Offer classes in infant care.

Have handouts and audiovisual aids available for parents to view at their own time.

Assess for level of knowledge in the area of growth and development, and provide information as needed.

Help parents understand the infant's cues and temperament.

See References/Bibliography for recommended printed material on parenting and child care.

When Immediate Separation of the Child from the Parents is Necessary Because of Prematurity or Illness, Provide for Bonding or Attachment Experiences, as Possible.

Allow parents to see and touch infant prior to transport.

Encourage father to visit the neonatal intensive care unit and
   bring back verbal reports of infant and pictures if possible.
Encourage earliest visiting for mother as feasible, with frequent
   phone contact with infant's caregivers if visiting is not
   possible.

Initiate Referrals as Needed.

Consult with community agencies for follow-up visits if
   indicated.
Refer parents to pertinent organizations.

▶ Parental Role Conflict

DEFINITION

The state in which a parent or primary caregiver experiences or
perceives a change in role in response to external factors (e.g.,
illness, hospitalization, divorce, separation, birth of child with
special needs).

▪▪▪▪ AUTHOR'S NOTE
This diagnosis describes a parent or parents whose previously effective functioning ability is challenged by external
factors. In certain situations, such as illness, role confusion and conflict are expected. This diagnosis differs from
Impaired Parenting, which describes a parent (or parents)
who demonstrates or is at high risk of demonstrating inappropriate parenting behaviors or lack of parental attachment.
If parents are not assisted in adapting their role to external
factors, *Parental Role Conflict* can lead to *Impaired Parenting*. The term *parent* refers to any individual defined as the
primary caregiver for a child.
   This diagnosis was developed by the Nursing Diagnosis
Discussion Group, Rainbow Babies' and Children's Hospital,
University Hospitals of Cleveland.

DEFINING CHARACTERISTICS
Major (Must Be Present, One or More)

Parent expresses concerns about changes in parental role.
Parent demonstrates disruption in care and/or caretaking
   routines.

Minor (May Be Present)

Parent expresses concerns/feelings of inadequacy to provide for child's physical and emotional needs during hospitalization or in the home.

Parent expresses concern about effect of child's illness on other children.

Parent expresses concerns about care of siblings at home.

Parent expresses concern about perceived loss of control over decisions relating to child.

RELATED FACTORS

Situational (Personal, Environmental)

Related to separation from child secondary to:

Birth of a child with a congenital defect or chronic illness

Hospitalization of a child with an acute or chronic illness

Change in acuity, prognosis, or environment of care (e.g., transfer to or from an intensive care unit)

Related to fear of involvement secondary to invasive or restrictive treatment modalities (e.g., isolation, intubation)

Related to interruption of family life secondary to:

Home care of a child with special needs (e.g., apnea monitoring, postural drainage, hyperalimentation)

Frequent visits to hospital

Addition of new family member (aging relative, newborn)

Related to change in ability to parent secondary to:

Illness of parent	Travel requirements
Work responsibilities	Divorce
Remarriage	Dating
Death	

NOC

See also *Parental Role Conflict*

Goals

The parent will demonstrate control over decision-making concerning the child and collaborate with health professionals in making decisions about the health/illness care of the child.

Indicators

• Relate information about the child's health status and treatment plan.

- Participate in caring for the child in the home/hospital setting to the extent he or she desires.
- Verbalize feelings about the child's illness and the hospitalization.
- Identify and use available support systems that allow parent time and energy to cope with ill child's needs.

NIC

See also *Parental Role Conflict*

Generic Interventions

Discuss what has influenced a change in role (e.g., divorce, remarriage, illness [child, parent], boarding away, family additions [newborn, aging parent]).

Allow parents to share frustrations.

Assist parents to determine the type of role desired and if realistic.

If indicated, refer for counseling for management of stressors and role changes.

For ill or hospitalized child:

Help parents adapt parenting behaviors to allow for continuation of parenting role during hospitalization or illness.

Provide information about hospital routines and policies, such as visiting hours, mealtimes, division routines, medical and nursing routines, rooming-in.

Explain procedures and tests to parents; help them interpret these activities to child; discuss child's age-appropriate range of responses.

Instruct parents to continue limit-setting strategies and demonstrations of caring behaviors (e.g., touching, hugging despite hospitalization and equipment).

Provide information to empower parents to adapt parenting role to the situation of hospitalization or the event of chronic illness of the child.

Foster open communication with parents, allowing time for questions, frequent repetition of information; provide direct and honest answers.

Approach parents with new information; do not make them assume the responsibility for seeking out the information.

When parents cannot be with their child, facilitate information-sharing through telephone calls; allow parents to call primary nurse or nurse caring for child.

Support continued decision-making of parents regarding child's care.

Provide parents opportunity to help formulate plan of care for their child.

Use parents as source of information about child; child's usual behaviors, reactions, and preferences.

Recognize parents as "experts" about their child.

Allow parents the choice to be present during treatments and procedures.

Allow parents to participate in caring for their child to the extent they desire.

Provide for 24-hour rooming-in for at least one parent and extended visiting for other family members.

Collaborate and negotiate with parents about parental tasks they want to continue to do, tasks they want others to assume, tasks they want to share, and tasks they want to learn to do; continually assess changes in their desired involvement in care.

Allow parents to have uninterrupted time with child.

Explore with parents their personal responsibilities (e.g., work schedule, sibling care, household responsibilities, responsibilities to extended family); assist them in establishing a schedule that allows sufficient caretaking time for child or visiting time with hospitalized child, without frustration in meeting other role responsibilities (e.g., if visiting is not possible until evening hours, delay child's bath time, and allow parent to bathe child then).

Support parents' ability to normalize the hospital/home environment for themselves and child.

Encourage parents to bring clothing and toys from home.

Allow parents to prepare home-cooked food or bring food from home if desired.

Encourage opportunities for families to eat meals together.

Encourage opportunities for parents to take child on leaves from the hospital, including visits home, as possible.

Help parents verbalize feelings about child's illness or hospitalization and adaptation of the parenting role to the situation.

Provide for parents' physical and emotional needs.

Assess and facilitate parents' ability to meet self-care needs (e.g., rest, nutrition, activity, privacy).

Allow parents an opportunity to determine the caregiving schedule to correspond with a schedule to meet their own needs.

Assess support systems: parent to parent, family, friends, minister, etc.

Initiate referrals if indicated: chaplain, social service, community agencies (respite care), parent self-help groups.

PERIPHERAL NEUROVASCULAR DYSFUNCTION, RISK FOR

DEFINITION

A state in which an individual is at risk of experiencing a disruption in circulation, sensation, or motion of an extremity.

■■■■ AUTHOR'S NOTE

This diagnosis represents a situation that nurses can prevent by identifying who is at risk and implementing measures to reduce or eliminate the causative or contributing factors. If undetected, compromised neurovascular function can lead to compartment syndrome. Compartment syndrome requires medical intervention (e.g., fasciotomy and nursing care before and after surgery).

RISK FACTORS

Presence of risk factors (see Related Factors)

RELATED FACTORS

Pathophysiologic

Related to increased volume of (specify extremity) secondary to:
Bleeding (e.g., trauma, fractures)
Coagulation disorder
Venous obstruction/pooling
Arterial obstruction

Related to increased capillary filtration secondary to:
Trauma
Severe burns (thermal, electrical)
Hypothermia
Frostbite
Allergic response (e.g., insect bites)
Venomous bites (e.g., snake)
Nephrotic syndrome

Related to restrictive envelope secondary to:
Circumferential burns of extremities
Excessive pressure

Treatment-Related

Related to increased volume secondary to:
Infiltration of intravenous infusion
Excessive movement
Dislocated prosthesis (knee, hip)
Nonpatent wound drainage system

Related to increased capillary filtration secondary to:
Total knee replacement
Total hip replacement

Related to restrictive envelope secondary to:
Tourniquet
Blood pressure cuff
Cast
Brace
Restraints
Antishock trousers
Excessive traction
Circumferential dressings, Ace wraps
Air splints
Premature or tight closure of fascial defects

NOC
Neurologic Status

Goals

The individual will report changes in peripheral sensation or movement.

Indicators
- Have palpable peripheral pulses.
- Have warm extremities.
- Have capillary refill less than 3 seconds.

NIC
Peripheral Sensation Management, Positioning, Embolus Precautions

Generic Interventions

Assess and Evaluate Neurovascular Status at Least Every Hour for First 24 Hours. Compare with Unaffected Limb if Possible.

Peripheral pulses
Skin color, temperature
Capillary refill time

For Injured Arms

Assess for ability to:
Hyperextend thumbs, wrist, and four fingers
Abduct (fan out) all fingers
Touch thumb to small finger

Assess Sensation with Pressure from a Sharp Point.
Web space between thumb and index finger
Distal fat pad of small finger
Distal surface of the index finger

For Injured Legs:

Assess for Ability to:
Dorsiflex (upward movement) ankle and extend toes at
    metatarsal phalangeal joints
Plantarflex (downward movement) ankle and toes

Assess Sensation with Pressure from a Sharp Point:
Web space between great toe and second toe
Medial and lateral surfaces of the sole (upper third)

Instruct to Report Unusual, New, or Different Sensations (e.g., Tingling, Numbness, or Decreased Ability to Move Toes or Fingers; Pain with Passive Stretch; Unrelieved Pain).

Reduce Edema or Its Effects on Function.

Remove jewelry from affected limb.
Elevate limbs unless contraindicated.
Advise to move fingers or toes of affected limb two to four times
    per hour.
Apply ice bags around injured site. Place a cloth between ice bag
    and skin.
Monitor drainage (characteristics, amount) from wounds or
    incisional site.
Maintain patency of the wound drainage system.

Notify the Physician If the Following Occur:

Change in sensation
Change in movement ability
Pale, mottled, or cyanotic skin
Slowed capillary refill more than 3 seconds
Diminished or absent pulse

Increasing pain or pain not controlled by medication
Pain with passive stretching of muscle
Pain increased with elevation

If Previous Signs or Symptoms Occur, Discontinue Elevation and Ice Application.

Promote Circulation in Affected Limb.

Ensure hydration is optimal to maximize circulation.

Monitor traction apparatus and splints for pressure on vessels or
nerves.

If wrist or ankle restraints are used, monitor for pressure on
vessels or nerves. Remove at least every hour, and perform
range-of-motion (ROM) exercises.

Encourage active ROM exercises of unaffected body parts and
ambulation if permissible.

After Hip or Knee Joint Replacement, Maintain Correct Positioning to Prevent Prosthetic Dislocation.

Initiate Health Teaching As Indicated.

*Teach client and family to watch for and
report the following symptoms:*

Severe pain
Numbness or tingling
Swelling
Skin discoloration
Paralysis or reduced movement
Cool, white toes or fingertips
Foul odor, warm spots, soft areas, or cracks in the cast

Emphasize the importance of follow-up evaluations.

POST-TRAUMA SYNDROME

Post-Trauma Syndrome
Post-Trauma Syndrome, Risk for
Rape-Trauma Syndrome

DEFINITION

The state in which an individual experiences a sustained painful
response for more than 1 month to one or more overwhelming
traumatic events that have not been assimilated.

DEFINING CHARACTERISTICS

Major (Must Be Present, One or More)

Re-experiencing the traumatic event, this may be identified in cognitive, affective, or sensory-motor activities, such as:

- Flashbacks, intrusive thoughts
- Repetitive dreams/nightmares
- Excessive verbalization of the traumatic events
- Survival guilt or guilt about behavior required for survival
- Painful emotion, self-blame, shame, or sadness
- Vulnerability or helplessness, anxiety, or panic
- Fear of repetition, death, loss of bodily control
- Anger outburst/rage, startle reaction
- Hyperalertness or hypervigilance

Minor (May Be Present)

Psychic/Emotional Numbness

Impaired interpretation of reality, impaired memory

Confusion, dissociation, or amnesia

Vagueness about traumatic event

Narrowed attention or inattention/daze

Feeling of numbness, constricted affect

Feeling detached/alienated

Reduced interest in significant activities

Altered Lifestyle

Submissiveness, passiveness, or dependency

Self-destructiveness (e.g., alcohol/drug abuse, suicide attempts, reckless driving, illegal activities)

Thrill-seeking activities

Difficulty with interpersonal relationships

Development of phobia regarding trauma

Avoidance of situations or activities that arouse recollection of the trauma

Social isolation/withdrawal, negative self-concept

Sleep disturbances, emotional disturbances

Irritability, poor impulse control, or explosiveness

Loss of faith in people or the world/feeling of meaninglessness in life

Chronic anxiety or chronic depression

Somatic preoccupation/multiple physiologic symptoms

RELATED FACTORS

Situational (Personal, Environmental)

Related to traumatic events of natural origin, including:

Floods

Earthquakes

Volcanic eruptions

Storms

Avalanches

Epidemics (may be of
    human origin)

Other natural disasters,
    which are overwhelming
    to most people

Related to traumatic events of human origin, such as:

Wars

Airplane crashes

Serious car accidents

Large fires

Bombing

Concentration camp
    confinement

Torture

Assault

Rape

Related to industrial disasters (nuclear, chemical, or other life-threatening accidents)

NOC

Abuse Recovery, Coping, Fear Self Control

Goals

The person will assimilate the experience into a meaningful whole and go on to pursue his or her life, as evidenced by goal-setting.

Indicators
- Report a lessening of reexperiencing the trauma or numbing symptoms.
- Acknowledge the traumatic event and begin to work with the trauma by talking over the experience and expressing feelings such as fear, anger, and guilt.
- Identify and make connection with support persons/resources.

NIC

Counseling, Anxiety Reduction, Emotional Support, Family Support, Support System Enhancement, Coping Enhancement, Active Listening, Presence, Grief Work Facilitation, Referral

Generic Interventions

In a quiet room, explore with the person what happened. If the person is too anxious, discontinue assessment.

Communicate to the person that you are sorry that this happened, that he or she is not to blame, that you are glad he or she is alive, and that he or she is safe here.

Assist the person to decrease extremes of reexperiencing or numbing symptoms:

- Provide a safe, therapeutic environment where the person can regain control.
- Stay with the person, and offer support during an episode of high anxiety.
- Assist the person to control impulsive acting-out behavior by setting limits, promoting ventilation, and redirecting excess energy into physical exercise activity (e.g., going to the gym, walking, jogging).

Reassure the person that these feelings/symptoms are often experienced by individuals who underwent such traumatic events.

Assist the person to acknowledge the traumatic event and begin to work through the trauma by talking about the experience and expressing feelings, such as fear, anger, and guilt.

Assist the person to make connections with support and resources according to his or her needs.

Encourage the person to resume old activities and begin some new ones.

Assist family/significant others to understand what is happening to the victim.

Encourage ventilation of their feelings.

Provide counseling sessions, or link the person with appropriate community resources as necessary.

Explain to the person and significant others:
- Flashbacks, nightmares
- Avoidance behavior
- Detached behavior
- Hypervigilance
- Exaggerated startle reflex
- Angry outbursts

Provide or arrange follow-up treatment where the person/family can continue to work through the trauma and integrate the experience into new ego synthesis.

🔵 Pediatric Interventions

Assist Child to Understand and Integrate the Experience in Accordance with His or Her Developmental Stage.

Assist to describe the experience and to express feelings (e.g., fear, guilt, rage) in safe, supportive places, such as play therapy sessions.

Provide accurate information and explanations to child in terms child can understand.

Provide family counseling to promote family members' understanding of child's needs.

Assist Family/Significant Others.

Assist them to understand what is happening to child.

Encourage ventilation of their feelings.

Provide family counseling and/or link them with appropriate community resources, as necessary.

▶ Post-Trauma Syndrome, Risk for

DEFINITION

A state in which the individual is at risk to experience a sustained painful response to one or more overwhelming traumatic events that have not been assimilated.

RISK FACTORS

Refer to Related Factors in *Post-Trauma Syndrome*.

Goals

The person will continue to function appropriately after the traumatic event.

Indicators

• Identify signs or symptoms that necessitate professional consultation.

• Express feelings regarding traumatic event.

Generic Interventions

Refer to *Post-Trauma Syndrome*.

▶ Rape-Trauma Syndrome

DEFINITION

The state in which an individual experiences a forced, violent sexual assault (vaginal or anal penetration) against his or her will and without his or her consent. The trauma syndrome that develops from this attack or attempted attack includes an acute phase of disorganization of the victim and family's lifestyle and a long-term process of reorganization of lifestyle (Holmstrom & Burgess, 1975).

DEFINING CHARACTERISTICS

Major (Must Be Present)

Reports or evidence of sexual assault

Minor (May Be Present)

If the victim is a child, parents may experience similar responses.

Acute Phase

Somatic responses
Gastrointestinal irritability (nausea, vomiting, anorexia)
Genitourinary discomfort (pain, pruritus)
Skeletal muscle tension (spasms, pain)

Psychological Responses

Denial
Emotional shock
Anger
Fear of being alone or that the rapist will return (a child victim
  will fear punishment, repercussions, abandonment, rejection)
Guilt
Panic on seeing assailant or scene of attack

Sexual Responses

Mistrust of men (if victim is a woman)
Change in sexual behavior

Long-Term Phase

Any response of the acute phase may continue if resolution does
not occur.

Psychological Responses

Phobias
Nightmares or sleep disturbances
Anxiety
Depression

NOC

Abuse Protection, Abuse Recovery Coping

Goals

The person will return to precrisis level of functioning.
The child will express feelings concerning the assault and the
  treatment.

Indicators

- Share feelings.
- Describe rationale and treatment procedures.
- Identify members of support system, and use them appropri-
  ately.

The parents, spouse, or significant other will return to pre-crisis
level of functioning.

Short-Term Goals

- Share feelings.
- Describe rationale and treatment procedures.
- Identify members of support system and use them appropriately.

Long-Term Goals

- Report sleeping well.
- Report return to former eating pattern.
- Report no or occasional somatic reactions.
- Demonstrate calmness and relaxation.

NIC

Abuse Protection Support, Coping Enhancement, Rape-Trauma Treatment, Support Groups, Anxiety Reduction, Presence, Emotional Support, Calming Technique, Active Listening, Family Support, Grief Work Facilitation

Generic Interventions

Promote Trusting Relationship, and Stay with Person During Acute Stage or Arrange for Other Support.

Communicate.

Victim is safe here.
It was not his or her fault.
You are sorry this happened.
You are glad he or she is alive.

Provide This Analogy: "Every Time You Think You Are Responsible for This Rape, Think Instead that You Were Hit Over the Head with a Shovel (e.g., 'I Would Not Have Been Hit Over the Head with a Shovel if I Didn't Wear that Dress, Drink Too Much, Kiss Him, Walk Home . . .')." This May Help Effect the Realization that This Was a Crime of Violence and Control, Not Sex.

Explain the Care and Examination She or He Will Experience.

Conduct the examinations in an unhurried manner.
Explain every detail before action.
If this is the person's first pelvic examination, explain the position and the instruments.
Discuss the possibility of pregnancy and a sexually transmitted disease and treatments available.

Explain the Legal Issues and Police Investigation (Heinrich, 1987).

Explain the need to collect specimens for future possible court use.

Explain that the choice to report the rape is the victim's.

If the police interview is permitted:

- Negotiate with victim and police for an advantageous time.
- Explain to victim what kind of questions will be asked.
- Remain with the victim during the interview; do not ask questions or offer answers.

Record Presence and Location of Bruises, Lacerations, Edema, or Abrasion.

Whenever Possible, Provide Crisis Counseling Within 1 Hour of Rape-Trauma Event.

Before Person Leaves Hospital, Provide Card with Information about Follow-Up Appointments and Names and Telephone Numbers of Local Crisis and Counseling Centers.

Encourage Person to Recognize Positive Responses or Support from Sexual Partner or Members of Opposite Sex.

Pediatric Interventions

Addressing the child's developmental level, elicit the child's reaction.

Explain what happened. Reinforce that the child did not deserve this.

Use play therapy with puppets or dolls with genitalia.

Evaluate the risk for suicide, especially in adolescent boys.

For adolescents:

- Educate the individual and family that rape is a violent crime.
- Discourage focusing on "what if . . ." or "I should have. . . ."
- Discourage violent, destructive, or irrational retribution toward rapist.
- Help family to be supportive of individual.

Refer child and caregivers for counseling.

Geriatric Interventions

Assess for change in behavior in cognitively impaired (elderly, developmentally delayed):

- Fearful behavior toward men
- Avoidance behavior with men

- Withdrawal behavior
- Staying near nurses' station
- Lying in fetal position

POWERLESSNESS

Powerlessness
Powerlessness, Risk for

DEFINITION

The state in which an individual or group perceives a lack of personal control over certain events or situations, which affects outlook, goals, and lifestyle.

▪▪▪ AUTHOR'S NOTE

Most individuals are subject to feelings of powerlessness in varying amounts in various situations. This diagnosis can be used to describe individuals who respond to loss of control with apathy, anger, or depression. Prolonged states of powerlessness may lead to hopelessness.

DEFINING CHARACTERISTICS

Major (Must Be Present)

Overt or covert expressions of dissatisfaction about inability to control situation (e.g., work, illness, prognosis, care, recovery rate) that is negatively affecting outlook, goals, and lifestyle

Minor (May Be Present)

Apathy	Passivity
Anger	Resignation
Violent behavior	Acting-out behavior
Anxiety	Depression
Unsatisfactory dependence on others	

RELATED FACTORS

Pathophysiologic

Any disease process—acute or chronic—can contribute to powerlessness. Some common sources are the following:

Related to inability to communicate secondary to: e.g.,
Cerebrovascular accident
Guillain-Barré syndrome
Intubation

Related to inability to perform activities of daily living secondary to: e.g., cerebrovascular accident, cervical trauma, myocardial infarction, or pain

Related to inability to perform role responsibilities secondary to: e.g., surgery, trauma, or arthritis

Related to progressive debilitating disease secondary to: for example, multiple sclerosis, terminal cancer, AIDS

Related to substance abuse

Situational (Personal, Environmental)

Related to feeling of loss of control and lifestyle restrictions secondary to (specify)

Related to change from curative status to palliative status

Related to overeating patterns

Related to personal characteristics that highly value control (e.g., internal locus of control)

Related to effects of hospital or institutional limitations

Related to lifestyle of helplessness

Related to fear of disapproval

Related to unmet dependency needs

Related to consistent negative feedback

Related to long-term abusive relationship

Maturational

Parents of Adolescent Children
Related to child-rearing problems

Older Adult

Related to multiple losses secondary to aging (e.g., retirement, sensory deficits, motor deficits, financial status, or significant others)

NOC

Depression Self Control, Health Beliefs: Perceived Control, Participation: Health Care Decisions

Goals

The person will verbalize ability to control/influence situations and outcomes.

Indicators
- Identify factors that can be controlled by him or her.
- Make decisions regarding his or her care, treatment, and future when possible.

NIC

Mood Management, Teaching: Individual, Decision-Making Support, Self-Responsibility Facilitation, Health System Guidance, Spiritual Support

Generic Interventions

Explore the effects of condition on:
- Occupation
- Leisure activities
- Role responsibilities
- Relationships

Allow to share losses (e.g., independence, roles, income).

Assist not to see self as helpless. Help to identify personal strengths and assets.

Explain all procedures, rules, and options. Allow time to answer questions; ask person to write questions down so as not to forget them.

Keep person informed about condition, treatments, and results. Anticipate questions/interest, and offer information.

While being realistic, point out positive changes in person's condition.

Provide opportunities for person to control decisions.

Allow person to manipulate surroundings, such as deciding what is to be kept where (shoes under bed, picture on window).

Record person's specific choices on care plan to ensure that others on staff acknowledge preferences ("Dislikes orange juice." "Takes showers." "Plan dressing change at 7:30 prior to shower.").

Provide daily recognition of progress.

For the person with chronic helplessness:
- Encourage to take responsibility for self-care.
- Assist to set realistic goals.
- Help to differentiate areas of life that she or he can and cannot control.
- Provide opportunities for person to be successful.

👥 Pediatric Interventions

Explore with child perceptions of the situation.
Use play therapy to help gain mastery of stressful situations.

Encourage personal possessions.

Explain all procedures. Allow child some aspect of control or choices.

Actively encourage child to ask questions.

If possible, elicit information from child rather than parent or caregiver.

C Geriatric Interventions

Involve in discussing plans and options early.

Provide time to adjust to changes.

Listen carefully to person's perceptions of the situation.

◗ Powerlessness, Risk for

DEFINITION

The state in which an individual or group is at risk to perceive a lack of personal control over certain events or situations that affects outlook, goals, and lifestyle.

RISK FACTORS

Refer to Related Factors in *Powerlessness*.

Goals

The person will continue to make decisions regarding his or her life, health care, and future.

Indicators
- Engage in discussions of options.
- Raise questions regarding choices.

Generic Interventions

Refer to *Powerlessness*.

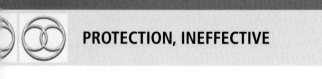

PROTECTION, INEFFECTIVE

Protection, Ineffective
Tissue Integrity, Impaired
Skin Integrity, Impaired

Risk for Impaired Skin Integrity
Oral Mucous Membrane, Impaired

DEFINITION

The state in which an individual experiences a decrease in the ability to guard against internal or external threats, such as illness or injury.

AUTHOR'S NOTE

Ineffective Protection represents a broad diagnostic category under which several specific nursing diagnoses are clustered: *Impaired Tissue Integrity*, *Impaired Oral Mucous Membrane*, and *Impaired Skin Integrity*. These diagnoses are more clinically useful than *Ineffective Protection*.

The nurse should be cautioned concerning the substitution of *Ineffective Protection* as a new name for compromised immune system, AIDS, disseminated intravascular coagulation, diabetes mellitus, etc. The nurse should focus on the functional abilities of the individual that are or may be compromised because of altered protection, such as *Fatigue*, *Risk for Infection*, and *Risk for Loneliness*. The nurse should also focus on the physiologic complications of altered protection that require nursing and medical interventions for management (i.e., collaborative problems, such as *Risk for Complications of Thrombocytopenia* or *Risk for Complications of Sepsis*).

DEFINING CHARACTERISTICS

Major (Must Be Present, One or More)

Deficient immunity
Impaired healing
Altered clotting
Maladaptive stress response
Neurosensory alterations

Minor (May Be Present)

Chilling	Cough
Perspiration	Itching
Dyspnea	Restlessness
Insomnia	Immobility
Fatigue	Disorientation
Anorexia	Pressure sores
Weakness	

▶ Tissue Integrity, Impaired

DEFINITION

The state in which an individual experiences or is at risk for altered integumentary, corneal, or mucous membranous tissues of the body.

▪▪▪▪ AUTHOR'S NOTE

Impaired Tissue Integrity is the broad category under which the more specific nursing diagnoses of *Impaired Skin Integrity* and *Impaired Oral Mucous Membranes* fall. Because tissue is composed of epithelium and connective muscle and nervous tissue, *Impaired Tissue Integrity* correctly describes some pressure ulcers that are deeper than dermal. *Impaired Skin Integrity* should be used to describe potential or actual disruptions of epidermal and dermal tissue only.

When a pressure ulcer is stage IV, necrotic, or infected, it may be more appropriate to label the diagnosis a collaborative problem as Risk for Complications of Stage IV pressure ulcer. This would represent a situation a nurse manages with physician- and nurse-prescribed interventions. When a stage II or III pressure ulcer needs a dressing that requires a physician's order in an acute care setting, the nurse should continue to label the situation a nursing diagnosis because other than hospital regulation, it would be appropriate and legal for a nurse to treat the ulcer independently (e.g., in the community).

If an individual is at risk for damage to corneal tissue, the nurse can use the diagnosis *Risk for Impaired Corneal Tissue Integrity related to*, for example, corneal drying and reduced lacrimal production secondary to unconscious state. If an individual is immobile and multiple systems—respiratory, circulatory, musculoskeletal, and integumentary—are threatened, the nurse can use *Disuse Syndrome* to describe the entire situation.

DEFINING CHARACTERISTICS

Major (Must Be Present, One or More)

Disruptions of corneal, integumentary, or mucous membranous tissue or invasion of body structure (incision, dermal ulcer, corneal ulcer, oral lesion)

Minor (May Be Present)

Lesions (primary, secondary)	Dry mucous membrane
Edema	Leukoplakia
Erythema	Coated tongue

RELATED FACTORS

Pathophysiologic

Related to inflammation of dermal-epidermal junctions secondary to:

Autoimmune Alterations

Lupus erythematosus	Scleroderma

Metabolic and Endocrine Alterations

Diabetes mellitus	Jaundice
Hepatitis	Cancer
Cirrhosis	Thyroid dysfunction
Renal failure	

Bacterial (impetigo, folliculitis, cellulitis)

Viral (herpes zoster [shingles], herpes simplex, gingivitis, AIDS)

Fungal (ringworm [dermatophytosis], athlete's foot, vaginitis)

Related to decreased blood and nutrients to tissues secondary to:

Diabetes mellitus	Anemia
Peripheral vascular alterations	Cardiopulmonary disorders
Venous stasis	Edema
Arteriosclerosis	Emaciation
Hyperthermia	Malnutrition
Obesity	Nutritional alterations
Dehydration	

Treatment-Related

Related to decreased blood and nutrients to tissues secondary to: NPO status, therapeutic extremes in body temperature, or surgery

Related to imposed immobility related to sedation

Related to mechanical trauma (e.g., therapeutic fixation devices, wired jaw, traction, casts, orthopedic devices/braces)

Related to effects of radiation on epithelial and basal cells

Related to effects of mechanical irritants or pressure secondary to:

Inflatable or foam "donuts"	External urinary catheters
Tourniquets	Nasogastric tubes

Foot boards
Restraints
Dressings, tape, solutions

Endotracheal tubes
Oral prostheses/braces
Contact lenses

Situational (Personal, Environmental)

Related to chemical trauma secondary to: excretions, secretions, or noxious agents/substances

Related to environmental irritants secondary to:
Radiation—sunburn
Temperature
Humidity
Parasites

Bites (insect, animal)
Inhalants
Poisonous plants

Related to the effects of pressure or immobility secondary to pain; fatigue; motivation; cognitive, sensory, or motor deficits
Related to inadequate personal habits (hygiene, dental, dietary, sleep)
Related to impaired mobility secondary to (specify)
Related to thin body frame

Maturational

Older Adult
Related to dry, thin skin and decreased dermal vascularity secondary to aging

▶ Skin Integrity, Impaired

DEFINITION

The state in which an individual experiences or is at risk for altered epidermis and/or dermis.

DEFINING CHARACTERISTICS

Major (Must Be Present)

Disruptions of epidermal and dermal tissue

Minor (May Be Present)

Denuded skin
Erythema
Lesions (primary, secondary)
Pruritus

RELATED FACTORS

See *Impaired Tissue Integrity*.

NOC
Tissue Integrity: Skin and Mucous Membrane

Goals
The person will demonstrate progressive healing of tissue.

Indicators
- Participate in risk assessment.
- Express willingness to participate in prevention of pressure ulcers.
- Describe etiology and prevention measures.
- Explain rationale for interventions.

NIC
Pressure Management, Pressure Ulcer Care, Skin Surveillance, Positioning

Generic Interventions

Identify the Stage of Pressure Ulcer Development:
Stage I: Nonblanchable erythema of intact skin
Stage II: Ulceration of epidermis or dermis
Stage III: Ulceration involving subcutaneous fat
Stage IV: Extensive ulceration penetrating muscle, bone, or supporting structure

Assess Status of Ulcer
Size—measure longest and widest wound surface

Depth:
- No break in skin
- Abrasion or shallow crater
- Deep crater
- Necrosis

Edges:
- Attached
- Not attached
- Fibrotic

Undermining:
- <2 cm
- 2 to 4 cm
- More than 4 cm
- Tunneling

Necrotic tissue type (color, consistency, adherence) and amount

Exudate type, amount

Surrounding skin color

Presence of peripheral tissue edema, induration

Granulation tissue

Epithelialization

Wash Reddened Area Gently with a Mild Soap, Rinse Thoroughly to Remove Soap, and Pat Dry

Gently Massage Healthy Skin Around the Affected Area to Stimulate Circulation; Do Not Massage If Reddened

Protect the Healthy Skin Surface with One or a Combination of the Following:

Apply a thin coat of liquid copolymer skin sealant.

Cover area with moisture-permeable film dressing.

Cover area with a hydrocolloid wafer barrier, and secure with strips of 1-inch nonallergenic tape; leave in place for 2 to 3 days.

Increase Protein and Carbohydrate Intake to Maintain a Positive Nitrogen Balance; Weigh the Person Daily, and Determine Serum Albumin Level Weekly to Monitor Status

Devise Plan for Pressure Ulcer Management Using Principles of Moist Wound-Healing

Débride necrotic tissue (collaborate with physician).

Flush ulcer base with sterile saline solution.

Protect granulating wound bed from trauma.

Cover pressure ulcer with a sterile dressing that maintains a moist environment over the ulcer base (e.g., film dressing, hydrocolloid wafer dressing, moist gauze dressing).

Avoid the use of drying agents (heat lamps, magnesium hydroxide [Maalox], milk of magnesia).

Monitor for clinical signs of wound infection.

Consult with Nurse Specialist or Physician for Treatment of Stage IV Pressure Ulcers

Refer to Community Nursing Agency If Additional Assistance at Home Is Needed

▶ Risk for Impaired Skin Integrity

DEFINITION

Refer to *Impaired Skin Integrity*.

RISK FACTORS

Refer to Related Factors in *Impaired Skin Integrity*.

NOC

Tissue Integrity: Skin and Mucous Membrane

Goals

The person will demonstrate skin integrity free of pressure ulcers (if able).

Indicators

- Participate in risk assessment.
- Express willingness to participate in prevention of pressure ulcers.
- Describe etiology and prevention measures.
- Explain rationale for interventions.

NIC

Skin Surveillance, Positioning

Generic Interventions

Maintain sufficient fluid intake for adequate hydration (approximately 2500 mL daily, unless contraindicated); check mucous membranes in mouth for moisture, and check urine specific gravity.

Establish a schedule for emptying bladder (begin with every 2 hours). If person is confused, determine incontinence pattern, and intervene before incontinence occurs. Explain problem to person, and secure cooperation for plan.

When incontinent, wash perineum with a liquid soap that will not alter skin pH, and apply a protective barrier to the perineal region (incontinence film barrier spray or wipes).

Encourage range-of-motion exercises and weight-bearing mobility, when possible.

Turn or instruct person to turn or shift weight every 30 minutes to 2 hours, depending on other causative factors present and the ability of the skin to recover from pressure.

Frequency of turning should be increased if any reddened areas that appear do not disappear within 1 hour after turning.

Keep bed as flat as possible to reduce shearing forces; limit Fowler's position to 30 minutes at a time.

Use enough personnel to lift person up in bed or chair rather than pull or slide skin surfaces.

Instruct person to lift self using chair arms every 10 minutes if possible, or assist person in rising up off the chair every 10 to 20 minutes, depending on risk factors present.

Observe for erythema and blanching, and palpate for warmth and tissue sponginess with each position change.

Do not rub reddened areas or over bony prominences.

Increase protein and carbohydrate intake to maintain a positive nitrogen balance; weigh the person daily, and determine serum albumin level weekly to monitor status.

Instruct person and family in specific techniques to use at home to prevent pressure ulcers.

Ⓖ Geriatric Interventions

Explain high-risk age-related factors:
- Decreased subcutaneous fat
- Drier skin, decreased elasticity
- Slowed rate of dermal healing
- Decreased skin strength (loss of collagen)
- Proteins, vitamins, and mineral deficiencies
- Immobility
- Urinary or bowel incontinence

▶ Oral Mucous Membrane, Impaired

DEFINITION

The state in which an individual experiences or is at risk of experiencing disruptions in the oral cavity.

DEFINING CHARACTERISTICS

Major (Must Be Present)

Disrupted oral mucous membranes

Minor (May Be Present)

Coated tongue   Edema
Xerostomia (dry mouth)   Hemorrhagic gingivitis

Stomatitis	Purulent drainage
Leukoplakia	Taste changes

RELATED FACTORS

Pathophysiologic

Related to inflammation secondary to:

Diabetes mellitus	Periodontal disease
Oral cancer	Infection

Treatment-Related

Related to drying effects of:
NPO status for 24 hours
Radiation to head or neck
Prolonged use of steroids or other immunosuppressives
Use of antineoplastic drugs

Related to mechanical irritation secondary to: endotracheal or nasogastric intubation

Situational (Personal, Environmental)

Related to chemical irritants secondary to: acidic foods, drugs, noxious agents, alcohol, or tobacco

Related to mechanical trauma secondary to: broken or jagged teeth, ill-fitting dentures, braces

Related to malnutrition

Related to dehydration

Related to mouth breathing

Related to inadequate oral hygiene

Related to lack of knowledge of oral hygiene

Related to decreased salivation

NOC

Oral Tissue Integrity, Oral Health

Goals

The person will demonstrate integrity of the oral cavity.

Indicators

- Be free of harmful plaque to prevent secondary infection.
- Be free of oral discomfort during food and fluid intake.
- Demonstrate optimal oral hygiene.

NIC

Oral Health Restoration, Chemotherapy Management, Oral Health Maintenance

Generic Interventions

Discuss the importance of daily oral hygiene and periodic dental examinations.

Evaluate ability to perform oral hygiene.

Teach correct oral care:

- Remove and clean dentures and bridges daily.
- Floss teeth (every 24 hours).
- Brush teeth (after meals and before sleep).
- Inspect mouth for lesions, sores, or excessive bleeding.

Perform oral hygiene on person who is unconscious or at risk for aspiration, as often as needed.

Teach preventive oral hygiene to individuals at risk of developing mucositis:

- Perform the regimen after meals and before sleep (if there is excessive exudate, also perform regimen before breakfast).
- Floss teeth only once in 24 hours.
- Omit flossing if excessive bleeding occurs, and use extreme caution with persons with platelet counts of less than 50,000.
- Avoid mouthwashes with high alcohol content, lemon/glycerine swabs, or prolonged use of hydrogen peroxide.

Use an oxidizing agent to loosen thick, tenacious mucus (gargle and expectorate); for example, hydrogen peroxide and water quarter strength (avoid prolonged use), or sodium bicarbonate 1 teaspoon in 8 oz warm water (can flavor these with mouthwash or one drop of oil of wintergreen).

Rinse mouth with saline solution after gargling.

Apply lubricant to lips every 2 hours and as needed (e.g., lanolin, A&D ointment, petroleum jelly).

If person cannot tolerate brushing or swabbing, teach to irrigate mouth (every 2 hours and as needed):

- With baking soda solution (4 teaspoons in 1 L warm water) using an enema bag (labeled for oral use only) with a soft irrigation catheter tip
- By placing catheter tip in mouth and slowly increasing flow while standing over a basin or having a basin held under chin
- Removing dentures before irrigation and not replacing in person with severe stomatitis

Inspect oral cavity three times daily with tongue blade and light; if mucositis is severe, inspect mouth every 4 hours. Teach client to inspect mouth.

Ensure that oral hygiene regimen is done every 2 hours while awake and every 6 hours (4 if severe) during the night.

Instruct individual to:

- Avoid commercial mouthwashes, citrus fruit juices, spicy foods, extremes in food temperature (hot, cold), crusty or rough foods, alcohol, mouthwashes with alcohol.
- Eat bland, cool foods (sherbets).
- Drink cool liquids every 2 hours and as needed.

Consult with physician or advanced practice nurse for an oral pain-relief solution.

Use lidocaine (Xylocaine Viscous) 2% oral swish and expectorant every 2 hours and before meals (if throat is sore, the solution can be swallowed; if swallowed, lidocaine produces local anesthesia and may affect the gag reflex). The dose of viscous xylocaine is not to exceed 25 ml per day.

Mix equal parts of lidocaine, 0.5 aqueous diphenhydramine (Benadryl) solution, and magnesium hydroxide; swish and swallow 1 oz of mixture every 2 to 4 hours as needed.

Mix equal parts of 0.5 aqueous diphenhydramine solution and kaolin (Kaopectate); swish and swallow every 2 to 4 hours as needed.

Teach person and family the factors that contribute to the development and progression of stomatitis.

Have individual describe or demonstrate home care regimen.

🏃 Pediatric Interventions

If thrush (oral candidiasis) is present:

- Rinse mouth with plain water after each feeding.
- Boil nipples and bottles for at least 20 minutes.
- Boil pacifiers once a day.
- Apply topical medication as prescribed.

Explain the need to teach 2-year-olds how to brush their teeth after meals and before bedtime.

Encourage parent to have toddler accompany him or her to dentist office to meet personnel.

Discuss the importance of routine dental examinations every 6 months beginning at 3 to 4 years old.

🤰 Maternal Interventions

Stress the importance of good oral hygiene and dental examinations.

Remind to advise dentist of pregnancy.

Explain that gum hypertrophy and tenderness are normal during pregnancy.

C Geriatric Interventions

Explain high-risk age-related factors (Miller, 2009):

- Degenerative bone disease
- Diminished oral blood supply
- Dry mouth
- Vitamin deficiencies

Explain that some medications cause dry mouth:

- Laxatives
- Antibiotics
- Antidepressants
- Analgesics
- Iron sulfate
- Cardiovascular
- Anticholinergics

Determine the presence of barriers to dental care:

- Financial
- Mobility
- Dexterity
- Lack of knowledge

RELOCATION STRESS (SYNDROME)

Relocation Stress (Syndrome)
Risk for Relocation Stress (Syndrome)

DEFINITION

A state in which an individual experiences physiologic and/or psychological disturbances as a result of transfer from one environment to another.

███ **AUTHOR'S NOTE**

Relocation represents a disruption for all parties involved. It can accompany a transfer from one unit to another or from one facility to another. It can involve a permanent move to a long-term care facility or to a new home. All age groups involved are disturbed by the relocation. When physiologic

(continued)

AUTHOR'S NOTE *(Continued)*
and psychological disturbances compromise functioning, the nursing diagnosis *Relocation Stress (Syndrome)* is appropriate.

The optimal nursing approach to relocation stress is to initiate preventive measures, using *Risk for Relocation Stress* as the diagnosis.

NANDA has accepted this diagnosis as a syndrome diagnosis. *Relocation Stress* as a syndrome diagnosis does not fit the criteria for a syndrome diagnosis, which is a cluster of actual or high-risk nursing diagnoses as defining characteristics. The defining characteristics associated with *Relocation Stress* are observable or reportable cues consistent with *Relocation Stress*, not *Relocation Stress Syndrome*. The author recommends deleting "syndrome" from the label.

Other terms found in the literature that describe relocation stress include admission stress, post-relocation crisis, relocation crisis, relocation shock, relocation trauma, transfer stress, transfer trauma, translocation syndrome, and transplantation shock.

DEFINING CHARACTERISTICS (HARKULICH & BRUGLER, 1988)

Major (80% to 100%)

Responds to transfer or relocation with:

Loneliness	Apprehension
Depression	Anxiety
Increased confusion (older adult population)	Anger

Minor (50% to 79%)

Change in eating habits
Change in sleep patterns
Demonstration of dependency
Demonstration of insecurity
Demonstration of lack of trust
Gastrointestinal disturbances
Increased verbalization of needs
Need for excessive reassurance
Restlessness
Sad affect
Unfavorable comparison of post-transfer with pretransfer staff
Verbalization of being concerned/upset about transfer

Verbalization of insecurity in new living situation
Vigilance
Weight change
Withdrawal

RELATED FACTORS

Pathophysiologic

Related to compromised ability to adapt to changes secondary to:

Decreased Physical Health Status
Decreased Psychosocial Health Status
Increased/perceived stress before relocation
Depression
Decreased self-esteem

Situational (Personal, Environmental)

Related to moderate to high amount of environmental change secondary to:

Decreased control of individual care
Decrease and/or change in available caregivers
Decrease/increase in client-monitoring equipment
Increased noise/activities in post-transfer environment
Loss of privacy

Related to negative history with previous transfers secondary to:

Involuntary moves
Frequent moves within short time spans
Transfers occurring at evenings/nights

Related to concurrent, recent, and past interpersonal losses secondary to:

Negative experiences dealing with earlier separations (for adults as well as children)
Loss of social and familial ties
Abandonment
Perceived/actual rejection by caregivers
Anticipation of lengthy and/or permanent stay in new environment
Threat to financial security
Change in relationship with family members

Related to little or no preparation for the impending move

Lack of predictability in new environment
Little or no time between notification and move

Unrealistic expectations of individual/family members regarding facility and staff

Lack of decision-making and control on behalf of the person who is moving

Maturational

School-Age and Adolescents

Related to losses associated with moving secondary to fear of rejection, loss of peer group, or school-related problems

Related to decreased security in new adolescent peer group and school

NOC

Anxiety Control, Coping, Loneliness, Psychosocial Adjustment: Life Changes, Quality of Life

Goals

The person will:

- Verbalize positive statements about acceptance of the new environment and reasons for leaving the previous environment
- Adjust to the new environment without physiologic and/or psychological disturbance

Indicators

- Participate in decision-making activities regarding the new environment.
- Establish bonds in the new environment.
- Become involved in activities in the new environment.
- Voice concerns regarding the move.
- Describe realistic expectations of the new environment.

NIC

Anxiety Reduction, Coping Enhancement, Counseling, Family Involvement Promotion, Support System Enhancement, Anticipatory Guidance, Family Integrity Promotion

Generic Interventions

Reduce environmental differences between old and new settings; promote continuity of care in new environment:

- Maintain person on same activity level and diet through pre-transfer and post-transfer units.

- Transfer person to similar, proximal area when possible.
- Wean any monitoring equipment gradually before transfer.
- Transfer all personal items (e.g., mobility aids, eyeglasses, hearing aids, dentures, prostheses, and belongings) with the person.
- Transfer person during daytime hours.

Offer person decision-making opportunities throughout relocation experience.

Promote person's input about new environment when possible, such as use of decorations and arrangement of furniture.

Encourage family members to share their perceptions of relocation with one another.

Offer person help in maintaining contact with significant others by telephone calls, writing letters, and visits with previous roommates when applicable.

Provide follow-up visit with nurse from pretransfer unit to person on post-transfer unit.

Retain highly anxious person in pretransfer unit until anxiety decreases, when possible.

Identify individuals at high risk for selected physiologic responses:
- Musculoskeletal/neurologic deficits
- Advanced age
- Infections
- Changes in orientation
- Cardiovascular deficits

Assess vital signs and level of orientation prior to relocation.

🏃 Pediatric Interventions

Teach parents to assist their child with the move:
- Remain positive about the move before, during, and after, with the acceptance that child may not be optimistic.
- Explore options with child on how to communicate with friends/families in previous environment.
- Keep regular routines in the new environment.
- Acknowledge the difficulty of peer losses with the adolescent.
- Join the organizations to which child previously belonged (e.g., Girl Scouts, sports).
- Plan a trip to school during a class and lunch period to reduce fear of unknown.
- Ask teacher or counselor at new school to introduce child to a student who recently relocated to that school.

Ⓒ Geriatric Interventions

Promote integration after transfer into a long-term care nursing facility:

- Allow as many choices as possible.
- Encourage person to bring familiar objects from home.
- Encourage person to interact with other individuals in new facility.
- Assist person to maintain previous interpersonal relationships.

▶ Risk for Relocation Stress (Syndrome)

DEFINITION

A state in which an individual is at risk to experience physiologic and/or psychological disturbances as a result of transfer from one environment to another.

RISK FACTORS

Refer to Related Factors in *Relocation Stress*.

NOC

Anxiety Control, Coping, Psychosocial Adjustment: Life Change

Goals

The person/family will continue to report adjustment to the new environment.

Indicators

- Verbalize positive aspects of relocation.
- Engage in decision-making regarding new environment.

NIC

Coping Enhancement, Counseling, Family Involvement Promotion, Anticipatory Guidance

Generic Interventions

Refer to *Relocation Stress*.

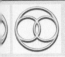
Resilience, Impaired Individual
Risk for Impaired Individual Resilience

DEFINITION

The state in which an individual has a decreased ability to sustain a pattern of positive responses to an adverse situation or crisis.

DEFINING CHARACTERISTICS

Decreased interest in academic activities
Decreased interest in vocational activities
Depression
Guilt
Isolation
Low self-esteem
Lower perceived health status
Renewed elevation of distress
Shame
Social isolation
Using maladaptive coping skills (i.e., drug use, violence, etc.)

RELATED FACTORS

Demographics that increase chance of maladjustment
Drug use
Gender
Inconsistent parenting
Low intelligence
Low maternal education
Large family size
Minority status
Parental mental illness
Poor impulse control
Poverty
Psychological disorders
Vulnerability factors which encompass indices that exacerbate
    the negative effects of the risk condition
Violence
Violence in neighborhood

■■■■ **AUTHOR'S NOTE**
This new NANDA-I diagnosis does not represent a nursing diagnosis. The defining characteristics are not defining resilience but in fact a variety of coping problems or mental disorders. Most of the related factors are prejudicial, pejorative and cannot be changed by interventions. One related factor listed—poor impulse control is a sign/symptom of hyperactivity disorders and some mental disorders.

Resilience is a strength that can be taught and nurtured in children. Resilient individuals and families can cope in adverse situations and crises. They problem solve and adapt their functioning to the situation. For example, when a mother of a family of five had to undergo chemotherapy, the family formulated a plan together to divide the responsibilities previously managed by the mother.

When an individual or family has inadequate resilience, they are at risk for ineffective coping. Refer to *Ineffective Coping, Compromised or Disabled Family Coping* for Key Concepts, Goals and Interventions/Rationale.

▶ Risk for Compromised Resilience

DEFINITION

The state in which an individual is at risk for decreased ability to sustain a pattern of positive responses to an adverse situation or crisis.

RISK FACTORS

Chronicity of existing crises
Multiple coexisting adverse situations
Presence of additional new crisis (e.g., unplanned pregnancy, death of spouse, loss of job, illness, loss of housing, death of family member

■■■■ **AUTHOR'S NOTE**
This new NANDA-I diagnosis does not represent a nursing diagnosis. Resilience is a strength that can be taught and nurtured in children. Resilient individuals and families can cope in adverse situations and crises. They problem solve and adapt their functioning to the situation. For example,

(continued)

■■■ **AUTHOR'S NOTE** *(Continued)*
when a mother of a family of five had to undergo chemotherapy, the family formulated a plan together to divide the
responsibilities previously managed by the mother.

When an individual or family is experiencing a chronic,
multiple adverse situation or a new crisis, refer to *Risk for
Ineffective Coping*. In situations involving loss of family member, significant other or friend, refer to *Grieving* for Key
Concepts, Goals, and Interventions/Rationale.

RESPIRATORY FUNCTION, RISK FOR INEFFECTIVE

Respiratory Function, Risk for Ineffective*
Dysfunctional Ventilatory Weaning Response
Dysfunctional Ventilatory Weaning Response, Risk for
Ineffective Airway Clearance
Ineffective Breathing Patterns
Impaired Gas Exchange
Inability to Sustain Spontaneous Ventilation

DEFINITION

The state in which an individual is at risk of experiencing a threat
to the passage of air through the respiratory tract and to the exchange of gases (O_2 and CO_2) between the lungs and vascular
system.

■■■ **AUTHOR'S NOTE**
The author has added this diagnosis to describe a state in
which the entire respiratory system may be affected, not

(continued)

---

*This diagnosis is not currently on the NANDA list, but has been included for
clarity or usefulness.

just isolated areas, such as airway clearance or gas exchange. Smoking, allergy, and immobility are examples of factors that affect the entire system and thus make it incorrect to use *Impaired Gas Exchange related to immobility*, because immobility also affects airway clearance and breathing patterns. It is advised that *Risk for Impaired Respiratory Function* not be used to describe an actual problem, which is a collaborative problem, not a nursing diagnosis.

The diagnoses *Ineffective Airway Clearance* and *Ineffective Breathing Patterns* can be used when the nurse can definitively alter the contributing factors that are influencing respiratory function—for example, ineffective cough, immobility, or stress. The nurse is cautioned not to use this diagnosis to describe acute respiratory disorders, which are the primary responsibility of physicians and nurses together (i.e., a collaborative problem). This can be labeled *Risk for Complications of Hypoxemia* or *Risk for Complications of Pulmonary Edema*.

RISK FACTORS

Presence of risk factors that can change respiratory function (see Related Factors)

RELATED FACTORS

Pathophysiologic

Related to excessive or thick secretions secondary to: infection, cystic fibrosis, or influenza

Related to immobility, stasis of secretions, and ineffective cough secondary to:

Diseases of the nervous system (e.g., Guillain-Barré syndrome, multiple sclerosis, myasthenia gravis)

Central nervous system depression/head trauma, spinal trauma

Quadriplegia

Treatment-Related

Related to immobility secondary to: sedating effects of medications (specify); anesthesia, general or spinal

Related to suppressed cough reflex secondary to (specify)

Situational (Personal, Environmental)

Related to immobility secondary to: surgery or trauma, pain, fear, anxiety, fatigue, or perceptual/cognitive impairment

NOC

Aspiration Control, Respiratory Status

Goals

The person will achieve maximum pulmonary function.

Indicators

• Relate the importance of hourly deep-breathing exercises (sigh) and cough sessions.

NIC

Airway Management, Cough Enhancement, Positioning, Respiratory Monitoring

Generic Interventions

Assess for optimal pain relief with minimal period of fatigue or respiratory depression.

Encourage ambulation as soon as consistent with plan of care.

If client cannot walk, establish a regimen for being out of bed in a chair several times a day (e.g., 1 hour after meals and 1 hour before bedtime).

Increase activity gradually, explaining that respiratory function will improve and dyspnea will decrease with practice.

Assist client to reposition, turning frequently from side to side (hourly if possible).

Encourage deep-breathing and controlled-coughing exercises five times every hour.

Teach client to use blow bottle or incentive spirometer every hour while awake (with severe neuromuscular impairment, the person may have to be awakened during the night as well).

Auscultate lung field every 8 hours; increase frequency if altered breath sounds are present.

🧑 Pediatric Interventions

Observe for nasal flaring, retractions, or cyanosis.

Allow child to select the color of water in blow bottles.

Monitor intake, output, and urine specific gravity.

Provide age-appropriate explanation for deep-breathing exercises.

▶ Dysfunctional Ventilatory Weaning Response

DEFINITION

A state in which an individual cannot adjust to lowered levels of mechanical ventilator support, which interrupts and prolongs the weaning process.

■■■ **AUTHOR'S NOTE**
Dysfunctional Ventilatory Weaning Response (DVWR) is a specific diagnosis within the category of *Risk for Impaired Respiratory Function. Ineffective Airway Clearance, Ineffective Breathing Patterns*, and *Impaired Gas Exchange* also can be encountered in the weaning situation, either as indicators of lack of weaning readiness or as factors related to the onset of *DVWR. DVWR* is a separate client state. Its distinctive etiologies and treatments arise from the process of separating the client from the mechanical ventilator.

DEFINING CHARACTERISTICS

DVWR is a progressive state, and experienced nurses have identified three levels of defining characteristics that can occur in response to weaning (Logan & Jenny, 1991):

Mild

Major (Must Be Present, One or More)
Restlessness
Slight increase in respiratory rate from baseline

Minor (May Be Present)
Expressed feelings of increased oxygen need, breathing discomfort, fatigue, warmth
Queries about possible machine dysfunction
Increased concentration on breathing

Moderate

Major (Must Be Present, One or More)
Slight increase in blood pressure <20 mm Hg or less from baseline
Slight increase in heart rate <20 beats/min or less from baseline
Increase in respiratory rate <5 breaths/min or less from baseline

Minor (May Be Present)
Hypervigilance to activities
Inability to respond to coaching
Inability to cooperate
Apprehension
Diaphoresis
Eye-widening (wide-eyed look)
Decreased air entry heard on auscultation
Skin color changes: pale, slight cyanosis
Slight respiratory accessory muscle use

Severe

Major (Must Be Present, One or More)
Agitation
Significant deterioration in arterial blood gases from baseline
Increase in blood pressure >20 mm Hg from baseline
Increase in heart rate >20 beats/min from baseline
Rapid, shallow breathing >25 breaths/min

Minor (May Be Present)
Full respiratory accessory muscle use
Shallow, gasping breaths
Paradoxical abdominal breathing
Adventitious breath sounds
Cyanosis
Profuse diaphoresis
Discoordinated breathing with the ventilator
Decreased level of consciousness

RELATED FACTORS

Pathophysiologic

Related to muscle weakness and fatigue secondary to:
Unstable hemodynamic status
Decreased level of consciousness
Anemia
Infection
Metabolic abnormalities or acid-base imbalance
Fluid or electrolyte imbalances
Severe disease process
Chronic respiratory disease
Chronic neuromuscular disability
Multisystem disease
Chronic nutritional deficit

Debilitated condition

Related to ineffective airway clearance

Treatment-Related

Related to obstructed airway

Related to muscle weakness and fatigue secondary to:
Excess sedation, analgesia
Uncontrolled pain

Related to inadequate nutrition (deficit in calories, excess carbohydrates, inadequate fat and protein intake)
Related to prolonged ventilator dependence (>1 week)
Related to previous unsuccessful ventilator weaning attempt(s)
Related to too-rapid pacing of the weaning process

Situational (Personal, Environmental)

Related to insufficient knowledge of the weaning process
Related to excessive energy demands (self-care activities, diagnostic and treatment procedures, visitors)
Related to inadequate social support
Related to insecure environment (noisy, upsetting events, busy room)
Related to fatigue secondary to interrupted sleep patterns
Related to inadequate self-efficacy
Related to moderate to high anxiety related to breathing efforts
Related to fear of separation from ventilator
Related to feelings of powerlessness
Related to feelings of hopelessness

NOC

Anxiety Control, Respiratory Status, Vital Signs Status, Knowledge: Weaning, Energy Conservation

Goals

The person will:

- Achieve progressive weaning goals
- Remain extubated *or*
- Demonstrate a positive attitude toward the next weaning trial

Indicators
- Collaborate willingly with the weaning plan.
- Communicate comfort status during the weaning process.
- Attempt to control the breathing pattern.
- Try to control emotional responses.

NIC

Anxiety Reduction, Preparatory Sensory Information, Respiratory Monitoring, Ventilation Assistance, Presence, Endurance

Generic Interventions

If Applicable, Assess Causative Factors for Previous Unsuccessful Weaning Attempts

Inadequate energy substrates: oxygen, nutrition, and rest
Inadequate comfort status
Excessive activity demands
Decreased self-esteem, confidence, feelings of control
Lack of knowledge of role in weaning
Lack of trust relationship with staff
Negative emotional state
Adverse weaning environment

Determine Readiness for Weaning (Geisman, 1989)

Oxygen concentration of 50% or less on the ventilator
Positive end-expiratory pressure less than 5 cm of water pressure
Respiratory rate less than 30 breaths/min
Minute ventilation of less than 10 L/min
Low dynamic and static pressures, with compliance of at least 35 cm of water pressure
Adequate respiratory muscle strength
Rested, controlled discomfort
Willingness to try weaning

If Readiness for Weaning is Determined to Be Present, Engage Client in Establishing the Plan

Explain the weaning process.
Jointly negotiate progressive weaning goals.
Explain that these goals will be reexamined daily with the client.

Refer to Unit Protocols for Specific Weaning Procedures

Explain Client's Role in the Weaning Process

Strengthen feelings of self-esteem, self-efficacy, and control.

Demonstrate confidence in client's ability to wean.

Maintain client's confidence by adopting a weaning pace (may require a doctor's order) that will ensure success and minimize setbacks.

Promote trust in the staff and environment.

Reduce Negative Effects of Anxiety and Fatigue

Monitor status frequently to prevent undue fatigue and anxiety.

Provide regular periods of rest before fatigue is advanced.

If the client is starting to get agitated, try to help him or her calm down while remaining at the bedside.

If weaning trial is discontinued, address client's perceptions of weaning failure. Reassure him or her that the trial was good exercise and a useful form of training.

Create a Positive Weaning Environment, Which Increases the Client's Feelings of Security

Coordinate Necessary Activities to Promote Adequate Time for Rest or Relaxation

Coordinate Analgesia Schedule with the Weaning Schedule

Start Weaning Trial When the Client Is Rested, Usually in the Morning after a Night's Sleep

Discuss Elements of the Weaning Process with Other Clinicians to Maximize the Probability of Weaning Success:

Starting time

Pace of the weaning

Adherence to the care plan

Diversional activities (e.g., trips outside the unit)

Scheduling of activities and rest periods

👫 Pediatric Interventions

Withhold oral feedings 2 hours before weaning attempts and after extubation.

▶ Dysfunctional Ventilatory Weaning Response, Risk for

DEFINITION

The state in which an individual is at risk for experiencing an inability to adjust to lowered levels of mechanical ventilator support during the weaning process, related to physical or psychological unreadiness to wean.

RISK FACTORS

Pathophysiologic

Related to airway obstruction

Related to muscle weakness and fatigue secondary to:

Impaired respiratory
    functioning
Anemia
Decreased level of
    consciousness
Infection
Metabolic abnormalities
Fluid or electrolyte
    imbalances

Unstable hemodynamic status
Dysrhythmia
Mental confusion
Fever
Acid-base abnormalities
Severe disease process
Multisystem disease

Treatment-Related

Related to ineffective airway clearance
Related to excess sedation, analgesia
Related to uncontrolled pain
Related to fatigue
Related to inadequate nutrition (deficit in calories, excess carbohydrates, inadequate fat and protein intake)
Related to prolonged ventilator dependence of more than 1 week
Related to previous unsuccessful ventilator weaning attempt(s)
Related to too-rapid pacing of the weaning process

Situational (Personal, Environmental)

Related to muscle weakness and fatigue secondary to:
Chronic nutritional deficit
Obesity
Ineffective sleep patterns

Related to deficient knowledge related to the weaning process
Related to inadequate self-efficacy related to weaning

Related to moderate to high anxiety related to breathing efforts
Related to fear of separation from ventilator
Related to feelings of powerlessness
Related to depressed mood
Related to feelings of hopelessness
Related to uncontrolled energy demands (self-care activities, diagnostic and treatment procedures, visitors)
Related to inadequate social support
Related to insecure environment (noisy, upsetting events, busy room)

NOC

Refer to *Dysfunctional Ventilatory Weaning Response*

Goals

The person will demonstrate a willingness to start weaning.

Indicators
- Demonstrate a positive attitude about ability to succeed.
- Maintain emotional control.
- Collaborate with planning of the weaning.

NIC

Refer to *Dysfunctional Ventilatory Weaning Response*

Generic Interventions

Assess for Causative and Contributory Factors of Inadequate Self-Efficacy About Weaning Readiness

Verbalizes continued need for ventilator support
Uses excuses for delaying the start of weaning
Displays concern about ability to adjust to lowered level of ventilator support or about the probability of success of weaning
Is agitated when weaning is mentioned
Has elevated blood pressure, pulse, and respirations when weaning is discussed

Reduce Risk Factors

Negotiate with the medical staff for a delayed start and a weaning plan with a slow pace that ensures success at each stage.
See *Dysfunctional Ventilatory Weaning Response*.

▶ Ineffective Airway Clearance

DEFINITION

The state in which an individual experiences a threat to respiratory status related to inability to cough effectively.

DEFINING CHARACTERISTICS

Major (Must Be Present, One or More)

Ineffective or absent cough
Inability to remove airway secretions

Minor (May Be Present)

Abnormal breath sounds
Abnormal respiratory rate, rhythm, depth

RELATED FACTORS

See *Risk for Impaired Respiratory Function.*

NOC

Aspiration Control, Respiratory Status

Goals

The person will not experience aspiration.

Indicators

• Demonstrate effective coughing.
• Demonstrate increased air exchange in lungs.

NIC

Cough Enhancement, Airway Suctioning, Positioning, Energy Management

Generic Interventions

Instruct person on the proper method of controlled coughing.

• Breathe deeply and slowly while sitting up as high as possible.
• Use diaphragmatic breathing.
• Hold breath for 3 to 5 seconds and then slowly exhale as much of this breath as possible through the mouth (lower rib cage and abdomen should sink down).
• Take a second breath, hold, and cough forcefully from the chest (not from the back of the mouth or throat), using two short forceful coughs.

Assess present analgesic regimen. Is the client too lethargic? Is he or she still in pain?

Initiate coughing when client appears to have best pain relief with optimal level of alertness and physical performance.

Splint abdominal or chest incisions with hand, pillow, or both.

Maintain adequate hydration (increase fluid intake to 2 to 3 quarts a day if not contraindicated by decreased cardiac output or renal disease).

Maintain adequate humidity of inspired air.

Plan for rest periods (after coughing, before meals).

Vigorously coach and encourage coughing, using positive reinforcement.

Proceed with health teaching with constant reinforcement in principles of care.

Acknowledge and encourage good individual effort and progress.

👥 Pediatric Interventions

Position to prevent aspiration.
Suction secretions from airway as needed.
Provide humidified atmosphere.

▶ Ineffective Breathing Patterns

DEFINITION

The state in which an individual experiences an actual or potential loss of adequate ventilation related to an altered breathing pattern.

▪▪▪ AUTHOR'S NOTE

This diagnosis has limited clinical utility except to describe situations that nurses definitively treat, such as hyperventilation. For individuals with chronic pulmonary disease with *Ineffective Breathing Patterns*, refer to *Activity Intolerance*. Individuals with periodic apnea and hypoventilation have a collaborative problem that can be labeled *Risk for Complications of Hypoxemia* to indicate that they are to be monitored for various respiratory dysfunctions. If the person is more vulnerable to a specific respiratory complication, the nurse can write the collaborative problem as *Risk for Complications of Pneumonia* or *Risk for Complications of Pulmonary Embolism*. Hyperventilation is a manifestation of anxiety or fear. The nurse can use *Anxiety* or *Fear related to (specify event) as manifested by hyperventilation* as a more descriptive diagnosis.

DEFINING CHARACTERISTICS

Major (Must Be Present, One or More)

Changes in respiratory rate or pattern (from baseline)
Changes in pulse (rate, rhythm, quality)

Minor (May Be Present)

Orthopnea
Tachypnea, hyperpnea, hyperventilation
Dysrhythmic respirations
Splinted/guarded respirations

RELATED FACTORS

See *Risk for Impaired Respiratory Function*.

NOC
Respiratory Status, Vital Signs Status, Anxiety Control

Goals

The person will demonstrate an effective respiratory rate and experience improved gas exchange in the lungs.

Indicators
• Relate the causative factors, if known.
• Relate adaptive ways of coping with causative factors.

NIC
Respiratory Monitoring, Progressive Muscle Relaxation, Teaching, Anxiety Reduction

Generic Interventions

For Hyperventilation:

Reassure person that measures are being taken to ensure safety.
Distract person from thinking about anxious state by having him or her maintain eye contact with you. Say, "Now look at me, and breathe slowly with me like this."
Consider use of paper bag as means of rebreathing expired air.
Stay with person, and coach in taking slower, more effective breaths.
Explain that one can learn to overcome hyperventilation through conscious control of breathing, even when the cause is unknown.

Discuss possible causes, physical and emotional, and methods of coping effectively (see *Anxiety*).

Pediatric Interventions

If child is prone to bronchospasm, medication may be indicated.

▶ Impaired Gas Exchange

DEFINITION

The state in which an individual experiences an actual or potential decreased passage of gases (oxygen and carbon dioxide) between the alveoli of the lungs and the vascular system.

■■■ AUTHOR'S NOTE

This diagnosis does not represent a situation for which nurses prescribe definitive treatment. Nurses do not treat *Impaired Gas Exchange*, but nurses can treat the functional health patterns that decreased oxygenation can affect, such as activity, sleep, nutrition, and sexual function. Thus, *Activity Intolerance related to insufficient oxygenation for activities of daily living* better describes the nursing focus. If an individual is at risk for or has experienced respiratory dysfunction, the nurse can describe the situation as *Risk for Complications of Ineffective Respiratory Function* or be even more specific with *Risk for Complications of Pulmonary Embolism*.

DEFINING CHARACTERISTICS

Major (Must Be Present)

Dyspnea on exertion

Minor (May Be Present)

Confusion/agitation
Tendency to assume a three-point position (sitting, one hand on each knee, bending forward)
Pursed-lip breathing with prolonged expiratory phase
Lethargy and fatigue
Increased pulmonary vascular resistance (increased pulmonary artery/right ventricular pressure)
Decreased gastric motility, prolonged gastric emptying
Decreased oxygen content, decreased oxygen saturation, increased Pco_2, as measured by blood gas studies
Cyanosis

RELATED FACTORS

See *Risk for Impaired Respiratory Function*.

▶ Inability to Sustain Spontaneous Ventilation

DEFINITION

A state in which an individual is unable to maintain adequate breathing to support life. This is measured by deterioration of arterial blood gases, increased work of breathing, and decreasing energy.

■■■ **AUTHOR'S NOTE**

This diagnosis represents respiratory insufficiency with corresponding metabolic changes that are incompatible with life. This situation requires rapid nursing and medical management, specifically resuscitation and mechanical ventilation. *Inability to Sustain Spontaneous Ventilation* is not appropriate as a nursing diagnosis; it is hypoxemia, a collaborative problem. Hypoxemia is insufficient plasma oxygen saturation from alveolar hypoventilation, pulmonary shunting, or ventilation-perfusion inequality. As a collaborative problem, physicians prescribe the definitive treatments; however, both nursing and medical-prescribed interventions are required for management. The nursing accountability is to monitor status continuously and to manage changes in status with the appropriate interventions using protocols. (For interventions refer to *Risk for Complications of Hypoxemia*, in Section 3 in Carpenito-Moyet, L. J. [2009]. *Nursing diagnosis: Application to clinical practice* [13th ed.]. Philadelphia: Lippincott Williams & Wilkins.)

DEFINING CHARACTERISTICS

Major (Must Be Present)

Dyspnea   Increased metabolic rate

Minor (May Be Present)

Increased restlessness   Increased heart rate
Apprehension   Decreased Po_2
Increased use of accessory muscles   Increased Pco_2
Decreased tidal volume   Decreased cooperation
    Decreased Sao_2

ROLE PERFORMANCE, INEFFECTIVE

DEFINITION

The state in which an individual experiences or is at risk of experiencing a disruption in the way he or she perceives that his or her role performance matches norms or expectations.

AUTHOR'S NOTE

This nursing diagnosis previously had been a subcategory under *Disturbed Self-Concept*. The use of this diagnosis in its present state may prove problematic. If a woman were unable to continue her household responsibilities because of illness and other family members assumed these responsibilities, the situations that might arise would better be described as *Risk for Disturbed Self-Concept related to recent loss of role responsibility secondary to illness* and *Risk for Impaired Home Maintenance Management related to lack of knowledge of family members*. Until clinical research defines this diagnosis more definitively, the nurse should use *Ineffective Role Performance* as a cause of *Disturbed Self-Concept* or *Risk for Impaired Home Maintenance*. If the role disturbance relates to parenting, the nurse should consider *Parental Role Conflict*.

DEFINING CHARACTERISTICS

Major (Must Be Present)

Conflict related to role perception or performance

Minor (May Be Present)

Change in self-perception of role
Denial of role
Change in others' perception of role
Change in physical capacity to resume role
Lack of knowledge of role
Change in usual patterns of responsibility

SEDENTARY LIFESTYLE

DEFINITION

The state in which an individual or group reports a habit of life that is characterized by a low physical activity level.

■■■ **AUTHOR'S NOTE**
This is the first nursing diagnosis submitted by a nurse from another country and accepted by NANDA. Congratulations to J. Adolf Gulirao-Goris of Valencia, Spain.

DEFINING CHARACTERISTICS

Major (Must Be Present, One or More)

Chooses a daily routine lacking physical exercise
Demonstrates physical deconditioning
Verbalizes preference for activities low in physical activity

RELATED FACTORS

Pathophysiologic

Related to decreased endurance secondary to obesity

Situational (Personal, Environment)

Related to inadequate knowledge of health benefits of physical activity
Related to inadequate knowledge of exercise routines
Related to insufficient resources (money, facilities)
Related to perceived lack of time
Related to lack of motivation
Related to lack of interest
Related to lack of injury

NOC

Knowledge: Health Behaviors, Physical Fitness

Goals

The person will verbalize intent to or engage in increased physical activity.

Indicators

- Sets a goal for weekly exercise.
- Identifies a desired activity or exercise.

NIC

Exercise Promotion, Exercise Therapy

Generic Interventions

Discuss Benefits of Exercise.

Reduces caloric absorption
Preserves lean muscle mass
Reduces depression, anxiety, stress
Improves body posture
Provides fun, recreation, diversion
Suppresses appetite
Increases oxygen uptake

Increases caloric expenditure
Maintains weight loss
Increases metabolic rate
Improves self-esteem
Increases restful sleep
Increases resistance to age-related degeneration

Assist Client to Identify Realistic Exercise Program.

Personality
Time of day
Safety
Physical size
Lifestyle
Season

Costs
Physical condition
Time factor
Occupation
Age

Discuss Aspects of Starting the Exercise Program.

Start slow and easy. Obtain clearance from physician.
Choose an activity that uses many body parts and is vigorous enough to cause "healthful fatigue."
Read, consult experts, and talk with friends/coworkers who exercise.
Plan a daily walking program:

- Start at 5 to 10 blocks for 0.5 to 1 mile/day; increase 1 block or 0.1 mile/week.
- Gradually increase rate and length of walk; remember to progress slowly.

Stop immediately if any of the following occur:
Tightness or pain in chest   Dizziness

Severe breathlessness
Lightheadedness

Loss of muscle control
Nausea

If pulse is 120 beats/minute (bpm) at 5 min or 100 bpm at 10 min after stopping exercise, or if shortness of breath occurs 10 min after exercise, slow down either the rate or the distance of walking.

If client cannot walk 5 blocks or 0.5 mile without signs of overexertion, decrease length of walking for 1 week to point before signs appear and then start to add 1 block/0.1 mile each week.

Walk at same rate; time with stopwatch or second hand on watch; after reaching 10 blocks (1 mile), try to increase speed.

Remember, increase only the rate or the distance of walking at one time.

Establish a regular time for exercise, with the goal of three to five times/week for 15 to 45 min and a heart rate of 80% of stress test or gross calculation (170 bpm for 20 to 29 years of age; decrease 10 bpm for each additional decade [e.g., 160 bpm for 30 to 39 years of age, 150 bpm for 40 to 49 years of age]).

Encourage significant others also to engage in walking program.

Add supplemental activity (e.g., parking far from destination, gardening, using stairs, spending weekends at activities that require walking).

Work up to 1 h of exercise per day at least 4 days per week.

Avoid lapses of more than 2 days between exercise sessions.

Assist Client to Increase Interest and Motivation.

Develop contract listing realistic short- and long-term goals.

Keep intake/activity records.

Increase knowledge by reading and talking with health-conscious friends and coworkers.

Make new friends who are health conscious.

Get a friend to also follow program or be a source of support.

Be aware of rationalization (e.g., a lack of time may be a lack of prioritization).

Keep a list of positive outcomes.

SELF-CARE DEFICIT SYNDROME

Self-Care Deficit Syndrome
Feeding Self-Care Deficit
Bathing Self-Care Deficit
Dressing Self-Care Deficit
Toileting Self-Care Deficit
Instrumental Self-Care Deficit*

DEFINITION

The state in which the individual experiences an impaired motor function or cognitive function, causing a decreased ability to perform each of the five self-care activities.

◼◼◼ AUTHOR'S NOTE

Self-care encompasses the activities needed to meet daily needs, usually called *activities of daily living*. Activities of daily living are learned and become life-long habits. Enmeshed in the broad category of self-care activities are tasks that *are* to be done (hygiene, bathing, dressing, toileting, feeding), *how* these tasks are done, and *when*, *where*, and *with whom* they are to be done. *Self-Care Deficit Syndrome*, not currently on the NANDA list, has been added to describe a person with compromised ability in all five self-care activities. The nurse will assess functioning in each of the five areas and identify the level of participation of which the person is capable. The goal will be to maintain that functioning or to increase participation and independence. The syndrome distinction will cluster all five self-care deficits together to provide clustering of interventions when indicated (e.g., to ensure that the individual is wearing the corrective lenses required). It also will permit specialized interventions for one of the five activities (e.g., to lay out clothes in the order in which they will be put on by the person).

The danger of *Self-Care Deficit* diagnoses is that the nurse could prematurely label a person as unable to participate at any level. This would eliminate a rehabilitation focus. The nurse must classify the client's functional level to promote independence.

*This diagnosis is not currently on the NANDA list, but has been included for clarity or usefulness.

DEFINING CHARACTERISTICS*

Major (One Deficit Must Be Present in Each Activity)

Self-Feeding Deficits
Unable to cut food or open packages
Unable to bring food to mouth

**Self-Bathing Deficits (Includes Washing Entire
Body, Combing Hair, Brushing Teeth, Attending
to Skin and Nail Care, and Applying Makeup)**
Unable or unwilling to wash body or body parts
Unable to obtain a water source
Unable to regulate temperature or water flow
Inability to perceive need for hygienic measures

**Self-Dressing Deficits (Including Donning
Regular or Special Clothing, Not Nightclothes)**
Impaired ability to put on or take off clothing
Unable to fasten clothing
Unable to groom self satisfactorily
Unable to obtain or replace articles of clothing

Self-Toileting Deficits
Unable or unwilling to get to toilet or commode
Unable or unwilling to carry out proper hygiene
Unable to transfer to and from toilet or commode
Unable to handle clothing to accommodate toileting
Unable to flush toilet or empty commode

Instrumental Self-Care Deficits
Difficulty using telephone
Difficulty accessing transportation
Difficulty laundering, ironing
Difficulty preparing meals
Difficulty shopping
Difficulty managing money
Difficulty with medication administration

*Evaluate each of the activities of daily living using the following coding scale:
  0 = Completely independent
  1 = Requires use of assistive device
  2 = Needs minimal help
  3 = Needs assistance or some supervision
  4 = Needs total supervision
  5 = Needs total assistance or unable to assist

RELATED FACTORS

Pathophysiologic

Related to lack of coordination secondary to (specify)
Related to spasticity or flaccidity secondary to (specify)
Related to muscular weakness secondary to (specify)
Related to partial or total paralysis secondary to (specify)
Related to atrophy secondary to (specify)
Related to muscle contractures secondary to (specify)
Related to visual disorders secondary to (specify)
Related to nonfunctioning or missing limb(s)
Related to regression to an earlier level of development
Related to excessive ritualistic behavior
Related to somatoform deficits (specify)

Treatment-Related

Related to external devices (specify), e.g., cast, splints, braces, IV equipment
Related to postoperative fatigue and pain

Situational (Personal, Environmental)

Related to cognitive deficits
Related to pain
Related to decreased motivation
Related to fatigue
Related to confusion
Related to disabling anxiety

Maturational

Older Adult
Related to decreased visual and motor ability, muscle weakness

ASSESSMENT

Subjective/Objective Data

Observed or reported inability or difficulty in performing some activity in each of the five areas of self-care.

NOC

See *Bathing, Feeding, Dressing, Toileting,* and/or *Instrumental Self-Care Deficit*

Goals

The person will participate in feeding, dressing, toileting, bathing activities

Indicators

- Identify preferences in self-care activities (e.g., time, products, location).
- Demonstrate optimal hygiene after assistance with care.

NIC

See *Feeding, Bathing, Dressing, Toileting,* and/or *Instrumental Self-Care Deficit*

Generic Interventions

Assess Causative or Contributing Factors.

Visual deficits
Impaired cognition
Decreased motivation
Impaired mobility
Lack of knowledge
Inadequate social support
Regression
Excessive ritualistic behavior

Promote Optimal Participation.

Promote Self-Esteem and Self-Determination.

During self-care activities, provide choices and request preferences.

Evaluate Ability to Participate in Each Self-Care Activity.

Encourage Client to Express Feelings About Self-Care Deficits.

For Self-Care Deficits Associated with Mental Disorders:

Encourage independence and involvement. Praise involvement.
Provide assistance with self-care activities. Remain nonjudgmental.
Avoid increasing person's dependency by doing for the person when he or she has demonstrated the ability to do independently.

Explore person's feelings about his or her disability and the need for help. Gently explore the disability and its purpose.

Refer to Interventions Under Each Diagnosis (Feeding, Bathing, Dressing, Toileting, and Instrumental Self-Care Deficit), as Indicated.

▶ Feeding Self-Care Deficit

DEFINITION

A state in which the individual experiences an impaired ability to perform or complete feeding activities for himself or herself.

DEFINING CHARACTERISTICS

Unable to cut food or open packages
Unable to bring food to mouth

RELATED FACTORS

See *Self-Care Deficit Syndrome*.

NOC

Nutritional Status, Self-Care: Eating, Swallowing Status

Goals

The person will demonstrate increased ability to feed self or report that he or she needs assistance.

Indicators

- Demonstrate ability to make use of adaptive devices, if indicated.
- Demonstrate increased interest and desire to eat.
- Describe rationale and procedure for treatment.
- Describe causative factors for feeding deficit.

NIC

Feeding, Self-Care Assistance: Feeding, Swallowing Therapy, Teaching: Aspiration Precautions

Generic Interventions

Ascertain from Person or Family Members What Foods the Person Likes or Dislikes.

Have Client Take Meals in the Same Setting, with Pleasant Surroundings that Are Not Too Distracting.

Maintain Correct Food Temperatures (Hot Foods Hot, Cold Foods Cold).

Provide Pain Relief, Because Pain Can Affect Appetite and Ability to Feed Self.

Provide Good Oral Hygiene Before and After Meals.

Encourage Person to Wear Dentures and Eyeglasses.

Place Person in the Most Normal Eating Position Suited to His or Her Physical Disability (Best is Sitting in a Chair at a Table).

Provide Social Contact During Eating.

For Perceptual Deficits:

Choose different-colored dishes to help distinguish items (e.g., red tray, white plates).

Ascertain person's usual eating patterns and provide food items according to preference (or arrange food items in clocklike pattern); record on care plan the arrangement used (e.g., meat, 6 o'clock; potatoes, 9 o'clock; vegetables, 12 o'clock).

Encourage eating of "finger foods" (e.g., bread, bacon, fruit, hot dogs) to promote independence.

To Enhance Maximum Independence, Provide Necessary Adaptive Devices:

Plate guard to avoid pushing food off plate
Suction device under plate or bowl for stabilization
Padded handles on utensils for a more secure grip
Wrist or hand splints with clamp to hold eating utensils
Special drinking cup
Rocker knife for cutting

Assist with Setup if Necessary, Opening Containers, Napkins, Condiment Packages; Cutting Meat; Buttering Bread.

For People with Cognitive Deficits:

Provide isolated, quiet atmosphere until person can attend to eating and is not easily distracted from the task.

Orient person to location and purpose of feeding equipment.

Place person in the most normal eating position he or she is physically able to assume.

Encourage person to attend to the task, but be alert for fatigue, frustration, or agitation.

For People Who Are Fearful of Being Poisoned:

Allow person to open canned foods.
Eat one cookie first.
Have family-style meals.

Assess to Ensure that Both Person and Family Understand the Reason for and Purpose of All Interventions.

▶ Bathing Self-Care Deficit

DEFINITION

A state in which the individual experiences an impaired ability to perform or complete bathing/activities for himself or herself.

DEFINING CHARACTERISTICS

Self-bathing deficits (including washing entire body, combing hair, brushing teeth, attending to skin and nail care, and applying makeup)
Unable or unwilling to wash body or body parts
Unable to obtain a water source
Unable to regulate temperature or water flow
Inability to perceive need for hygienic measures

RELATED FACTORS

See *Self-Care Deficit Syndrome*.

NOC

Self-Care: Activities of Daily Living, Self-Care: Bathing, Self-Care: Hygiene

Goals

The person will perform bathing activity at expected optimal level or report satisfaction with accomplishments despite limitations.

Indicators

• Relate feeling of comfort and satisfaction with body cleanliness.

- Demonstrate ability to use adaptive devices.
- Describe causative factors of bathing deficit.

NIC

Self-Care Assistance: Bathing/Hygiene, Teaching:
Individual

Generic Interventions

**Encourage Person to Wear Prescribed
Corrective Lenses or Hearing Aid.**

**Keep Bathroom Temperature Warm; Ascertain
Client's Preferred Water Temperature.**

Provide for Privacy During Bathing Routine.

Provide All Bathing Equipment Within Easy Reach.

**Provide for Safety in the Bathroom
(Nonslip Mats, Grab-Bars).**

When person is physically able, encourage use of either tub or
shower stall, depending on which facility is at home (the person
should practice in the hospital in preparation for going home).

Provide for Adaptive Equipment as Needed.

Chair or stool in bathtub or shower
Long-handled sponge to reach back or lower extremities
Grab-bars on bathroom walls where needed to assist in mobility
Bath board for transferring to tub chair or stool
Safety treads or nonslip mat on floor of bathroom, tub, and
    shower
Washing mitts with pocket for soap
Adapted toothbrushes
Shaver holders
Hand-held shower spray

For People with Visual Deficits:

Place bathing equipment in location most suitable to individual.
Keep call bell within reach if person is to bathe alone.
Give the visually impaired individual the same degree of privacy
    and dignity as any other person.
Verbally announce yourself before entering or leaving the
    bathing area.
Observe the person's ability to locate all bathing utensils.

Observe the person's ability to perform mouth care, hair combing, and shaving tasks.

Provide place for clean clothing within easy reach.

For People With Affected or Missing Limbs:

Bathe early in morning or before bed at night to avoid unnecessary dressing and undressing.

Encourage person to use a mirror during bathing to inspect the skin of paralyzed areas.

Encourage person with amputation to inspect remaining foot or stump for good skin integrity.

Provide only the amount of supervision or assistance necessary for relearning the use of extremity or adaptation to the handicap.

For People with Cognitive Deficits:

Provide a consistent time for the bathing routine as part of a structured program to help decrease confusion.

Keep instructions simple and avoid distractions; orient to purpose of bathing equipment.

If person is unable to bathe the entire body, have the individual bathe one part until it is done correctly; give positive reinforcement for success.

Supervise activity until person can safely perform the task unassisted.

Encourage attention to the task, but be alert for fatigue that may increase confusion.

Evaluate Bathing Facilities at Home, and Assist in Determining if There Is Any Need for Adaptations; Refer to Occupational Therapy or Social Services for Help in Obtaining Needed Home Equipment.

▶ Dressing Self-Care Deficit

DEFINITION

A state in which the individual experiences an impaired ability to perform or complete dressing and grooming activities for himself or herself.

DEFINING CHARACTERISTICS

Self-dressing deficits (including donning regular or special clothing, not nightclothes)

Impaired ability to put on or take off clothing
Unable to fasten clothing
Unable to groom self satisfactorily
Unable to obtain or replace articles of clothing

RELATED FACTORS

See *Self-Care Deficit Syndrome.*

NOC

Self-Care: Activities of Daily Living, Self-Care: Dressing,
Self-Care: Grooming

Goals

The person will demonstrate increased ability to dress self or the
need for having someone else assist him or her in performing the
task.

Indicators

- Demonstrate ability to learn how to use adaptive devices to fa-
  cilitate optimal independence in the task of dressing.
- Demonstrate increased interest in wearing street clothes.
- Describe causative factors for dressing deficit.
- Relate rationale and procedures for treatments.

NIC

Self-Care Assistance: Dressing/Grooming, Teaching:
Individual Dressing

Generic Interventions

**Encourage Person to Wear Prescribed
Corrective Lenses or Hearing Aid.**

**Promote Independence in Dressing Through
Continual and Unaided Practice.**

**Choose Clothing that is Loose-Fitting, With Wide
Sleeves and Pant Legs and Front Fasteners.**

**Allow Sufficient Time for Dressing and Undressing,
Because the Task May Be Tiring, Painful, or Difficult.**

**Plan for Person to Learn and Demonstrate One
Part of an Activity Before Progressing Further.**

Lay Clothes Out in the Order in Which They Will Be Needed to Dress.

Provide Dressing Aids as Necessary (Some Commonly Used Aids Include Dressing Stick, Swedish Reacher, Zipper Pull, Buttonhook, Long-Handled Shoehorn, and Shoe Fasteners Adapted With Elastic Laces, Velcro Closures, or Flip-Back Tongues; All Garments with Fasteners May Be Adapted with Velcro Closures).

Encourage Person to Wear Ordinary or Special Clothing Rather Than Nightclothes.

Provide for Privacy During Dressing Routine.

For People with Visual Deficits:

Allow person to ascertain the most convenient location for clothing, and adapt the environment to accomplish the task (e.g., remove unnecessary barriers).

Verbally announce yourself before entering or leaving the dressing area.

For People with Cognitive Deficits:

Establish a consistent dressing routine to provide a structured program to decrease confusion.

Keep instructions simple, and repeat them frequently; avoid distractions.

Introduce one article of clothing at a time.

Encourage attention to the task; be alert for fatigue, which may increase confusion.

Assess Understanding and Knowledge of Individual and Family for Above Instructions and Rationale.

▶ Toileting Self-Care Deficit

DEFINITION

A state in which the individual experiences an impaired ability to perform or complete toileting activities.

DEFINING CHARACTERISTICS

Unable or unwilling to get to toilet or commode
Unable or unwilling to carry out proper hygiene
Unable to transfer to and from toilet or commode

Unable to handle clothing to accommodate toileting
Unable to flush toilet or empty commode

RELATED FACTORS

See *Self-Care Deficit Syndrome*.

NOC

Self-Care: Activities of Daily Living, Self-Care: Hygiene,
Self-Care: Toileting

Goals

The person will demonstrate increased ability to toilet self or report the need to have someone assist him or her to perform the task.

Indicators

- Demonstrate ability to make use of adaptive devices to facilitate toileting.
- Describe causative factors for toileting deficit.
- Relate rationale and procedures for treatment.

NIC

Self-Care Assistance: Toileting, Self-Care Assistance:
Hygiene, Teaching: Individual, Mutual Goal Setting

Generic Interventions

**Encourage Person to Wear Prescribed
Corrective Lenses or Hearing Aid.**

**Obtain Bladder and Bowel History from
Client or Significant Other (See Constipation
or Impaired Urinary Elimination).**

**Ascertain Communication System Person
Uses to Express the Need to Toilet.**

**Maintain Bladder and Bowel Record
to Determine Toileting Patterns.**

**Avoid Development of "Bowel Fixation"
by Less Frequent Discussion and Inquiries
About Bowel Movements.**

Be Alert to Possibility of Falls When Toileting Person (Be Prepared to Ease Him or Her to Floor Without Injuring Either of You).

Achieve Independence in Toileting by Continual and Unaided Practice.

Allow Sufficient Time for Toileting to Avoid Fatigue (Lack of Sufficient Time to Use the Toilet May Cause Incontinence or Constipation).

Avoid Use of Indwelling Catheters and Condom Catheters to Expedite Bladder Continence (if Possible).

For People with Visual Deficits:

Keep call bell easily accessible so person can quickly obtain help to get to toilet; answer call bell promptly to decrease anxiety.

If bedpan or urinal is necessary for toileting, be sure it is within person's reach.

Verbally announce yourself before entering or leaving toileting area.

Observe person's ability to obtain equipment or get to the toilet unassisted.

Provide for a safe and clear pathway to toilet area.

For People with Affected or Missing Limbs:

Provide only the amount of supervision and assistance necessary for relearning or adapting to the prosthesis.

Encourage person to look at affected area or limb and use it during toileting tasks.

Encourage useful transfer techniques taught by occupational or physical therapy (the nurse should familiarize himself or herself with planned mode of transfer).

Provide the necessary adaptive devices to enhance independence and safety (commode chairs, spill-proof urinals, fracture bedpans, raised toilet seats, support side rails for toilets).

Provide for a safe and clear pathway to toilet area.

For People with Cognitive Deficits:

Offer toileting reminders every 2 hours, after meals, and before bedtime.

When person is able to indicate the need to use toilet, begin toileting at 2-hour intervals, after meals, and before bedtime.

Answer call bell immediately to avoid frustration and incontinence.

Encourage wearing ordinary clothes (many confused individuals are continent while wearing regular clothing).

Avoid the use of bedpans and urinals; if physically possible, provide a normal atmosphere of elimination in bathroom (the toilet used should remain constant to promote familiarity).

Give verbal cues as to what is expected of the individual, and give positive reinforcement for success.

See *Impaired Urinary Elimination* for additional information on incontinence.

Ascertain Home Toileting Needs, and Refer to Occupational Therapy or Social Services for Help in Obtaining Necessary Equipment.

▶ Instrumental Self-Care Deficit

DEFINITION

A state in which the individual experiences an impaired ability to perform certain activities or access certain services essential for managing a household.

> **AUTHOR'S NOTE**
> *Instrumental Self-Care Deficit* describes problems in performing certain activities or accessing certain services needed to live in the community (e.g., telephone use, shopping, money management). This diagnosis is important to consider in discharge planning and during assessment by the community nurse.

DEFINING CHARACTERISTICS

Major (Must Be Present, One or More)

Observed or reported difficulty in:
- Using a telephone
- Accessing transportation
- Laundering, ironing
- Preparing meals
- Shopping (food, clothes)
- Managing money
- Medication administration

RELATED FACTORS

See *Self-Care Deficit Syndrome*.

NOC
Self-Care: Instrumental Activities of Daily Living

Goals

The person, family will report satisfaction with household management.

Indicators
- Demonstrate use of adaptive devices (e.g., telephone, cooking aids).
- Describe a method to ensure adherence to medication schedule.
- Report ability to call on and answer telephone.
- Report regular laundering by self or others.
- Report daily intake of two nutritious meals.
- Identify transportation options to stores, physician, house of worship, social activities.
- Demonstrate management of simple money transactions.
- Identify individuals who will assist with money matters.

NIC
Teaching: Individual, Family Involvement Promotion

Generic Interventions

Assess for Causative and Contributing Factors.

Visual, hearing deficits
Impaired cognition
Impaired mobility
Lack of knowledge
Inadequate social support

Assist Client to Identify Self-Help Devices.

Promote Self-Care and Safety with Clients Who Have Cognitive Deficits.

Evaluate activities that are achievable.
Evaluate ability to procure, select, and prepare nutritious food daily.
Teach hints for adherence to medicine schedule (e.g., 7-day pill holder, separate pill for each time to be taken).
Evaluate ability to understand money, budget money, and pay bills.

Determine Sources of Transportation (e.g., Church Groups, Neighbors).

Determine Sources of Social Support (Transportation, Laundry, Money Matters).

Discuss the Importance of Identifying Need for Assistance (e.g., Department of Social Services, Agency on Aging).

SELF-CONCEPT, DISTURBED

Disturbed Self-Concept*
Disturbed Body Image
Disturbed Personal Identity
Disturbed Self-Esteem
Chronic Low Self-Esteem
Situational Low Self-Esteem
Risk for Situational Low Self-Esteem

DEFINITION

The state in which an individual experiences, or is at risk of experiencing, a negative state of change about the way he or she feels, thinks, or views himself or herself. It may include a change in body image, self-esteem, or personal identity (Boyd, 2005).

■■■■ **AUTHOR'S NOTE**
Disturbed Self-Concept represents a broad category under which more specific categories fall. Initially the nurse may not have sufficient clinical data to validate a more specific diagnosis such as *Chronic Low Self-Esteem* or *Disturbed Body Image*; thus, he or she can use *Disturbed Self-Concept* until more specific diagnoses can be supported with data.

DEFINING CHARACTERISTICS

This diagnosis reflects a broad diagnostic category which can be used initially until more specific assessment data can support a specific nursing diagnosis such as *Disturbed Body Image* or *Disturbed Self-Esteem*.

*This diagnosis is not currently on the NANDA list, but has been included for clarity or usefulness.

Some examples observed or reported:
- Verbal or nonverbal negative responses to actual or perceived change in structure and/or function (e.g., shame, embarrassment, guilt, revulsion)
- Expressions of shame or guilt
- Rationalizes away or rejects positive feedback and exaggerates negative feedback about self
- Hypersensitivity to slight criticism
- Episodic occurrence of negative self-appraisal in response to life events in a person with a previously positive self-evaluation
- Verbalization of negative feelings about self (helplessness, uselessness)
- Displaying hostility toward the healthy
- Showing change in ability to estimate relationship of body to environment

RELATED FACTORS

A self-concept disturbance can occur as a response to a variety of health problems, situations, and conflicts. Some common sources include the following.

Pathophysiologic

Related to change in appearance, lifestyle, role, and response of others secondary to:

Loss of body part(s)	Chronic disease
Loss of body function(s)	Pain
Severe trauma	

Situational (Personal, Environmental)

Related to feelings of abandonment or failure secondary to:
Divorce, separation from, or death of significant other
Loss of job or ability to work

Related to immobility or loss of function
Related to unsatisfactory relationships (parental, spousal)
Related to change in usual patterns of responsibilities

Maturational

Older Adult
Related to multiple losses (job, roles, etc.)

NOC

Quality of Life, Coping, Depression, Violence Control, Self-Esteem

Goals

The person will demonstrate healthy adaptation and coping skills.

Indicators
- Appraise situations in a realistic manner without distortions.
- Verbalize and demonstrate increased positive feelings.

NIC

Hope Instillation, Mood Management, Values Clarification, Counseling, Referrals, Support Group, Coping Enhancement

Generic Interventions

Encourage Person to Express Feelings, Especially About the Way Person Feels, Thinks, or Views Self.

Encourage Person to Ask Questions about Health Problem, Treatment, Progress, Prognosis.

Provide Reliable Information and Reinforce Information Already Given.

Elicit Areas that He or She Would Like to Change. Encourage to Consider Options.

Clarify Any Misconceptions the Person Has About Self, Care, or Caregivers.

Avoid Criticism.

Provide Privacy and a Safe Environment.

If Indicated, Refer to **Disturbed Self-Esteem** or **Disturbed Body Image** for Interventions.

Teach Person What Community Resources Are Available, If Needed (e.g., Mental Health Centers, Self-help Groups Such as Reach for Recovery, Make Today Count).

Pediatric Interventions

Allow the Child to Bring His or Her Own Experiences Into the Situation (e.g., Some Children Say that an Injection Feels Like a Insect Sting, and Some Say They Don't Feel Anything). "After We Do This, You Can Tell Me How It Felt."

Avoid Using "Good" or "Bad" to Describe Behavior. Be Specific and Descriptive (e.g., "You Really Helped Me by Holding Still. Thank You for Helping.").

Connect a Previous Experience with the Present One (e.g., "The X-ray Camera Will Look Different from the Last Time. You Will Have to Hold Real Still Again. The Table Will Move Too.").

Convey Optimism with Positive Self-talk (e.g., "I Am So Busy Today. I Wonder if I Will Get All My Work Done? I Bet I Can." "When You Come Back from Surgery, You Will Need to Stay in Bed. What Would You Like to Do When You Come Back?").

Help the Child Plan Playtime with Choices. Encourage Crafts that Produce a Product.

Encourage Interaction with Peers and Supportive Adults.

Encourage Decoration of Room with Crafts and Personal Items.

▶ Disturbed Body Image

DEFINITION

The state in which an individual experiences, or is at risk to experience a disruption in the way he/she perceives his/her body.

DEFINING CHARACTERISTICS

Major (Must Be Present)

Verbal or nonverbal negative response to actual or perceived change in structure or function (e.g., shame, embarrassment, guilt, revulsion)

Minor (May Be Present)

Not looking at body part
Not touching body part
Hiding or overexposing body part
Change in social involvement
Negative feelings about body, feelings of helplessness, hopelessness, powerlessness, vulnerability
Preoccupation with change or loss
Refusal to verify actual change

Depersonalization of part or loss
Self-destructive behaviors (e.g., mutilation, suicide attempts, overeating, undereating)

RELATED FACTORS

Pathophysiologic

Related to changes in appearance secondary to:
Chronic disease
Loss of body part
Loss of body function
Severe trauma

Related to unrealistic perceptions of appearance secondary to:
Psychoses
Anorexia nervosa or bulimia

Treatment-Related

Related to changes in appearance secondary to:
Hospitalization
Surgery
Chemotherapy or radiation

Situational

Related to physical trauma secondary to:
Sexual abuse or rape (perpetrator known or unknown)

Related to effects of (specify) on appearance (e.g., obesity, pregnancy, immobility)

Maturational

Related to developmental changes

NOC

Body Image, Child Development (specify age), Grief Resolution, Psychosocial Adjustment, Life Change, Self-Esteem

Goals

The person will implement new coping patterns and verbalize and demonstrate acceptance of appearance (grooming, dress, posture, eating patterns, presentation of self).

Indicators

• Demonstrate a willingness and ability to resume self-care/role responsibilities.

- Initiate new or reestablish contacts with existing support systems.

NIC

Self-Esteem Enhancement, Counseling, Presence, Active Listening, Body Image Enhancement, Grief Work Facilitation, Support Group Referral

Generic Interventions

Encourage Person to Express Feelings, Especially about the Way He or She Feels, Thinks, or Views Self.

Encourage Person to Ask Questions About Health Problem, Treatment, Progress, Prognosis.

Provide Reliable Information, and Reinforce Information Already Given.

Clarify Any Misconceptions the Person Has About Self, Care, or Caregivers.

Prepare Significant Others for Physical and Emotional Changes. Support Family Members as They Adapt.

Encourage Visits from Peers and Significant Others. Advise Them to Share with the Person How Important He or She Is to Them.

Encourage Contact (Letters, Telephone) with Peers and Family.

Provide Opportunity to Share with People Going Through Similar Experiences.

For Loss of Body Part or Function:

Assess the meaning of the loss for the individual and significant others, as related to visibility of loss, function of loss, and emotional investment.

Expect the individual to respond to the loss with denial, shock, anger, and depression.

Be aware of the effect of the responses of others to the loss; encourage sharing of feelings among significant others.

Allow individual to ventilate feelings and grieve.

Use role-playing to assist with sharing.

Explore realistic alternatives and provide encouragement.

Explore strengths and resources with person.

Assist with the Resolution of a Surgically Created Alteration of Body Image.

Replace the lost body part with prosthesis as soon as possible.
Encourage viewing of site.
Encourage touching of site.

For Changes Associated with Chemotherapy (Cooley et al., 1986):

Discuss the possibility of hair loss, absence of menses, temporary or permanent sterility, decreased estrogen levels, vaginal dryness, mucositis.

Encourage person to share concerns, fears, and perception of the impact of these changes on his or her life.

Explain where hair loss may occur (head, eyelashes, eyebrows, and axillary, pubic, and leg hair).

Explain that hair will grow back after treatment but may change in color and texture.

Have person select a wig and wear it before hair loss. Consult a beautician for tips on how to vary the look of the wig (e.g., combs, clips).

Encourage the wearing of scarves, turbans when wig is not on.

Teach to minimize the amount of hair loss:

- Avoid excessive shampooing; use a conditioner twice weekly.
- Pat hair dry gently.
- Avoid electric curlers, dryers, and curling irons.
- Avoid pulling hair with bands, clips, or bobby pins.
- Avoid hair spray and hair dye.
- Use a wide-tooth comb; avoid vigorous brushing.

Refer to American Cancer Society for information regarding new or used wigs. Inform that the wig is a tax-deductible item.

Discuss the Difficulty that Others (Spouse, Friends, Coworkers) May Have with Visible Changes.

Allow Significant Others Opportunities to Share Feelings and Fears.

Assist Significant Others to Identify Positive Aspects of the Client and Ways This Can Be Shared.

Teach Person What Community Resources Are Available if Needed (e.g., Mental Health Centers, Self-Help Groups Such as Reach for Recovery, Make Today Count).

👫 Pediatric Interventions

Discuss with Parents How Body Image Develops and What Interactions Contribute to Their Child's Self-Perceptions.

Teach the names and functions of body parts.
Acknowledge changes (e.g., height).
Allow some choices of what to wear.

Ask Child to Draw a Picture of His or Her Body Just after a Bath (Naked). Ask to Describe Picture.

Focus Child on Body Changes (e.g., "What Can You Do Now That You Couldn't Do When You Were Little?").

Adolescent Interventions

Discuss with Parents the Adolescent's Need to "Fit In."
Do not dismiss adolescent's concerns too quickly.
Be flexible and compromise when possible (e.g., clothes are temporary, tattoos are not).
Negotiate a time to think about it (e.g., 4 to 6 weeks).
Provide reasons for denying a request. Elicit adolescent's reasons. Compromise if possible (e.g., curfew parents want, 11:00; adolescent, 12:00; compromise 11:30).

Provide Opportunities to Discuss Concerns When Parents Are Not Present.

Ask to Describe Best Features and Those He or She Dislikes.

Prepare for Impending Developmental Changes.

👫 Maternal Interventions

Teach Couples about Anticipated Physiologic Changes and Possible Changes In Sexual Response.

Allow Woman Opportunities to Discuss Her Feelings Regarding Body Changes.

▶ Disturbed Personal Identity

DEFINITION

The state in which an individual experiences, or is at risk of experiencing, an inability to distinguish between self and nonself.

AUTHOR'S NOTE
Disturbed Personal Identity is a very complex diagnosis and should not be used to relabel autism. It may be more useful in nursing to use *Anxiety* or *Impaired Social Interactions* for a nursing focus

DEFINING CHARACTERISTICS (VARCAROLIS, 2007, P. 2040)

Appears unaware of or uninterested in others or their actions
Unable to identify parts of the body or body sensations, e.g., enuresis
Excessively imitates another's actions or words
Fails to distinguish parent/caretakers as a whole person
Becomes distressed with body contact with others
Spends long periods of time in self stimulating behaviors (touching self, sucking, rocking)
Needs ritualistic behaviors and sameness to control anxiety
Cannot tolerate being separated from parent/caregiver

RELATED FACTORS (VARCAROLIS, 2007, P. 103)

Pathophysiologic

Related to biochemical imbalance
Related to impaired neurological development or dysfuction

Maturational

Related to failure to develop attachment behaviors resulting in fixation at autisitic phase of development
Related to separation anxiety secondary to interrupted or incompleted separation/individualization process
Interventions/rationale
Refer to chronic low self-esteem

▶ Disturbed Self-Esteem

DEFINITION

The state in which an individual experiences, or is at risk of experiencing, negative self-evaluation about self or capabilities.

■■■ **AUTHOR'S NOTE**
Self-esteem is one of the four components of self-concept. *Disturbed Self-Esteem* is the general diagnostic category. *Chronic Low Self-Esteem* and *Situational Low Self-Esteem* represent specific types of *Disturbed Self-Esteem*, thus involving more specific interventions. Initially, the nurse may not have sufficient clinical data to validate a more specific diagnosis, such as *Chronic Low Self-Esteem* or *Situational Low Self-Esteem*. Refer to the major defining characteristics under these diagnoses for validation.

DEFINING CHARACTERISTICS

Overt or Covert:
Self-negating verbalization
Expressions of shame or guilt*
Evaluation of self as unable to deal with events*
Rationalizing away/rejecting positive feedback and exaggerating negative feedback about self*
Inability to set goals
Indecisiveness
Lack of/poor problem-solving
Signs of depression (sleeping, eating)
Seeking approval or reassurance excessively
Poor body presentation (posture, eye contact, movements)
Self-abusive behavior (mutilation, suicide attempts, nail biting, substance abuse, becoming a victim)
Hesitation to try new things/situations*
Denial of problems obvious to others
Projection of blame/responsibility for problems*
Rationalization of personal failures*
Hypersensitivity to slight criticism*
Grandiosity*

RELATED FACTORS

Disturbed Self-Esteem can be either an episodic event or a chronic problem. Failure to resolve a problem or multiple sequential

---

*Norris, J., & Kunes-Connell, M. (1987). Self-esteem disturbance: A clinical validation study. In A. McLane (Ed.), *Classification of nursing diagnoses: Proceedings of the seventh NANDA national conference*. St. Louis: C. V. Mosby.

stresses can result in *Chronic Low Self-Esteem*. Factors that occur with time and are associated with *Chronic Low Self-Esteem* are indicated by CLSE.

Pathophysiologic

Related to change in appearance secondary to:
Loss of body part(s)
Loss of body function(s)
Disfigurement (trauma, surgery, birth defects)
Related to biochemical/neurophysiologic imbalance

Situational (Personal, Environmental)

Related to unmet dependency needs
Related to lack of positive feedback

Related to feelings of abandonment secondary to:
Death of significant other
Child abduction/murder
Separation from significant other

Related to feelings of failure secondary to:
Unemployment
Financial problems
Loss of job or ability to work
Relationship problems
Marital discord
Separation
Step-parents
In-laws
Increase/decrease in weight
Premenstrual syndrome

Related to failure in school
Related to history of ineffective relationship with own parents (CLSE)
Related to history of abusive relationships (CLSE)
Related to unrealistic expectations of child by parent (CLSE)
Related to unrealistic expectations of self (CLSE)
Related to unrealistic expectations of parent by child (CLSE)
Related to parental rejection (CLSE)
Related to inconsistent punishment (CLSE)
Related to feelings of helplessness or failure secondary to: institutionalization (e.g., mental health facility, jail, orphanage, halfway house)
Related to history of numerous failures (CLSE)

Maturational

Infant/Toddler/Preschooler
Related to lack of stimulation or closeness (CLSE)
Related to separation from parents/significant others (CLSE)
Related to continual negative evaluation by parents
Related to inadequate parental support (CLSE)
Related to inability to trust significant other (CLSE)

School Age
Related to failure to achieve grade-level objectives
Related to loss of peer group
Related to repeated negative feedback (CLSE)

Adolescent
Related to loss of independence and autonomy secondary to (specify)
Related to disruption of peer relationships
Related to scholastic problems
Related to loss of significant others

Middle Age
Related to changes associated with aging

Older Adult
Related to losses (people, function, financial, retirement)

NOC
Refer to *Chronic Low Self-Esteem*

Goals

The person will express a positive outlook for the future and resume previous level of functioning.

Indicators
- Identify source of threat to self-esteem and work through that issue.
- Identify positive aspects of self.
- Analyze own behavior and its consequences.
- Identify one positive aspect of change.

NIC
Refer to *Chronic Low Self-Esteem*

Generic Interventions

Establish a Trusting Nurse–Client Relationship.

Encourage person to express feelings, especially about way he or she thinks or views self.

Encourage person to ask questions about health problem, treatment, progress, prognosis.

Provide reliable information and reinforce information already given.

Clarify any misconceptions the person has about self, care, or caregivers. Avoid criticism.

Promote Social Interaction.

Assist person to accept help from others.

Avoid overprotection while still limiting the demands made on the individual.

Encourage movement.

Explore Strengths and Resources with Person.

Discuss Expectations.

Explore realistic alternatives.

Refer to Community Resources as Indicated (e.g., Counseling, Assertiveness Courses).

▶ Chronic Low Self-Esteem

DEFINITION

The state in which an individual experiences a long-standing negative self-evaluation about self or capabilities.

DEFINING CHARACTERISTICS (NORRIS & KUNES-CONNELL, 1987)

Major (80% to 100%)

Long-Standing or Chronic:
Self-negating verbalization
Expressions of shame/guilt
Evaluation of self as unable to deal with events
Rationalizing away/rejecting positive feedback and exaggerating negative feedback about self
Hesitation to try new things/situations

Minor (50% to 79%)

Frequent lack of success in work or other life events
Overly conforming, dependent on opinions of others
Poor body presentation (eye contact, posture, movements)
Nonassertive/passive
Indecisive
Excessively seeking reassurance

RELATED FACTORS

See *Disturbed Self-Esteem*.

NOC

Depression Level, Self-Esteem, Quality of Life,
Depression self-control

Goals

The individual will identify positive aspects of self and a realistic
appraisal of limitations.

Indicators

- Modify excessive and unrealistic self-expectations.
- Verbalize acceptance of limitations.
- Verbalize nonjudgmental perceptions of self.
- Cease self-abusive behavior.
- Begin to take verbal and behavioral risks.

NIC

Hope Instillation, Anxiety Reduction, Self-Enhancement,
Coping Enhancement, Socialization Enhancement,
Referral

Generic Interventions

Assist the Person to Reduce Anxiety Level.

Assist to indentify cognitive distortions that
increase negative self-appraisal (Varcarolis, 2007)

With overgeneralization, teach to
focus on each event as separate

With self-blame, teach to evauate if he/
she is really responsible and why.

If Mind-reading, Advise to Clarify Verbally
What He/She Thinks Is Happening.

Teach Not To Discount Positive Responses of
Others by Simple Responding with Thank You.

Provide Encouragement as a Task or Skill
Is Attempted. Allow Person to Perform
as Independently as Possible.

Assist Person in Expressing Thoughts and Feelings.

Encourage Visits/Contact with Peers and
Significant Others (Letters, Telephone).

Be a Role Model in One-to-One Interactions.

Involve in Activities, Especially When
Strengths Can Be Used.

Do Not Allow Person to Isolate Self (Refer to
Social Isolation for Further Interventions).

Set Limits on Problematic Behavior, Such as
Aggression, Poor Hygiene, Ruminations, and
Suicidal Preoccupation. Refer to **Risk for Suicide** or
Risk for Violence if these are assessed as problems.

Encourage Activities That Exercise Large
Muscles (e.g., Walking, Biking, Swimming).

Avoid Competitive Activities.

Provide for Development of Social
and Vocational Skills.

Refer for Vocational Counseling If Indicated.

Pediatric Interventions

Provide opportunities for child to be successful and needed.
Personalize the child's environment with pictures, possessions,
   and crafts made.
Provide structured and unstructured playtime.
Ensure continuance of academic experiences in the hospital or
   home. Provide uninterrupted time for school work.

Geriatric Interventions (Miller, 2009)

Acknowledge person by name.
Use tone of voice that you would use for own peer group.
Avoid words associated with babies (e.g., diapers).

Ask about family pictures, personal items, and past experiences.
Avoid attributing disabilities to "old age."
Knock on door of bedrooms and bathrooms.
Allow person enough time to accomplish tasks at own pace.

▶ Situational Low Self-Esteem

DEFINITION

The state in which an individual who previously had positive self-esteem experiences negative feelings about self in response to an event (loss, change).

▦▰▰ AUTHOR'S NOTE

Although *Situational Low Self-Esteem* is an episodic event, repeated occurrences or the continuation of these negative self-appraisals over time can lead to *Chronic Low Self-Esteem*.

DEFINING CHARACTERISTICS (NORRIS & KUNES-CONNELL, 1987)

Major (80% to 100%)

Episodic occurrence of negative self-appraisal in response to life events in a person with a previously positive self-evaluation
Verbalization of negative feelings about self (helplessness, uselessness)

Minor (50% to 79%)

Self-negating verbalizations
Expressions of shame/guilt
Evaluation of self as unable to handle situations/events
Difficulty making decisions
Self-neglect
Social isolation

RELATED FACTORS

See *Disturbed Self-Esteem*.

NOC

Decision Making, Grief Resolution, Psychosocial Adjustment, Life Change, Self-Esteem

Goals

The person will express a positive outlook for the future and resume previous level of functioning.

Indicators

- Identify source of threat to self-esteem and work through that issue.
- Identify positive aspects of self.
- Analyze own behavior and its consequences.
- Identify one positive aspect of change.

NIC

Active Listening, Presence, Counseling, Cognitive Restructuring, Family Support, Support Group, Coping Enhancement

Generic Interventions

Assist the Individual In Identifying and Expressing Feelings.

Practice Self-Talk (Murray, 2000).

Write a brief description of the change and the consequence that it has created (e.g., "My spouse has had an affair. I am betrayed.").

Write three things that may be useful about this situation.

Communicate that the Person Can Handle the Change.

Challenge the Person to Imagine Positive Futures and Outcomes.

Examine and Reinforce Positive Abilities and Traits (e.g., Hobbies, Skills, School, Relationships, Appearance, Loyalty, Industriousness).

Encourage an Activity that Exercises Large Muscles (e.g., Walking, Swimming, Biking). Avoid Competitive Situations.

Encourage Examination of Current Behavior and Its Consequences (e.g., Dependency, Procrastination, Isolation).

Help to Identify Negative Automatic Thoughts and Overgeneralizing.

Assist in Identifying Own Responsibility
and Control in a Situation (e.g., When
Continually Blaming Others for Problems).

Refer to Community Resources as
Indicated (e.g., Reach for Recovery).

▶ Risk for Situational Low Self-Esteem

DEFINITION

The state in which an individual who previously had a positive
self-esteem is at risk to experience negative feelings about self in
response to an event (loss, change).

RISK FACTORS

Refer to *Situational Low Self-Esteem*.

NOC

See *Situational Low Self-Esteem*

Goals

The person will continue to express a positive outlook for the future and to identify positive aspects of self.

Indicators
- Identify threats to self-esteem.
- Identify one positive aspect of change.

NIC

See *Situational Low-Self-Esteem*

General Interventions

Refer to *Situational Low Self-Esteem*.

SELF-HARM, RISK FOR*

Risk for Self-Harm
Self-Mutilation
Risk for Self-Mutilation
Risk for Suicide†

DEFINITION

A state in which an individual is at risk for inflicting direct harm on himself or herself. This may include one or more of the following: self-abuse, self-mutilation, suicide.

> ### ■■■ AUTHOR'S NOTE
> *Risk for Self-Harm* represents a broad diagnosis that can encompass self-abuse, self-mutilation, or risk for suicide. Although initially they may appear the same, the distinction lies in the intent. "Self-mutilation and self-abuse are pathological attempts to relieve stress (temporary reprieve), whereas suicide is an attempt to die (to relieve stress permanently)" (Carscadden, 1993; personal communication). *Risk for Self-Harm* can also be a useful early diagnosis when insufficient data are present to differentiate one from the other.

DEFINING CHARACTERISTICS

Major (Must Be Present, One or More)

Expresses desire or intent to harm self
Expresses desire to die or commit suicide
Has history of attempts to harm self

Minor

Reports or Observed:

Depression   Hopelessness
Poor self-concept   Helplessness

---

*This diagnosis is not currently on the NANDA list but has been included for clarity or usefulness.

†This diagnosis is not currently on the NANDA list but has been included for clarity or usefulness.

Hallucinations/delusions
Substance abuse
Poor impulse control
Agitation

Lack of support system
Emotional pain
Hostility

RELATED FACTORS

Risk for Self-Harm can occur as a response to a variety of health problems, situations, and conflicts. Some sources are listed below.

Pathophysiologic

Related to feelings of helplessness, loneliness, or hopelessness secondary to:
Disabilities
Chemical dependency
Terminal illness
Substance abuse
Chronic illness
Mental impairment (organic or traumatic)
Chronic pain
Psychiatric disorder
   Schizophrenia
   Bipolar disorder
   Post-traumatic stress
    disorder

   Personality disorder
   Adolescent adjustment disorder
   Somatoform disorders

New diagnosis of positive HIV status

Treatment-Related

Related to unsatisfactory outcome of treatment (medical, surgical, psychological)

Related to prolonged dependence on, e.g., dialysis, insulin injections, chemotherapy/radiation, ventilator

Situational (Personal, Environmental)

Related to:
Depression
Ineffective individual coping skills
   Substance abuse in family

Child abuse (present, past)
Parental/marital conflict

Related to real or perceived loss secondary to:
Finances/job
Threat of abandonment
Death of significant others

Status/prestige
Separation/divorce
Someone leaving home

Related to wish for revenge on real or perceived injury (body or self-esteem)

Related to multiple losses associated with AIDS

Maturational

Adolescent

Related to feelings of abandonment
Related to unrealistic expectations of child by parents
Related to peer pressure or rejection
Related to depression
Related to relocation
Related to significant loss

Older Adult

Related to multiple losses secondary to retirement, social isolation, significant loss, or illness

NOC

Aggression Control, Impulse Control

Goals

The person will choose alternatives that are not harmful.

Indicators

- Acknowledge self-harm thoughts.
- Admit to use of self-harm behavior if it occurs.
- Be able to identify personal triggers.
- Learn to properly identify and tolerate uncomfortable feelings.

NIC

Presence, Anger Control, Environmental Management: Violence Prevention, Behavior Modification, Security Enhancement, Therapy Group, Coping Enhancement, Impulse Control Training, Crisis Intervention

Generic Interventions

Demonstrate an Acceptance of the Individual as a Worthwhile Person Through the Use of Nonjudgmental Statements and Behavior.

Actively listen or provide support by just being there if the person is silent.
Label the behavior, not the person.

Assist in Recognizing the Presence of Hope and the Element of Alternatives.

Orient Individual as Required. Point Out Sensory or Environmental Misperceptions Without Belittling Fears or Indicating Disapproval of Verbal Expressions.

Help Reframe Old Thinking/Feeling Patterns.

Assist in identifying thought–feeling–behavior concept.
Help assess payoffs and drawbacks to self-harm.
Encourage identification of personal triggers.
Facilitate the development of new behaviors.

Validate Good Coping Skills Already in Existence.

Encourage the Use of Positive Affirmations, Meditation and Relaxation Techniques, and Other Esteem-Building Exercises.

Encourage Journaling, Keeping a Diary of Triggers, Thoughts, and Feelings, and Alternatives That Do or Do Not Work.

Assist in Developing Body Awareness as a Method of Ascertaining Triggers and Determining Levels of Impending Self-Harm.

Introduce "Contracting" to Individual.

Assist in Role-Playing to Solve Problems in Situations/Relationships.

Reduce Excessive Stimuli.

Intervene at Earliest Stages to Assist Person to Regain Control, Prevent Escalation, and Allow Treatment in the Least Restrictive Manner.

Promote the Use of Alternatives.

Stress that there are always alternatives.
Stress that self-harm is a choice, not something uncontrollable.
Allow opportunities for verbal expression of thoughts and
    feelings.
Provide acceptable physical outlets.

Initiate Support Systems to Community When Indicated.

Teach Family:

Constructive expression of feelings
How to recognize levels of impending self-harm
How to assist with appropriate interventions
How to deal with self-harm behavior/results

Supply Phone Number of 24-Hour Emergency Hotlines.

Recommend Counseling, as Appropriate.

Leisure/vocational counseling
Halfway houses
Other community resources

❱ Self-Mutilation

DEFINITION

The state in which an individual has performed a deliberate act on the self with the intent to injure, not kill, that produces immediate tissue damage.

DEFINING CHARACTERISTICS

Expresses desire or intent to harm self
Past history of attempts to harm self, including:

Cutting	Scratching
Slashing	Picking
Stabbing	Gouging

RELATED FACTORS

See *Risk for Self-Harm.*

Goals

See *Risk for Self-Harm.*

Generic Interventions

See *Risk for Self-Harm.*

❱ Risk for Self-Mutilation

DEFINITION

A state in which an individual is at risk to perform a deliberate act upon the self with the intent to injure, not kill, which produces immediate tissue damage to the body.

DEFINING CHARACTERISTICS

Major (Must Be Present, One or More)

Expresses desire or intent to harm self
History of attempts to harm self, e.g.:

- Cutting, slashing
- Stabbing, picking
- Scratching
- Gouging

RELATED FACTORS

See *Risk for Self-Harm*.

Goals

See *Risk for Self-Harm*.

Generic Interventions

See *Risk for Self-Harm*.

▶ Risk for Suicide

DEFINITION

The state in which an individual is at risk for killing himself or herself.

▰▰▰ AUTHOR'S NOTE

Risk for Suicide is not currently on the NANDA list but has been added for clarity. *Risk for Self-Directed Violence* is included under *Risk for Violence*. The term *violence* is described as a swift and intense force or a rough or injurious physical force. Suicide can be violent, but it can also be nonviolent (overdose of barbiturates). Using the term *violence* unfortunately can cause the risk for suicide to be undetected because of the belief that an individual is not capable of violence. *Risk for Suicide* clearly denotes an individual at high risk for suicide and the need for protection. The treatment of the diagnosis comprises validation, contracting, and protection. The treatment of the underlying depression and hopelessness should be addressed with other nursing diagnoses (e.g., *Ineffective Coping*, *Hopelessness*).

RISK FACTORS

Major (Must Be Present, One or More)

Suicidal ideation
Previous suicidal attempts

Refer to Table II.3 on p. 417.

Minor (May Be Present)

See *Risk for Self-Harm.*

RELATED FACTORS

See *Risk for Self-Harm.*

NOC

Impulse Control, Suicide Self-Restraint

Goals

The person will not commit suicide.

Indicators

- State the desire to live.
- Verbalize feelings of anger, loneliness, hopelessness.
- Identify persons to contact if suicidal thoughts occur.
- Identify alternative coping mechanisms.

NIC

Active Listening, Coping Enhancement, Suicide Prevention, Impulse Control Training, Behavior Control Training, Behavior Management: Self-Harm, Hope Instillation, Contracting, Surveillance: Safety

Generic Interventions

Assess Level of Risk (Table II.3) (High, Moderate, Low).

Assess Level of Long-Term Risk: Lifestyle, Lethality of Plan, Usual Coping Mechanisms, Support Available.

Provide Closely Supervised Environment for High-Risk Person.

Restrict glass, nail files, scissors, nail polish remover, mirrors, needles, razors, soda cans, plastic bags, lighters, electrical equipment, belts, hangers, knives, tweezers, alcohol, guns.

Meals should be provided in a closely supervised area.

When administering oral medications, check to ensure that all medications are swallowed.

Provide checks on the person per institution policy.

Restrict the individual to the unit unless specifically ordered by physician. When off unit, provide a staff member to accompany the person.

TABLE II.3 ASSESSING THE DEGREE OF SUICIDAL RISK

Behavior or Symptom	Intensity of Risk		
	LOW	MODERATE	HIGH
Anxiety	Mild	Moderate	High or panic state
Depression	Mild	Moderate	Severe
Isolation/withdrawal	Some feelings of isolation; no withdrawal	Some feelings of hopelessness, withdrawal	Hopeless, withdrawn, and self-deprecating; isolation
Daily functioning	Effective Good grades in school Close friends No prior suicide attempt Stable job	Moody Variable grades Some friends Prior suicidal thoughts	Depressed Poor grades Few or no close friends Prior suicide attempts Erratic or poor work history
Lifestyle	Stable	Moderately stable	Unstable
Alcohol/drug use	Infrequently to excess	Frequently to excess	Continual abuse
Previous suicide attempts	None or of low lethality (few pills)	One or more (pills, superficial wrist slash)	One or more (entire bottle of pills, gun, hanging)

(continued)

417

TABLE II.3 ASSESSING THE DEGREE OF SUICIDAL RISK (Continued)

Behavior or Symptom	Intensity of Risk		
	LOW	MODERATE	HIGH
Associated events	None or an argument	⚔ Disciplinary action ⚔ Failing grades Work problems Family illness	Relationship breakup Death of a loved one Loss of job Pregnancy
Purpose of act	None or not clear	Relief of shame or guilt To punish others To get attention	Wants to die Escape to join deceased Debilitating disease
Family's reaction and structure	Supportive Intact family Good coping and mental health No history of suicide	Mixed reaction Divorced/separated Usually copes and understands	Angry and unsupportive Disorganized Rigid/abusive History of suicide in family
Suicide plan (method, location, time)	No plan	Frequent thoughts, occasional ideas about a plan	Specific plan

⚔ Applies only to children and adolescents.
(Adapted from Hatton, C. L., & McBride, S. [1984]. *Suicide: Assessment and intervention.* Norwalk, CT: Appleton-Century-Crofts and Jackson, D. B., & Saunders, R. B. [1993]. *Child health nursing.* Philadelphia: J. B. Lippincott.)

Instruct visitors on restricted items.

The acutely suicidal person may be required to wear a hospital gown to prevent unauthorized leaving.

Room searches should be done periodically per institution policy.

Use seclusion and restraint if necessary (refer to *Risk for Violence* for discussion).

Notify police if the person leaves and is at risk for suicide.

Notify All Staff that This Person Is at Risk for Suicide.

Make a No-Suicide Contract with the Individual (Include Family If Person Is at Home).

Written contract
Mutual agreement

Encourage Appropriate Expression of Anger and Hostility.

Set Limits on Ruminations about Suicide or Previous Attempts.

Assist in Recognizing Predisposing Factors: "What Was Happening Before You Started Having These Thoughts?"

Facilitate Examination of Life Stresses and Past Coping Mechanisms.

Explore Alternative Behaviors.

Anticipate Future Stresses and Assist in Planning Alternatives.

Involve Person in Planning the Treatment Goals and Evaluating Progress.

Instruct Significant Others in How to Recognize an Increase in Risk: Change in Behavior, Verbal, Nonverbal Communication, Withdrawal, Signs of Depression.

Supply Phone Numbers of 24-hour Emergency Hotlines.

Refer to Community Agency for Ongoing Therapy.

🚸 Pediatric Interventions

Take All Suicide Threats Seriously.

Engage Parents, Friends, School Personnel, and the Individual in Behavior Contracts to "Keep Safe."

Explore Feelings and Reason for Suicidal Feelings.

Consult with a Psychiatric Expert Regarding the Most Appropriate Environment for Treatment.

Participate in Programs in Schools to Teach about the Symptoms of Depression and Signs of Suicidal Behavior.

Ⓖ Geriatric Interventions

Be Direct (e.g., "Are You Thinking of Hurting Yourself?").

Acknowledge the Intent with Concern; Remain Nonjudgmental.

Help to Identify Other Options.

Accept the Person's Feelings of Helplessness and Hopelessness.

Discuss the Problem with Family.

SELF-HEALTH MANAGEMENT, EFFECTIVE INDIVIDUAL

DEFINITION

A pattern in which the individual integrates into daily living a program for treatment of illness and its sequelae that is satisfactory for meeting health goals.

▮▮▮ AUTHOR'S NOTE

Effective Individual Self-Health Management describes an individual who is successfully managing an illness or condi-

(continued)

■■■■ **AUTHOR'S NOTE** (*Continued*)

tion. The concept of enhanced is appropriate. The nurse can assist the person to enhance his or her management. The focus would be one of anticipatory guidance (e.g., teaching the person what events could negatively impact his or her management and how to reduce the negative impact).

This diagnosis does not need related factors. Writing related factors would only repeat the characteristics of persons who manage their conditions well (e.g., motivated, knowledgeable).

DEFINING CHARACTERISTICS

Appropriate choices of daily activities for meeting the goals of a treatment or prevention program

Illness symptoms within a normal range of expectation

Verbalization of desire to manage the treatment of illness and prevention of sequelae

Verbalization of intent to reduce risk factors for progression of illness and sequelae

RELATED FACTORS

Refer to Author's Note for an explanation.

NOC

Compliance Behavior, Knowledge: Treatment Regimen, Participation: Health Care Decisions, Risk Control

Goals

The person will describe strategies to address progression or complication of his or her condition if it should arise.

Indicators

- Discuss situations that can challenge his or her continued successful management.
- Describe or demonstrate self-care techniques needed.

NIC

Behavior Modification, Mutual Goal Setting, Teaching: Individual, Decision-Making Support, Health System Guidance, Anticipatory Guidance

Generic Interventions

Discuss Possible Changes in Person's Condition that May Affect the Usual Management.

Exacerbation
Complications
Side effects of medication

Advise Early Contact with Care Provider to Discuss Possible Changes in Management Regimen.

Discuss How Increased Levels of Stress Can Negatively Affect Previous Successful Management and Possibly Decrease Resistance to Colds or Influenza.

Explore with the Person His or Her Evaluation of the Level of Stress with Which He or She Usually Lives.

Usual level of stress
Signs of overload

Discuss that Stress Comes with Favorable and Unfavorable Life Events (e.g., Marriage, Divorce, Birth, Death, Vacations, Work).

When Faced with Upcoming Additional Stresses, Plan to:

Reduce stress in other aspects of life, if possible.
Increase adherence to healthy habits:
- Sleep 7 to 8 hours.
- Eat breakfast.
- Exercise daily (at least a 30-minute brisk walk).
- Eliminate or minimize alcohol intake.
- Increase intake of complex carbohydrates/fiber.
- Decrease intake of fat.
- Decrease caffeine intake.

Increase spiritually related activities:
- Meditation
- Listening to relaxing music

- Nature walks (e.g., woods, near water, mountains).
- Reading poetry

Initiate Health Teaching and Referrals
Regarding Stress-Reduction Techniques.

SELF-HEALTH MANAGEMENT, INEFFECTIVE INDIVIDUAL

DEFINITION

A pattern in which the individual experiences or is at risk to experience difficulty integrating into daily living a program for treatment of illness and the sequelae of illness and reduction of risk situations (e.g., unsafe, pollution).

AUTHOR'S NOTE

Ineffective Self-Health Management is a useful diagnosis for nurses in most settings. Individuals and families experiencing a variety of health problems, acute or chronic, are usually faced with treatment programs that require changes in previous functioning or lifestyle. These regimens are activities or habits of medication therapy, treatments, diet, exercise, stress management, problem-solving, symptom management, and other strategies that improve health and well-being.

This diagnosis describes individuals or families who are experiencing difficulty in achieving positive outcomes. The nurse is the primary professional who, with the client, determines what choices are available and how success can be achieved. The primary nursing interventions are exploring available options with the client and family and teaching the client how to implement the selected option.

When an individual is faced with a complex regimen to follow or has compromised functioning that impedes successful management, the diagnosis *Risk for Ineffective Self-Health Management* is appropriate. In addition to teaching the client how to manage the regimen, the nurse must also assist him or her to identify the adjustments needed because of a functional deficit. *Risk for Ineffective Self-Health Management* is a useful diagnosis for discharge teaching.

DEFINING CHARACTERISTICS
Major (Must Be Present, One or More)

Verbalized desire to manage the treatment of illness and prevention of sequelae

Verbalized difficulty with regulation/integration of one or more prescribed regimens for treatment of illness and its effects or for prevention of complications

Minor (May Be Present)

Acceleration (expected or unexpected) of illness symptoms

Verbalization that client did not take action to include treatment regimens in daily routines

Verbalization that client did not take action to reduce risk factors for progression of illness and sequelae

RELATED FACTORS
Treatment-Related
Related to:

Complexity of therapeutic regimen

Financial cost of regimen

Complexity of health care system

Side effects of therapy

Unfamiliar treatments or techniques

Situational (Personal, Environmental)
Related to:

Decisional conflicts

Family conflicts

Mistrust of regimen

Mistrust of health care personnel

Health belief conflicts

Questions about seriousness of problem

Questions about susceptibility

Questions about benefits of regimen

Insufficient social support

Insufficient confidence

Previous unsuccessful experiences

Related to barriers to comprehension secondary to:

Cognitive deficits	Fatigue
Hearing impairments	Motivation
Anxiety	Memory problems

NOC

Compliance Behavior, Knowledge: Treatment Regimen,
Participation: Health Care Decisions, Treatment
Behavior: Illness or Dying

Goals

The person/family will relate an intent to practice health behaviors needed or desired for recovery from illness and prevention of recurrence or complications.

Indicators
- Relate less anxiety related to fear of the unknown, fear of loss of control, or misconceptions.
- Describe disease process, causes, and factors contributing to symptoms, and the regimen for disease or symptom control.

NIC

Decision-Making Support, Teaching Health System
Guidance

Generic Interventions

Identify Causative or Contributing Factors that Impede Effective Management:

Lack of trust

Insufficient confidence (self-efficacy)

Insufficient knowledge

Insufficient resources

Build Trust and Strength (Zerwich, 1992).

Gain entrance to family system. Do not take over.

Avoid impression of pressuring.

Listen to discover concerns, not to impose expectations.

Attempt to discover a match between expressed needs and services the nurse can provide.

Discover and affirm strengths.

Accept persons where they are.

Demonstrate persistence, but proceed slowly.

Demonstrate honesty, consistency, stability.

Maintain preestablished contacts in person or by phone.

Promote Confidence and Positive Self-Efficacy (Bandura, 1982).

Explore past successful management of problems.

Tell stories of other successes.

If appropriate, encourage opportunities to witness others successfully coping in a similar situation.

Encourage participation in self-help groups.

If high autonomic response (e.g., rapid pulse, diaphoresis) is reducing feeling of confidence, teach short-term anxiety interrupters (Grainger, 1990):

- Look up.
- Control breathing.
- Lower shoulders.
- Slow thoughts.
- Alter voice.
- Give self-directions (out loud, if possible).
- Exercise.
- "Scruff your face"—change facial expression.
- Change perspective (imagine watching the situation from a distance).

Identify Factors that Influence Learning.

Perception of seriousness
Susceptibility to complications
Prognosis
Perception of control of progression
Level of anxiety
Financial status
Support system
Past experiences
Physical status
Emotional status
Cognitive ability

Promote a Positive Attitude and Active Participation of the Person and Family.

Solicit expressions of feelings, concerns, and questions from person and family.

Encourage person/family to seek information and make informed decisions.

Explain responsibilities of person/family and how these can be assumed.

Explain and Discuss:

Disease process
Treatment regimen (medications, diet, procedures, exercises, equipment use)
Rationale of regimen

Expectations (client, family) of regimen
Side effects of regimen
Lifestyle changes needed
Methods to monitor condition
Follow-up care needed
Signs or symptoms of complications
Resources, support available
Home environment alterations needed

Explain that Changes in Lifestyle and Needed Learning Will Take Time to Integrate.

Provide printed material.
Explain whom to contact with questions.

Identify Referrals or Community Services Needed for Follow-Up.

Geriatric Interventions

To Promote Learning:

Avoid times of day when the person is fatigued.
Reduce distractions.
Relate information to prior experiences.
Use visual cues.
Provide outlines prior to class.

Allow Person to Self-Pace the Learning.

Create a List of Cues to Organize Activities.

SELF-HEALTH MANAGEMENT, INEFFECTIVE FAMILY

DEFINITION

A pattern in which the family experiences or is at risk to experience difficulty integrating into daily living a program for treatment of illness and the sequelae of illness and reduction of risk situations (e.g., safety, pollution).

■■■ **AUTHOR'S NOTE**
Refer to *Ineffective Self-Health Management*.

DEFINING CHARACTERISTICS

Major

Inappropriate family activities for meeting the goals of a
treatment or prevention program

Minor

Acceleration (expected or unexpected) of illness symptoms of a
family member

Lack of attention to illness and its sequelae

Verbalization of desire to manage the treatment of illness and
prevention of sequelae

Verbalization of difficulty with regulation/integration of one
or more prescribed regimens for treatment of illness and its
effects or prevention of complications

Verbalization that family did not take action to reduce risk
factors for progression of illness and sequelae

RELATED FACTORS

Refer to *Ineffective Self-Health Management*.

Generic Interventions

Refer to *Ineffective Self-Health Management*.

SELF-HEALTH MANAGEMENT, INEFFECTIVE COMMUNITY

DEFINITION

A pattern in which the community experiences or is at high risk to
experience difficulty integrating a program for prevention/treat-
ment of illness and the sequelae of illness and reduction of risk
situations (e.g., safety, pollution).

■■■■ **AUTHOR'S NOTE**
This diagnosis describes a community that has evidence that a population is underserved because of insufficient availability of, access to, or knowledge of health care resources. The community nurse, using the results of a community assessment, can identify at-risk groups and overall community needs. In addition, the nurse will assess health systems, transportation, social services, and access.

DEFINING CHARACTERISTICS
Major

Verbalized difficulty in meeting health needs in communities
Acceleration (expected or unexpected) of illness(es)
Morbidity, mortality rates above the norm

RELATED FACTORS
Situational (Environmental)

Related to availability of community programs for (specify):

Prevention of diseases	Screening for diseases
Immunizations	Dental care
Accident prevention	Fire safety
Smoking cessation	Substance abuse
Alcohol abuse	Child abuse

Related to problem accessing program secondary to, for example, inadequate communication, limited hours, no transportation, insufficient funds

Related to complexity of population's needs

Related to lack of awareness of availability

Related to presence of environmental or occupational health hazards

Related to multiple needs of vulnerable groups (specify):
Homeless
Pregnant teenagers
Persons living below poverty level
Home-bound individuals

Related to unavailable or insufficient health care agencies

NOC

Participation: Health Care Decisions, Risk Control, Risk Detection

Goals

The community will promote the use of community resources for health problems.

Indicators
- Identify community resources that are needed.
- Participate in program development as needed.

NIC

Decision-Making Support, Health System Guidance, Risk Identification, Community Health Development

Generic Interventions

Create a Survey to Determine:

Health problem identification
Awareness of health services
Use of health services
Interest in health-promotion programs
Recommendation for funding sources

Survey Samples of the Target Population:

Mail survey
One-to-one survey at community center, sports field, supermarket
Group survey (e.g., church groups, clubs)
Survey of key community leaders

Design the Survey for Easy Reading and Answering (e.g., Circle the Number that Best Describes Your Answer: 1—No Concern; 2—Medium; 3—High).

How concerned are you about, e.g.:
- Hypertension
- Stress
- Alcohol misuse
- Violence
- Nutrition
- HIV

Organize the Response Data.

Analyze the Findings.

What are the overall health problems reported?
What are the health concerns of:
- Elderly population
- Households with children up to age 20 years
- Single-parent households
- Respondents younger than 45 years
- Individuals below the poverty level

Evaluate Community Resources.

What resources are available for the health problems identified?
Are there use or access problems with the services?
How does the population know of services?
Identify problems that do not have community services available.

If Services Are Available but Are Underused, Evaluate:

Hours of operation (convenient?)
Location of services (access, esthetics)
Efficiency and atmosphere
Advertising strategies

If Services Are Unavailable, Pursue Program Development.

Examine and evaluate similar programs in other communities:
- Basic information
- Purpose, goals
- Services available
- Funding
- Cost to participants
- Availability of services
- Accessibility of services
- Satisfaction (citizen, employees)

Meet with appropriate persons to discuss findings (survey, on-site visits).
Address the following:
- Presence of community support
- Available expertise and technology in community
- Financial support

Identify appropriate community sources of assistance (e.g., hospital departments, schools of nursing, private foundations).
Plan the program (refer to *Readiness for Enhanced Community Coping* for interventions for community planning).

Evaluate Vulnerable Population's Access to Health Care and Knowledge of Risk Factors.

Rural families, elderly
Migrant workers
New immigrants
Homeless
Individuals and groups below the poverty level

Make a Priority of Ensuring that Basic Needs for Food, Shelter, Clothing, and Safety Are Met Before Attempting to Address Higher Health Needs.

Provide Information Regarding Illness Prevention, Health Promotion, and Health Services to Vulnerable Populations.

DISTURBED SENSORY PERCEPTION

DEFINITION

The state in which an individual/group experiences, or is at risk of experiencing, a change in the amount, pattern, or interpretation of incoming stimuli.

AUTHOR'S NOTE

The diagnosis *Disturbed Sensory Perception* describes a person with altered perception and cognition influenced by physiologic factors (e.g., pain, sleep deprivation, immobility, and excessive or decreased meaningful stimuli from the environment). *Disturbed Sensory Perception* results when barriers or factors interfere with a person's ability to interpret stimuli accurately.

The diagnosis *Disturbed Sensory Perception* has six subcategories: visual, auditory, kinesthetic, gustatory, tactile, and olfactory. When a person has a visual or hearing deficit, how does the nurse intervene with the diagnosis *Disturbed Sensory Perception: Visual related to effects of glaucoma*? What would the goals be? The nurse should assess for the individual's response to the visual loss and specifically label the response, not the deficit.

(continued)

■■■ **AUTHOR'S NOTE** *(Continued)*
 The diagnosis *Disturbed Sensory Perception* is more
clinically useful without the addition of the specific sense.
Examples of responses to sensory deficits may be:

Visual
   Risk for Injury   *Self-Care Deficit*
Auditory
   Impaired Communication   *Social Isolation*
Kinesthetic
   Risk for Injury
Olfactory
   Imbalanced Nutrition
Tactile
   Risk for Injury
Gustatory
   Imbalanced Nutrition

DEFINING CHARACTERISTICS

Major (Must Be Present, One or More)

Inaccurate interpretation of environmental stimuli *and/or*
Negative change in amount or pattern of incoming stimuli

Minor (May Be Present)

Disorientation about time or
  place
Auditory or visual
  hallucinations
Altered problem-solving
  ability
Altered behavior or
  communication pattern

Restlessness
Disorientation about people
Irritability
Poor concentration

RELATED FACTORS

Many factors in an individual's life can contribute to *Disturbed
Sensory Perception*. Some common factors are listed below.

Pathophysiologic

Related to misinterpretations secondary to:

Sensory Organ Alterations
Visual, gustatory, auditory, olfactory, and tactile deficits

Neurologic Alterations

Cerebrovascular accident   Neuropathies
Encephalitis/meningitis

Metabolic Alterations

Fluid and electrolyte   Acidosis
   imbalances   Alkalosis
Elevated blood urea nitrogen

Impaired Oxygen Transport

Cerebral   Respiratory
Cardiac   Anemia

Related to mobility restrictions secondary to paraplegia or quadriplegia

Treatment-Related

Related to misinterpretations secondary to:
Medications (sedatives, tranquilizers)
Surgery (glaucoma, cataract, detached retina)
Related to physical isolation (reverse isolation, communicable disease, prison)
Related to immobility
Related to mobility restrictions (bed rest, traction, casts, Stryker frame, CircOlectric bed)

Situational (Personal, Environmental)

Related to misinterpretations secondary to pain or stress
Related to socially restricted environment
Related to excessive noise
Related to complex environment (noise, lights, constant changes, excess activity, frequent demands)
Related to monotonous environment
Related to loss of socialization

NOC

Cognitive Orientation, Distorted Thought Control

Goals

The person will demonstrate decreased symptoms of sensory overload as evidenced by (specify).

Indicators

- Identify and eliminate the potential risk factors, if possible.
- Describe the rationale for the treatment modality.

NIC

Cognitive Stimulation, Reality Orientation

Generic Interventions

Reduce Excess Noise or Light.

Share with Person the Source of the Noise.

Discuss the Use of a Radio with Earplugs
to Provide Soft, Relaxing Music.

Share with Personnel the Need to Reduce Noise
and Provide Individuals with Uninterrupted
Sleep for at Least 2 to 4 Hours.

Attempt to Reduce Fears and Concerns by
Explaining Equipment, Its Purpose, and Noises.

Encourage Person to Share Perceptions of Noises.

Orient to All Three Spheres (Person, Place, Time).

Offer Simple Explanations of Each Task.

Allow Person to Participate in Task,
Such as Washing Own Face.

Promote Movement In and Out of Bed.

Avoid Isolation of the Person; Change
Environment Daily (e.g., Move Into Hall).

Provide at Least Four Undisturbed Sleep and
Rest Periods for 100 Minutes Every 24 Hours.

Use a Variety of Methods to Stimulate Senses (e.g.,
Perfume, Pet Therapy, Ambulate to Window).

Ask Family to Bring in Familiar Possessions.

Limit Use of Sedation.

If at Risk for Injury, Refer to **Risk for Injury**.

Sexuality Patterns, Ineffective
Sexual Dysfunction

DEFINITION

The state in which an individual experiences, or is at risk of experiencing, a change in sexual health. Sexual health is the integration of somatic, emotional, intellectual, and social aspects of sexual being in ways that are enriching and that enhance personality, communication, and love.

AUTHOR'S NOTE

The diagnoses *Ineffective Sexuality Patterns* and *Sexual Dysfunction* are difficult to differentiate. *Ineffective Sexuality Patterns* is a broad diagnosis of which sexual dysfunction can be one part. Sexual health is the integration of somatic, emotional, intellectual, and social aspects of sexual being in ways that are enriching and that enhance personality, communication, and love (World Health Organization).

Sexual Dysfunction may be more appropriately used by a nurse with advanced preparation in sex therapy. Until *Sexual Dysfunction* is differentiated from *Ineffective Sexuality Patterns*, it is unnecessary for most nurses to use this diagnosis.

DEFINING CHARACTERISTICS

Major (Must Be Present)

Actual or anticipated negative changes in sexual functioning or sexual identity

Minor (May Be Present)

Expression of concern about sexual functioning or sexual identity
Inappropriate sexual verbal or nonverbal behavior
Changes in primary and/or secondary sexual characteristics

RELATED FACTORS

Altered sexuality patterns can occur as a response to a variety of health problems, situations, and conflicts. Some common sources are listed below.

Pathophysiologic

Related to biochemical effects on energy and libido secondary to:

Endocrine

Diabetes mellitus	Hyperthyroidism
Decreased hormone production	Addison's disease
Acromegaly	Myxedema

Genitourinary

Chronic renal failure

Neuromuscular and Skeletal

Arthritis

Multiple sclerosis

Amyotrophic lateral sclerosis

Disturbances of the nerve supply to the brain, spinal cord, sensory nerves, and autonomic nerves

Cardiorespiratory

Myocardial infarction	Congestive heart failure
Peripheral vascular disorders	Chronic respiratory disorders

Related to fears associated with (specify) (sexually transmitted diseases)

HIV/AIDS	Genital warts
Herpes	Chlamydia
Syphilis	Gonorrhea

Related to the effects of alcohol on performance

Related to decreased vaginal lubrication secondary to (specify)

Related to fear of premature ejaculation

Related to painful intercourse

Treatment-Related

Related to the effects of medications or radiation treatment

Related to altered self-concept from change in appearance (trauma, radical surgery)

Situational (Personal, Environmental)

Related to partner problem (specify), for example, unwilling, uninformed, abusive, not available, separated, divorced
Related to no privacy
Related to stressors secondary to job problems, financial worries, conflicting values, or religious conflict
Related to misinformation or lack of knowledge
Related to fatigue
Related to fear of rejection secondary to obesity
Related to pain
Related to fear of sexual failure
Related to fear of pregnancy
Related to depression
Related to anxiety
Related to guilt
Related to history of unsatisfactory sexual experiences

Maturational

Adolescent

Related to ineffective role models
Related to negative sexual teaching
Related to absence of sexual teaching

Adult

Related to adjustment to parenthood
Related to effects of pregnancy on energy levels and body image
Related to values conflict

NOC

Body Image, Self-Esteem, Role Performance, Sexual Identity

Goals

The person will resume previous sexual activity or engage in alternative satisfying sexual activity.

Indicators

- Identify impact of stressors, loss, or change on sexual functioning.
- Modify behavior to reduce stressors.
- Identify limitations on sexual activity caused by health problem.

- Identify appropriate modifications in sexual practices in response to these limitations.
- Report satisfying sexual activity.

NIC

Behavioral Management: Sexual, Counseling, Emotional Support, Active Listening, Teaching: Sexuality

Generic Interventions

Acquire a Sexual History.

Usual sexual pattern
Satisfaction (individual, partner)
Sexual knowledge
Problems (sexual, health)
Expectations
Mood, energy level

Encourage Client to Ask Questions About Sexuality or Sexual Functioning that May Be Disturbing Him or Her.

Explore His or Her Relationship with Partner.

If Stressors or a Stressful Lifestyle Have Decreased Functioning:

Assist person in modifying lifestyle to reduce stress.
Encourage identification of present stressors in life; group as those the person can control and those the person cannot, e.g.:
Can control:
- Personal lateness
- Involvement in community activities
Cannot control:
- Report due
- Daughter's illness

Initiate a Regular Exercise Program for Stress Reduction. See **Health-Seeking Behaviors** for Interventions.

Identify Alternative Methods for Dispersing Sexual Energy When Partner Is Unavailable or Unwilling.

Use masturbation, if acceptable to individual.
Teach the physical and psychological benefits of regular physical activity (at least three times a week for 30 minutes).

If partner is deceased, explore opportunities to meet and socialize with others (night school, singles club, community work).

If a Change or Loss of Body Part Has Decreased Functioning:

Assess the stage of adaptation of the individual and partner to the loss (denial, depression, anger, resolution; see *Grieving*).

Explain the normality of the foregoing responses to loss.

Explain the need to share concerns with partner:

- Imagined response of partner
- Fear of rejection
- Fear of future losses
- Fear of physically hurting partner

Encourage the Partner to Discuss the Strengths of Their Relationship and to Assess the Influence of the Loss on Their Strengths.

Encourage Person to Resume Sexual Activity as Close to Previous Pattern as Possible.

Identify Barriers to Satisfying Sexual Functioning (e.g., Hypoxia, Pain, Impaired Mobility, Pregnancy, Side Effects of Medications).

Teach Techniques to:

Reduce oxygen consumption.

Use oxygen during sexual activity if indicated.

Engage in sexual activity after intermittent positive-pressure breathing treatment or postural drainage.

Plan sexual activities for time of day person is most rested.

Use positions for intercourse that are comfortable and permit unrestricted breathing.

Reduce Cardiac Workload.

Clients with Cardiac Problems Should Avoid Sexual Activity:

In extremes of temperature

Directly after eating or drinking

When intoxicated

When tired

With unfamiliar partner

Rest before engaging in sexual activity (mornings are best)

Clients with Cardiac Problems Should Terminate Sexual Activity if Chest Discomfort or Dyspnea Occurs.

Reduce or Eliminate Pain.

If vaginal lubrication is decreased, use a water-soluble lubricant.
Take medication for pain before beginning sexual activity.
Use whatever relaxes individual before beginning sexual activity
  (hot packs, hot shower).

Initiate Health Teaching and Referrals As Indicated; Discuss with Individuals or Couples the Availability of Self-Help Groups (e.g., Reach for Recovery, United Ostomy Association).

🚶 Pediatric Interventions

Clarify the Confidentiality of the Discussion.

Strive to Be Open, Warm, Objective, Unembarrassed, and Reassuring.

Explore Feelings and Sexual Experiences. Encourage Questions. Dispel Myths.

Discuss How Bacteria Are Transferred (Vaginally, Anally, Orally).

For Young Women, Explain the Relationship of Sexually Transmitted Diseases and Pelvic Inflammatory Disease, Infertility, and Ectopic Pregnancies.

Show a Diagram of Reproductive Structures.

Emphasize that Most Sexually Transmitted Diseases Have No Symptoms Initially.

Discuss Abstinence from Sexual Perspective (e.g., Right to Say No, Commitment, Unwanted Pregnancies, Sexually Transmitted Diseases).

Discuss Contraceptive Methods Available (e.g., Pill, Depo-Provera, Intrauterine Device, Condoms, Foam, Diaphragm, Spermicides):

How it works
Effectiveness

Cost
Prevention of sexually transmitted diseases

Explain and Provide Written Instructions for Method Chosen.

👫 **Maternal Interventions**

Discuss Body Changes During Pregnancy.

Encourage Couple to Share Their Feelings.

Reassure that Unless Problems Exist (Preterm Labor, Previous Early Loss, Bleeding or Rupture of Membranes) Intercourse Is Allowed Until Labor Begins.

Suggest Alternative Sexual Positions for Later Pregnancy to Prevent Abdominal Pressure (e.g., Side-Lying, Woman Kneeling, Woman on Top).

Give Reassurance about Postpartum Changes. Reassure that This Is a Temporary State and Will Resolve in 2 to 3 Months.

Reassure that Sexual Attitudes Change Throughout Pregnancy from Feeling Very Desirous of Sex to Wanting Only to Be Cuddled.

Discuss Techniques to Enhance the Couple's Relationship (Polomeno, 1999).

Explore Fears and Anxieties (Separately).

Discuss Barriers to Disclosing Fears and Anxieties.

Role-Play Disclosure.

Encourage Client to Share the "Little Things" that Represent Caring.

Instruct on "Heart Talks." One Partner Talks for 5 Minutes with No Interruption or Argument. The Other Partner then Has a Chance to Talk. At the End the Couple Hugs and Says, "I Love You" (Polomeno, 1999).

Instruct on "Sexual Conversation" (Gray, 1995). Useful Questions Are:

What do you like about having sex with me?
Would you like more sex?
Would you like more or less foreplay?
Is there a way that you would like me to touch you?

Discuss Methods to Keep Romance Alive (Gray, 1995):

Set aside regular time with each other.
Hold hands.
Send messages that partner is appreciated.

Acknowledge Fatigue, Especially During First Trimester, Last Month, and Postpartum.

Encourage Person to Make Time for Her Relationship in Sexual and Other Contexts.

Teach Couples to Abstain from Any Sex Play or Intercourse and Seek the Advice of Their Health Care Provider If Any of the Following Situations Are Present (Pillitteri, 2007):

Vaginal bleeding
Multiple pregnancy
Placenta previa
History of premature
    delivery

Premature dilation
Engaged fetal head or
    lightening
Rupture of membranes
History of miscarriage

Ⓖ Geriatric Interventions

Explain that Normal Aging Affects Reproductive Abilities but Has Little Effect on Sexual Functioning.

Explore Interest, Activity, Attitude, and Knowledge Regarding Sexual Functioning.

If Pertinent, Discuss the Effects of Chronic Diseases on Functioning.

Explain the Effects of Certain Medications on Sexual Functioning (e.g., Cardiovascular, Antidepressants, Antihistamine, Gastrointestinal, Sedatives, Alcohol).

If Sexual Dysfunction Is Related to Medications, Explore Alternatives (e.g., Medication Change, Dose Reduction).

With Women, Discuss the Quality of Vaginal Lubrication and Available Water-Soluble Lubricants.

Encourage Questions. If Needed, Refer to Urologist or Other Specialist.

▌ Sexual Dysfunction

DEFINITION

The state in which an individual experiences, or is at risk of experiencing, a change in sexual function that is viewed as unrewarding or inadequate.

■■■■ **AUTHOR'S NOTE**
Refer to *Ineffective Sexuality Patterns*.

DEFINING CHARACTERISTICS

Major (Must Be Present, One or More)

Verbalization of problem with sexual function
Reports limitations on sexual performance imposed by disease or therapy

Minor (May Be Present)

Fears future limitations on sexual performance
Is misinformed about sexuality
Lacks knowledge about sexuality and sexual function

Has value conflicts involving sexual expression (cultural, religious)
Experiences altered relationship with significant other
Is dissatisfied with sex role (perceived or actual)

SHOCK, RISK FOR

DEFINITION (NANDA)

The state in which an individual is at risk for inadequate blood flow to the body's tissues which may lead to life-threatening cellular dysfunction.

RISK FACTORS (NANDA)

Hypertension
Hypovolemia
Hypoxemia
Hypoxia
Infection
Sepsis
Systemic inflammatory response syndrome

AUTHOR'S NOTE

This newly accepted diagnosis by NANDA-I represents several collaborative problems. In order to decide which of the following collaborative problems is appropriate for an individual client, determine what you are monitoring for. Which of the following describes the focus of nursing for this client:

- Risk for Complications of Hypertension
- Risk for Complications of Bleeding
- Risk for Complications of Hypovolemia
- Risk for Complications of Decreased Cardiac Output
- Risk for Complications of Hypoxemia

Interventions/goals

Refer to Section 3 for goals and interventions for each of the above collaborative problems.

SLEEP PATTERN, DISTURBED

Sleep Pattern, Disturbed
Insomnia
Sleep Deprivation

DEFINITION

The state in which an individual experiences or is at risk of experiencing a change in the quantity or quality of his or her rest pattern that causes discomfort or interferes with desired lifestyle.

DEFINING CHARACTERISTICS

ADULTS

Major (Must Be Present)

Difficulty falling or remaining asleep

Minor (May Be Present)

Fatigue on awakening or
during the day
Mood alterations

Agitation
Dozing during the day

CHILDREN

Sleep disturbances in children are frequently related to fear, enuresis, or inconsistent responses of parents to the child's requests for changes in sleep rules, such as requests to stay up late.
Reluctance to retire, desire to sleep with parents
Frequent awakening during the night

RELATED FACTORS

Many factors in life can contribute to *Disturbed Sleep Patterns.* Some common factors are listed below.

Pathophysiologic

Related to frequent awakenings secondary to:

Angina
Diarrhea, constipation
Urinary problems

Dyspnea
Gastric ulcers

Treatment-Related

Related to difficulty assuming usual position secondary to:
Casts, traction, pain, intravenous therapy

Related to excessive daytime sleeping secondary to medications, e.g.,

Tranquilizers, sedatives
Antidepressants
Barbiturates
Corticosteroids

Monoamine oxidase
  inhibitors
Antihypertensives
Amphetamines

Situational (Personal, Environmental)

Related to excessive hyperactivity secondary to:
Bipolar disorder
Attention-deficit disorder

Panic anxiety
Hyperthyroidism

Related to excessive daytime sleeping
Related to inadequate daytime activities
Related to fears and/or pain
Related to anxiety response, depression
Related to discomforts secondary to pregnancy
Related to lifestyle disruptions (e.g., occupational, emotional, social, sexual, financial)
Related to environmental changes (e.g., hospitalization [noise, disturbing roommate, fear] or travel)
Related to circadian rhythm changes

Maturational

Child
Related to fear of the dark

Adult Women
Related to hormonal changes (e.g., perimenopausal)

NOC

Rest, Sleep, Well-Being

Goals

The person will report an optimal balance of rest and activity.

Indicators
- Describe factors that prevent or inhibit sleep.
- Identify techniques to induce sleep.

NIC

Energy Management, Sleep Enhancement,
Environmental Management

Generic Interventions

**Organize Procedures to Provide the Fewest
Disturbances During Sleep Period (e.g., When
Individual Awakens for Medication, Also
Administer Treatments and Obtain Vital Signs).**

**If Voiding During the Night Is Disruptive, Have Person
Limit Nighttime Fluids and Void before Retiring.**

**Establish with Person a Schedule for a Daytime
Program of Activity (Walking, Physical Therapy).**

**Limit Amount and Length of Daytime
Sleeping If Excessive (i.e., >1 Hour).**

**Assess with Person, Family, or Parents the
Usual Bedtime Routine—Time, Hygiene
Practices, Rituals (Reading, Toy)—and
Adhere to It as Closely as Possible.**

**Limit Intake of Caffeinated Drinks
after Mid-Afternoon.**

**Explain to Person and Significant Others
the Causes of Sleep/Rest Disturbance and
Possible Ways to Avoid It (Boyd, 2005).**

Avoid alcohol.
Keep regular bedtimes and rising times.
Set a relaxing routine to prepare for sleep (e.g., herbal tea, warm
    bath).
Keep bedroom slightly cool.
Wear ear plugs if noise is a problem.
Do not exercise within 3 hours of bedtime.

👫 Pediatric Interventions

Explain Night to the Child (Stars and Moon).

**Discuss How Some Persons (Nurses,
Factory Workers) Work at Night.**

Compare the Contrast that When Night Comes for Him or Her, Day Is Coming for People in Other Countries.

If a Nightmare Occurs, Encourage the Child to Talk about it if Possible. Reassure Child that It Is a Dream, Even If It Seems Real. Share with Child that You Have Dreams Too.

Provide Child with a Night Light or a Flashlight to Use to Give Child Control Over the Dark.

Reassure Child that You Will Be Nearby All Night.

Explain the Possible Problems of Sleeping with Child.

👥 Maternal Interventions

Explain Some Reasons for Sleeping Difficulties During Pregnancy (e.g., Leg Cramps, Backache).

Teach How to Position Pillows in Side-Lying Position (One Between Legs, One Under Abdomen, One Under Top Arm, One Under Head).

Teach to Avoid Caffeine and Large Meals Within 2 to 3 Hours of Bedtime.

Advise to Exercise Daily and Take a Warm Bath at Bedtime.

▶ Insomnia

DEFINITION

The state in which a client reports a persistent pattern of difficulty falling asleep and frequent awakening that disrupts daytime life.

DEFINING CHARACTERISTICS

Major (Must Be Present)

Adults

Report persistent difficulty falling or remaining asleep

Minor (May Be Present)

Adults

Fatigue on awakening or during the day	Dozing during the day

RELATED FACTORS

Refer to *Disturbed Sleep Pattern*.

▶ Sleep Deprivation

DEFINITION

The state in which an individual experiences prolonged periods of time without sustained, natural, periodic states of relative unconsciousness.

AUTHOR'S NOTE

This diagnostic label represents a situation in which insufficient sleep is achieved. It is the most common type of sleep pattern disturbance and will probably be used for most clinical situations.

DEFINING CHARACTERISTICS

Refer to *Disturbed Sleep Pattern*.

RELATED FACTORS

Refer to *Disturbed Sleep Pattern*.

Goals

Refer to *Disturbed Sleep Pattern*.

SOCIAL INTERACTION, IMPAIRED

DEFINITION

The state in which an individual experiences, or is at risk of experiencing, negative, insufficient, or unsatisfactory responses from interactions.

DEFINING CHARACTERISTICS

Major (Must Be Present, One or More)

Reports inability to establish and/or maintain stable supportive relationships

Is dissatisfied with social network

Minor (May Be Present)

Social isolation
Superficial relationships
Blaming others for interpersonal problems
Feelings of rejection
Avoidance of others

Others reporting problematic patterns of interaction
Feelings of being misunderstood
Interpersonal difficulties at work

RELATED FACTORS

Impaired Social Interaction can result from a variety of situations and health problems that are related to the inability to establish and maintain rewarding relationships. Some common sources are as follows:

Pathophysiologic

Related to embarrassment or limited physical mobility or energy secondary to loss of body function, terminal illness, or loss of body part

Related to communication barriers secondary to hearing deficits, mental retardation, visual deficits, speech impediments, or chronic mental illness

Treatment-Related

Related to surgical disfigurement
Related to therapeutic isolation

Situational (Personal, Environmental)

Related to alienation from others secondary to:

Constant complaining
Rumination
Overt hostility
Manipulative behaviors
Mistrust or suspicions
Illogical ideas
Egocentric behavior
Emotional immaturity
Aggressive responses

High anxiety
Impulsive behavior
Delusions
Hallucinations
Disorganized thinking
Dependent behavior
Strong unpopular beliefs
Depressive behavior

Related to language/cultural barriers
Related to lack of social skills
Related to change in usual social patterns secondary to divorce, relocation, or death

Maturational

Child/Adolescent
Related to impulse control
Related to altered appearance
Related to speech impediments

Adult
Related to loss of ability to practice vocation

Older Adult
Related to change in usual social patterns secondary to:

Death of spouse
Retirement

Functional deficits

NOC

Family Functioning, Social Interaction Skills, Social Involvement

Goals

The person/family will report increased satisfaction with socialization.

Indicators

- Identify problematic behavior that deters socialization.
- Substitute constructive behaviors for disruptive social behaviors (specify).
- Describe strategies to promote effective socialization.

NIC

Anticipatory Guidance, Behavior Modification, Family Integrity: Promotion, Counseling, Behavior Management, Family Support, Self-Responsibility, Facilitation

Generic Interventions

Provide an Individual, Supportive Relationship.

Help to Identify How Stress Precipitates Problems.

Support Healthy Defenses.

Help to Identify Alternative Courses of Action.

Assist in Analyzing Approaches that Work Best.

Role Play Situations that Are Problematic. Discuss Feelings.

If in Group Therapy:

Focus on here and now.

Establish group norms that discourage inappropriate behavior.

Encourage testing of new social behavior.

Use snacks or coffee to decrease anxiety during sessions.

Role model certain accepted social behaviors (e.g., responding to a friendly greeting versus ignoring it).

Foster development of relationships among members through self-disclosure and genuineness.

Use questions and observations to encourage persons with limited interaction skills.

Encourage members to validate their perception with others.

Identify strengths among members and ignore selected weaknesses.

For Family Members of Persons with Chronic Mental Illness:

Assist in understanding and providing support.

Provide factual information concerning illness, treatment, and progress.

Validate feelings of frustration when dealing with daily problems.

Provide guidance on overstimulating or understimulating environments.

Allow families to discuss their feelings of guilt and how their behavior affects the person.

Develop an alliance with family.

Arrange for periodic respite care.

For Individuals with Chronic Mental Illness, Teach (McFarland & Wasli, 2000):

Responsibilities of his or her role as a client (making requests clearly known, participating in therapies)

How to outline activities of the day and focus on accomplishing them

How to approach others to communicate

How to identify which interactions encourage others to give him or her consideration and respect

How to identify how he or she can participate in formulating family roles and responsibility to comply

How to recognize signs of anxiety and methods to relieve them

How to identify his or her positive behavior and experience satisfaction with self in selecting constructive choices

As Indicated, Refer to Community Agencies (e.g., Social Service, Occupational Counseling, Family Therapy, Crisis Intervention).

Pediatric Interventions

If Impulse Control Is a Problem:

Set firm, responsible limits.

Do not lecture.

State limits simply and back them up.

Maintain routines.

Limit play to one playmate to learn appropriate play skills (e.g., relative, adult, quiet child).

Gradually increase number of playmates.

Provide immediate and constant feedback.

Teach Parents To:

Avoid harsh criticism.

Not disagree in front of child.

Establish eye contact before giving instructions and ask child to repeat what was said.

Teach Older Child to Self-Monitor Target Behaviors and to Develop Self-Reliance.

If Antisocial Behavior Is Present, Help To:

Describe behaviors that interfere with socialization.

Role play alternative responses.

Limit social circle to a manageable size.

Elicit peer feedback for positive and negative behavior.

SOCIAL ISOLATION

DEFINITION

The state in which an individual or group experiences or perceives a need or desire for increased involvement with others but is unable to make that contact.

■■■ **AUTHOR'S NOTE**

In 1994, NANDA added a new diagnosis, *Risk for Loneliness*. Although this diagnosis is only in stage 1 of a four-stage developmental process, it more accurately adheres to the NANDA definition of "response to." Social isolation is not a response but a cause of or contributing factor to loneliness. In addition, one can experience loneliness even with many persons around. I recommend deleting *Social Isolation* from clinical use and using *Loneliness* or *Risk for Loneliness*.

DEFINING CHARACTERISTICS

Because social isolation is a subjective state, all inferences made about a person's feelings of aloneness must be validated because the causes vary and people show their aloneness in different ways.

Major (Must Be Present, One or More)

Expresses feelings of aloneness, rejection
Desire for more contact with people
Reports insecurity in social situations*
Describes a lack of meaningful relationships*

Minor (May Be Present)

Time passing slowly ("Mondays are so long for me.")
Inability to concentrate and make decisions
Feelings of uselessness
Feelings of rejection
Underactivity (physical or verbal)
Appearing depressed, anxious, or angry
Failure to interact with others nearby
Sad, dull affect*

---

*Elsen, J., & Blegen, M. (1991). Social isolation. In M. Maas, K. Buckwalter, & M. Hardy (Eds.), *Nursing diagnoses and interventions for the elderly*. Redwood City, CA: Addison-Wesley Nursing.

Uncommunicative*
Withdrawn*
Poor eye contact*
Preoccupied with own thoughts and memories

RELATED FACTORS

A state of social isolation can result from a variety of situations and health problems that are related to a loss of established relationships or to a failure to generate these relationships. Some common sources follow.

Pathophysiologic

Related to fear of rejection secondary to:

Obesity
Cancer (disfiguring surgery of head or neck, superstitions of others)
Physical handicaps (paraplegia, amputation, arthritis, hemiplegia)
Emotional handicaps (extreme anxiety, depression, paranoia, phobias)
Incontinence (embarrassment, odor)
Communicable diseases (AIDS, hepatitis)
Psychiatric illness (schizophrenia, bipolar affective disorder, personality disorders)

Treatment-Related

Therapeutic isolation

Situational (Personal, Environmental)

Related to death of a significant other
Related to divorce
Related to disfiguring appearance

Related to fear of rejection secondary to:

Obesity
Hospitalization or terminal illness (dying process)
Unemployment
Extreme poverty

Related to moving to another culture (e.g., unfamiliar language)

Related to history of unsatisfying relationships secondary to:

Drug abuse
Immature behavior
Delusional thinking
Alcohol abuse
Unacceptable social behavior

Related to loss of usual means of transportation

Maturational

Child
Related to protective isolation or a communicable disease

Older Adult
Related to loss of usual social contacts

CHRONIC SORROW

DEFINITION

The state in which a person experiences, or is at risk of experiencing, permanent sadness, variable in intensity, in response to loss of a loved one or a loved one forever changed by an event or condition, and the ongoing losses of normality (Teel, 1991).

> ### AUTHOR'S NOTE
> *Chronic Sorrow* was identified in 1962 by Olchansky. *Chronic Sorrow* is different from *Grieving*. *Grieving* is time-limited and ends in adaptation to the loss. *Chronic Sorrow* will vary in intensity, but persists as long as the person with the disability or chronic sorrow condition lives (Eakes, 1995). Chronic sorrow can also occur in an individual with a chronic disease that regularly impairs the person's ability to live a "normal life" (e.g., paraplegia, AIDS, sickle cell disease).

DEFINING CHARACTERISTICS

Life-long episodic sadness due to the loss of a loved one or the loss of normality in a loved one who is disabled

Variable in intensity

RELATED FACTORS

Situational (Personal, Environmental)
Related to the chronic loss of normality secondary to child's condition

Autism	Mental retardation
Down syndrome	Psychiatric condition

Severe scoliosis   Spina bifida
HIV   Sickle cell disease
Type I diabetes mellitus

Related to lifetime losses associated with infertility
Related to ongoing losses associated with a degenerative
condition
Multiple sclerosis   Alzheimer's disease
Related to untimely loss of a loved one (e.g., child)
Related to losses associated with caring for a child with a fatal
illness

NOC

Depression Self Control, Coping, Mood Equilibrium
Acceptance: Health Status

Goals

The person will be assisted to anticipate developmental events
that can trigger heightened sadness.

Indicators

- Express sadness.
- Discuss the loss periodically.

NIC

Anticipatory Guidance, Coping Enhancement, Referral,
Active Listening, Presence, Resiliency Promotion

Generic Interventions

Explain the Difference Between Chronic Sorrow and Chronic Grieving:

Normal response
Focused on loss of normality
Not time-limited
Episodic and persists throughout life

Encourage to Share His or Her Feelings Since the Change (e.g., Birth of Child, Accident).

Gently Encourage to Share Lost Dreams or Hopes.

Assist to Identify Developmental Milestones that Will Exacerbate the Loss of Normality (e.g., School Play, Sports, Prom, Dating).

Encourage to Participate in Support Groups with Others Experiencing Chronic Sorrow.

Link the Family with Appropriate Services (e.g., Home Health, Respite Counselor).

Clarify that His or Her Feelings Will Fluctuate (Intensify, Diminish) Through the Years, But the Sorrow Will Not Disappear.

Stress the Importance of Maintaining Support Systems and Friendships.

Share the Difficulties of:

Living worried
Treating child like other children
Staying in the struggle
Refer also to *Caregiver Role Strain*.

SPIRITUAL DISTRESS

Spiritual Distress
Spiritual Distress, Risk for
Religiosity, Impaired
Religiosity, Risk for Impaired

DEFINITION

The state in which an individual or group experiences, or is at risk of experiencing, a disturbance in the belief or value system that provides strength, hope, and meaning to life.

DEFINING CHARACTERISTICS

Major (Must Be Present)

Experiences a disturbance in belief system

Minor (May Be Present)

Questions meaning of life, death, and suffering
Questions credibility of belief system
Demonstrates discouragement or despair
Chooses not to practice usual religious rituals

Has ambivalent feelings (doubts) about beliefs

Expresses that he or she has no reason for living

Feels a sense of spiritual emptiness

Shows emotional detachment from self and others

Expresses concern—anger, resentment, fear—about the meaning of life, suffering, death

Requests spiritual assistance for a disturbance in belief system

RELATED FACTORS

Pathophysiologic

Related to challenges to belief system or separation from spiritual ties secondary to:

Loss of body part or function

Pain

Terminal illness

Trauma

Debilitating disease

Miscarriage, stillbirth

Treatment-Related

Related to conflict between (specify prescribed regimen) and beliefs

Abortion

Surgery

Blood transfusion

Dietary restrictions

Isolation

Amputation

Medications

Medical procedures

Situational (Personal, Environmental)

Related to death or illness of significant other

Related to embarrassment at practicing spiritual rituals

Related to barriers to practicing spiritual rituals

Intensive care restrictions

Confinement to bed or room

Lack of privacy

Lack of availability of special foods/diet

Related to beliefs opposed by family, peers, health care providers

Related to divorce, separation from loved ones

NOC

Hope, Spiritual Well-Being

Goals

The person will express satisfaction with spiritual condition.

Indicators
- Continue spiritual practices not detrimental to health.
- Express decreasing feelings of guilt and anxiety.

NIC

Spiritual Growth Facilitation, Hope Instillation, Active Listening, Presence, Emotional Support, Spiritual Support

Generic Interventions

Communicate Acceptance of Various Spiritual Beliefs and Practices.

Convey Nonjudgmental Attitude.

Acknowledge Importance of Spiritual Needs.

Express Willingness of Health Care Team to Help in Meeting Spiritual Needs.

Provide Privacy and Quiet As Needed for Daily Prayer, Visit of Spiritual Leader, and Spiritual Reading and Contemplation.

Contact Spiritual Leader to Clarify Practices and Perform Religious Rites or Services if Desired.

Maintain Diet with Religious Restrictions When Not Detrimental to Health.

Encourage Spiritual Rituals Not Detrimental to Health.

Provide Opportunity for Individual to Pray with Others or Be Read to by Members of Own Religious Group or a Member of the Health Care Team Who Feels Comfortable with These Activities.

Give "Permission" to Discuss Spiritual Matters with Nurse by Bringing Up Subject of Spiritual Welfare if Necessary.

Use Questions about Past Beliefs and Spiritual Experiences to Assist Person in Putting this Life Event Into Wider Perspective.

Offer to Pray/Meditate/Read with Client If You Are Comfortable with This, or Arrange for Another Member of Health Care Team If More Appropriate.

Be Available and Willing to Listen When Client Expresses Self-Doubt, Guilt, or Other Negative Feelings.

Offer to Contact Other Spiritual Support Person (e.g., Pastoral Care, Hospital Chaplain) if Person Cannot Share Feelings with Usual Spiritual Leader.

Pediatric Interventions

Provide Child with Opportunity to Engage in Usual Spiritual Practices (e.g., Bedtime Prayers, Visit to Chapel).

Discuss if Being Sick Has Changed His or Her Beliefs (e.g., Prayer Requests).

Clarify that Accidents or Illnesses Are Not Punishments for "Bad" Acts.

Support an Adolescent Who May Be Struggling for Understanding of Spiritual Teachings.

For Parental Conflict About Treatment of Child:

If parents refuse treatment of child, encourage consideration of alternative methods of therapy (e.g., use of Christian Science nurses and practitioners; special surgeons and techniques for surgery without blood transfusions); support individual making informed decision even if decision conflicts with own values.

If treatment is still refused, physician or hospital administrator may obtain court order appointing temporary guardian to consent to treatment.

Call spiritual leader to support parents (and possibly child).

Encourage expression of negative feelings.

▶ Spiritual Distress, Risk for

DEFINITION

The state in which the individual or group is at risk of experiencing a disturbance in the belief or value system that provides strength, hope, and meaning to life.

RISK FACTORS

Refer to *Spiritual Distress* for related factors.

NOC

Hope, Spiritual Well-Being

Goals

The person will express continued spiritual harmony.

Indicators
- Continue to practice usual spiritual rituals.
- Describe increased comfort after assistance.

NIC

Refer to *Spiritual Distress*

Generic Interventions

Refer to *Spiritual Distress* for interventions.

▶ Religiosity, Impaired

DEFINITION

The state in which a person or group has impaired ability to exercise reliance on beliefs of a particular denomination or faith community and to participate in related rituals.

DEFINING CHARACTERISTICS

Individual experiences distress because of difficulty in adhering to prescribed religious rituals.

Examples
- Religious ceremonies
- Dietary regulations
- Certain clothing
- Prayer
- Request to worship
- Holiday observances
- Expresses emotional distress because of separation from faith community
- Expresses emotional distress regarding religious beliefs and/or religious social network

- Expresses a need to reconnect with previous belief patterns and customs
- Questions religious belief patterns and customs

RELATED FACTORS

Pathophysiologic

Related to sickness/illness
Related to suffering
Related to pain

Situational

Related to personal crisis related to activity
Related to fear of death
Related to embarrassment at practicing spiritual rituals
Related to barriers to practicing spiritual rituals
Intensive care restrictions
Confinement to bed or room
Lack of privacy
Lack of availability of special foods/diets

NOC

Spiritual Well-Being

Goal

The person will express satisfaction with spiritual condition.

Indicators

- Continue spiritual practices not detrimental to health.
- Express decreasing feelings of guilt and anxiety.

NIC

Spiritual Support, Presence

General Interventions

Explore Whether the Client Desires to Engage in an Allowable Religious or Spiritual Practice or Ritual; If So, Provide Opportunities To Do So.

Express Your Understanding and Acceptance of the Importance of the Client's Religious or Spiritual Beliefs and Practices.

Assess for Causative and Contributing Factors.

Hospital or nursing home environment

Limitations related to disease process or treatment regimen (e.g., cannot kneel to pray owing to traction; prescribed diet differs from usual religious diet)

Fear of imposing on or antagonizing medical and nursing staff with requests for spiritual rituals

Embarrassment over spiritual beliefs or customs (especially common in adolescents)

Separation from articles, texts, or environment of spiritual significance

Lack of transportation to spiritual place or service

Spiritual leader unavailable because of emergency or lack of time

Eliminate or Reduce Causative and Contributing Factors, If Possible.

Limitations Imposed by the Hospital or Nursing Home Environment

Provide privacy and quiet as needed for daily prayer, visit of spiritual leader, and spiritual reading and contemplation:

- Pull curtains or close door.
- Turn off television and radio.
- Ask desk to hold calls, if possible.
- Note spiritual interventions on Kardex and include in care plan.

Contact spiritual leader to clarify practices and perform religious rites or services, if desired:

- Communicate with spiritual leader concerning person's condition.
- Address Roman Catholic, Orthodox, and Episcopal priests as "Father," other Christian ministers as "Pastor," and Jewish rabbis as "Rabbi."
- Prevent interruption during visit, if possible.
- Offer to provide table or stand covered with clean white cloth.
- Chart visit and client's response.

Inform about religious services and materials available within the institution.

Limitations Related to Disease Process or Treatment Regimen

Encourage spiritual rituals not detrimental to health:

- Assist clients with physical limitations in prayer and spiritual observances (e.g., help to hold rosary; help to kneeling position, if appropriate).

- Assist in habits of personal cleanliness.
- Avoid shaving if beard is of spiritual significance.
- Allow client to wear religious clothing or jewelry whenever possible.
- Make special arrangements for burial of resected limbs or body organs.
- Allow family or spiritual leader to perform ritual care of body.
- Make arrangements as needed for other important spiritual rituals (e.g., circumcisions).

Maintain diet with spiritual restrictions when not detrimental to health:

- Consult with dietitian.
- Allow fasting for short periods, if possible.*
- Change therapeutic diet as necessary.*
- Have family or friends bring in special food, if possible.
- Have members of spiritual group supply meals to the person at home.
- Be as flexible as possible in serving methods, times of meals, and so forth.

Fear of Imposing or Embarrassment

Communicate acceptance of various spiritual beliefs and practices.

Convey nonjudgmental, respectful attitude.

Acknowledge importance of spiritual needs.

Express willingness of health care team to help in meeting spiritual needs.

Provide privacy and ensure confidentiality.

Separation from Articles, Texts, or Environment of Spiritual Significance

Question person about missing religious or spiritual articles or reading material.

Obtain missing items from clergy in hospital, spiritual leader, family, or members of spiritual group.

Treat these articles and books with respect.

Allow person to keep spiritual articles and books within reach as much as possible, or where they can be easily seen.

Protect from loss or damage (e.g., medal pinned to gown can be lost in laundry).

Recognize that articles without overt religious meaning may have spiritual significance for person (e.g., wedding band).

---

*May require a primary care professional's order.

Use spiritual texts in large print, in Braille, or on tape when appropriate.

Provide opportunity for person to pray with others or be read to by members of own religious group or member of the health care team who feels comfortable with these activities.

Jews and Seventh-Day Adventists would find Psalms 23, 24, 42, 63, 71, 103, 121, and 127 appropriate.

Christians would also appreciate I Corinthians 13, Matthew 5:3–11, Romans 12, and the Lord's Prayer.

Lack of Transportation

Take person to chapel or quiet environment on hospital grounds.

Arrange transportation to church or synagogue for person in home.

Provide access to spiritual programming on radio and television when appropriate.

Spiritual Leader Unavailable Because of Emergency or Lack of Time

Baptize critically ill newborn of Greek Orthodox, Episcopal, or Roman Catholic parents.

Perform other mandatory spiritual rituals, if possible.

▶ Religiosity, Risk for Impaired

DEFINITION

The state in which an individual is at risk for impaired ability to exercise reliance on beliefs of a particular denomination or faith community and to participate in related rituals.

RISK FACTORS

Refer to *Impaired Religiosity*.

NOC

Spiritual Well-being

Goals

The person will express continued satisfaction with religious activities.

Indicators

- Continue to practice religious rituals.
- Describe increased comfort after assessment.

Interventions

Refer to **Impaired Religiosity** for interventions.

STRESS OVERLOAD

DEFINITION

State in which an individual or group experiences overwhelming, excessive amounts and types of demands that require action.

DEFINING CHARACTERISTICS

Physiologic

Headaches
Indigestion
Sleep difficulties
Restlessness
Fatigue

Emotional

Crying
Edginess
Nervous
Overwhelmed

Anger
Impatience
Easily upset
Feeling sick

Cognitive

Memory loss
Forgetfulness
Difficulty making decisions

Constant worry
Loss of humor
Trouble thinking clearly

Behavioral

Isolation
Lack of intimacy
Excessive smoking

Intolerance
Compulsive eating
Resentment

RELATED FACTORS

The related factors for *Stress Overload* for one person can be multiple co-existing stressors which can be pathophysiologic, maturational, treatment related, situational, environmental, and/or personal.

Pathophysiologic

Related to coping with:
- Acute illness (myocardial infarction, fractured hip)
- Chronic illness (arthritis, depression, COPD)
- Terminal illness
- New diagnosis (cancer, genital herpes, HIV, multiple sclerosis, diabetes mellitus)
- Disfiguring condition

Situational (Personal, Environmental)

Related to actual or anticipated loss of a significant other secondary to:

Death, dying	Moving
Divorce	Military duty

Related to coping with:

Dying	War
Assault	

Related to actual or perceived change in socioeconomic status secondary to:

Unemployment	New job
Promotion	Illness
Destruction of personal property	

Related to coping with:

Family violence	New family member
Substance abuse	Relationship problems

Maturational

Related to coping with:

Retirement	Financial changes
Loss of residence	Functional losses

■■■ AUTHOR'S NOTE

This new diagnosis in 2006 represents a person in an overwhelming situation with multiple varied stressors. The person determines if he or she is in overload with the nurse's help. If *Stress Overload* is not reduced, the person can deteriorate and is in danger of injury and illness.

(continued)

■■■ **AUTHOR'S NOTE** *(Continued)*

In addition to *Stress Overload*, the nurse should assess for the presence of other nursing diagnoses that also may be present. For example, unrelenting caregiving responsibilities can cause *Caregiver Role Strain*. Individual or family member abuse of alcohol or drugs can cause *Ineffective Coping*, *Dysfunctional Family Processes*, and/or *Risk for Other-Directed Violence*. *Impaired Parenting* may be present.

If the person is also experiencing a loss of a significant person or situation such as divorce or loss of a job, *Grieving* may be an additional nursing diagnosis.

Even if other nursing diagnoses are present, *Stress Overload* is very useful to assist the person with problem-solving strategies and stress reduction activities such as exercise and sufficient sleep.

NOC

Well-Being, Health Beliefs, Anxiety Level, Coping, Knowledge: Health Promotion, Knowledge: Health Resources

Goal

The person will verbalize an intent to change two behaviors to decrease or manage stressors.

Indicators

- Identify stressors that can be controlled and those that cannot.
- Identify one behavior to reduce or eliminate, to increase successful stress management.

NIC

Anxiety Reduction, Behavior Modification, Exercise Promotion

Interventions

Assist the Person to Appraise Their Current Stressors as Extrinsic (No Control) or Intrinsic (Some Control).

Teach the Person How to Break the Cycle of His or Her Stress in a Traffic Jam and that There Is an Increase in Heart Rate and Respirations and Strong Feelings of Anger (Edelman & Mandle, 2006).

Purposefully distract yourself by thinking of something pleasant.

Engage in a diversional activity.

Initiate relaxation breaking: inhale through the nose, taking 4 seconds.

Refer to resources to learn relaxation techniques, such as audiotapes, printed material, yoga.

Ask the Person to List One or Two Changes He or She Would Like to Make in the Next Week.

Diet (eat one vegetable a day)

Exercise (walk one to two blocks each day)

If Sleep Disturbances Are Present, Refer to Disturbed Sleep Patterns.

Ask what activity brings them feelings of peace, joy, and happiness. Ask them to incorporate one of these activities each week.

If Spiritual Needs Are Identified as Deficient, Refer to Spiritual Distress.

Ask what is important, and if change is needed to include in life.

Assist to Set Realistic Goals to Achieve a More Balanced, Health-Promoting Lifestyle.

What is most important?

What aspects of your life would you like to change most?

What is the first step?

When?

Initiate Health Teaching and Referrals as Necessary.

If person is engaged in substance or alcohol abuse, refer him or her for drug and alcohol abuse.

If person has severe depression or anxiety, refer him or her for professional counseling.

If family functioning is disabled, refer him or her for family counseling.

SUDDEN INFANT DEATH SYNDROME, RISK FOR

DEFINITION
The state in which an infant younger than 1 year old is at risk to experience sudden death, unexpected by history and unexplained by postmortem examination.

RISK FACTORS (MCMILLAN ET AL., 1999)
Pathophysiologic
Related to increased vulnerability secondary to:

Cyanosis
Poor feeding
Tachycardia
Small for gestational age*
Hypothermia
Irritability
History of diarrhea, vomiting, or listlessness 2 weeks before death

Tachypnea
Prematurity*
Fever
Respiratory distress
Low birth weight*
Low Apgar score (<7)

Related to increased vulnerability secondary to prenatal maternal:

Anemia*
Sexually transmitted infections
Intrauterine hypoxia

Urinary tract infection
Poor weight gain

Situational (Personal, Environmental)
Related to increased vulnerability secondary to maternal:

Cigarette smoking,
Drug use* (cocaine, heroin)
Inadequate prenatal care
Low educational levels*
Nutritional deficiencies
Young maternal age (<20 years)*

Alcohol use
Lack of breastfeeding*
Single mother*
Shorter interval between pregnancies

*Widely accepted; general agreement among investigators.

Related to increased vulnerability secondary to:

Crowded living conditions*
Sleeping on side*
Infant/parent bed sharing
No pacifier
Cold environment
Previous SIDS death in
   family

Sleeping on stomach
   (prone)*
Sleeping on soft surface
Overheating
Smoking exposure
   (prenatal, postnatal)

Related to increased infant vulnerability secondary to

Male gender*
Native American origin*
Alaskan Native origin
Recent febrile illness
Growth failure

Multiple births
African descent*
Prematurity
Age 2-4 months

NOC

Knowledge: Maternal–Child Health, Risk Control:
Tobacco Use, Risk Control Knowledge: Infant Safety

Goals

The caregiver will reduce or eliminate risk factors that are
modifiable.

Indicators

- Position infant on back.
- Eliminate smoking in the home, near the infant, and during
  pregnancy.
- Participate in prenatal and newborn medical care.
- Improve maternal health (e.g., treat anemia, promote optimal
  nutrition).
- Enroll in drug and alcohol programs, if indicated.
- Avoid giving over-the-counter medications to infant.

NIC

Teaching: Infant Safety, Risk Identification

Generic Interventions

**Explain SIDS to Caregivers and
Identify Risk Factors Present.**

Reduce or Eliminate Risk Factors that Can Be Modified.

- Maintain room temperature that is not too hot or cold
- Position infant on back only
- Avoid tobacco smoke
- Do not sleep with infant, but have infant in the same room in own crib
- Avoid pillows, loose blankets, heavy blankets

Determine If Home Cardiorespiratory Monitoring Is Indicated. Consult With Pediatrician or Neonatal/Pediatric Nurse Practitioner (McMillan et al., 1999).

Teach Parents to Focus on the Infant When Alarm Sounds, Not the Machine.

Teach to Assess
Infant's color pink?
Infant's breathing

Initiate Health Teaching and Referrals as Indicated.

Provide instructions on use of home monitor, if appropriate.
Refer client to drug and alcohol treatment programs as indicated.
Discuss strategies to stop smoking (refer to the index under *Smoking*).
Provide emergency numbers as indicated.
Refer to social agencies as indicated.

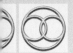

SURGICAL RECOVERY, DELAYED

DEFINITION

The state in which an individual experiences, or is at risk of experiencing, an extension of the number of postoperative days required to initiate and perform self-care activities.

■■■■ **AUTHOR'S NOTE**
This newly accepted diagnosis represents an individual who has not achieved recovery from a surgical procedure during the expected time period. As one reviews the defining characteristics from NANDA, there is some confusion regarding the difference between defining characteristics (signs and symptoms) and related factors. Those preceded by an asterisk (*) are not defining characteristics, but are factors that can cause or contribute to *Delayed Surgical Recovery*. Currently the diagnosis has not been developed sufficiently for clinical use. This author recommends utilizing other nursing diagnoses, such as *Self-Care Deficit*, *Acute Pain*, or *Imbalanced Nutrition*.

DEFINING CHARACTERISTICS (NANDA)

Postpones resumption of activities (home, work)
Perception that more time is needed to recover
Requires help to complete self-care
*Evidence of interrupted healing of surgical area
*Loss of appetite with or without nausea
*Difficulty in moving about
*Refer to Author's Note for explanation of asterisk.
*Reports pain or discomfort

THOUGHT PROCESSES, DISTURBED

Thought Processes, Disturbed
Memory, Impaired

DEFINITION

The state in which an individual experiences a disruption in such mental activities as conscious thought, reality orientation, problem solving, judgment, and comprehension related to coping, personality, and/or mental disorder.

AUTHOR'S NOTE

This diagnosis was deleted from the NANDA list in 2008 because significant revision work was not submitted to NANDA. This author will retain this diagnosis because of its clinical usefulness and because it has been developed by this author.

The diagnosis *Disturbed Thought Processes* describes an individual with altered perception and cognition that interferes with daily living. Causes are biochemical or psychological disturbances (e.g., depression, personality disorders). The focus of nursing is to reduce disturbed thinking and promote reality orientation.

The nurse should be cautioned when using this diagnosis as a "wastebasket" diagnosis for all clients with disturbed thinking or confusion. Frequently, confusion in older adults is erroneously attributed to aging. Confusion in the older adult can be caused by a single factor or multiple factors (e.g., dementia, medication side effects, depression, or metabolic disorder). Depression causes impaired thinking in older adults more frequently than dementia (Miller, 2009). Refer to *Confusion* for additional information.

DEFINING CHARACTERISTICS

Major (Must Be Present)

Inaccurate interpretation of stimuli, internal or external

Minor (May Be Present)

Cognitive deficits, including abstraction, problem solving, memory deficits
Suspiciousness
Delusions
Hallucinations
Phobias
Obsessions

Confusion/disorientation
Ritualistic behavior
Impulsivity
Inappropriate social behavior
Distractibility
Lack of consensual validation

RELATED FACTORS

Pathophysiologic

Related to physiologic changes secondary to:
Drug or alcohol withdrawal

Related to biochemical alterations

Situational (Personal, Environmental)

Related to emotional trauma

Related to abuse (physical, sexual, mental)

Related to torture

Related to childhood trauma

Related to repressed fears

Related to panic level of anxiety

Related to continued low levels of stimulation

Related to decreased attention span and ability to process information secondary to:

Depression	Anxiety
Fear	Grieving

Maturational

Older Adult

Isolation, late-life depression

NOC

Cognitive Ability, Cognitive Orientation, Concentration, Distorted Thought Control, Information Processing, Memory, Decision Making

Goals

The person will maintain reality orientation and communicate clearly with others.

Indicators

- Recognize changes in thinking/behavior.
- Identify situations that occur before hallucinations/delusions.
- Use coping strategies to deal effectively with hallucinations/delusions (specify).
- Participate in unit activities (specify).
- Express delusional material less frequently.

NIC

Cognitive Stimulation, Dementia Management, Reality Orientation, Family Support, Decision-Making Support, Hallucination Management, Anxiety Reduction, Memory Training, Environmental Management: Safety

Generic Interventions

Approach in a Calm, Nurturing Manner.

Recognize When Person Is Testing the Trustworthiness of Others.

Avoid Making Promises that Cannot Be Fulfilled.

Initial Staff Contact Should Be Minimal and Brief With Suspicious Person; Increase Time as Suspicion Decreases.

Verify Your Interpretation of What Person Is Experiencing ("I Understand You Are Fearful of Others.").

Use Communication that Helps Person Maintain Own Individuality (e.g., "I" Instead of "We").

For Hallucinations:

Observe for verbal and nonverbal hallucinations—inappropriate laughter, delayed verbal response, eye movements, moving lips without sound, increased motor movements, grinning.

Direct the focus from delusional expression to discussion of reality-centered situations.

Encourage differentiation of stimuli arising from inner sources from those from outside (e.g., in response to "I hear voices," say, "Those are the voices of persons on television" or "I hear no one speaking now; they are your own thoughts.").

Avoid the impression that you confirm or approve reality distortions; tactfully express doubt.

Set limits for discussing repetitive delusional material ("You've already told me about that; let's talk about something realistic.").

Identify the underlying needs being met by the delusions/hallucinations.

Help connect false beliefs with increased levels of anxiety.

Assist in Communicating More Effectively.

Ask for the meaning of what is said; do not assume that you understand.

Validate your interpretation of what is being said ("Is this what you mean?").

Clarify all global pronouns—we, they ("Who is *they*?").

Refocus when person changes the subject in the middle of an explanation or thought.

Tell the person when you are not following his or her train of thought.

Do not mimic or restate words or phrases that you do not understand.

Teach the person to validate consensually with others.

Ask yes, no, or multiple choice questions.

Keep sentences short and clear.

Assist Person to Set Limits on Own Behavior.

Discuss alternative methods of coping (e.g., taking a walk instead of crying).

Confront person with the attitude that regression is not acceptable behavior.

Help delay gratification (e.g., "I want you to wait 5 minutes before you repeat your request for help in making your bed.").

Encourage person to achieve realistic expectations.

Pace expectations to avoid frustration.

Encourage and Support Person in the Decision-Making Process.

Compliment the person who assumes more responsibility.

Provide opportunity for person to contribute to own treatment plan.

Help establish future goals that are realistic; examine problems in achieving a goal, and suggest various alternatives.

Assist Person to Differentiate Between Needs and Demands.

Explain the difference between needs and demands (e.g., food and clothing are needs; expectations that others dress and feed person, if he or she can do it, are demands).

Assist person to examine the effects of behavior on others; encourage a change in behavior if it evokes negative responses.

Help Person Recognize Behaviors that Stimulate Rejection.

Identify activities that reduce interpersonal anxiety (e.g., exercise, controlled-breathing exercises).

Set limits firmly and kindly on destructive behavior.

Allow expression of negative emotions, verbally or in constructive activity.

Help person accept responsibility for responses he or she elicits from others.

Encourage discussion of problems in relating after visits with family members.

Help person test new skills in relating to others in role-playing situations.

Anticipate Difficulties in Adjusting to Community Living; Discuss Concerns about Returning to Community, and Elicit Family Reaction to Individual's Discharge.

Provide Health Teaching that Will Prepare Person to Deal with Life Stresses (Methods of Relaxation, Problem-Solving Skills, How to Negotiate With Others, How to Express Feelings Constructively).

Inform Person of Social Agencies that Offer Help in Adjusting to Community Living.

Provide Sensory Input that Is Sufficient and Meaningful.

Keep person oriented to time and place:

- Refer to time of day and place each morning.
- Provide person with a clock and calendar large enough to see.
- Provide person with opportunity to see daylight and dark through a window, or take person outdoors.
- Single out holidays with cards or pins (e.g., wear a red heart for Valentine's Day).

Encourage family to bring in familiar objects from home (photographs, afghan).

Discuss current events, seasonal events (snow, water activities); share your interests (travel, crafts).

Assess if person can perform an activity with own hands (e.g., latch rugs, wood crafts):

- Provide reading materials, audio tapes, puzzles (manual, computer, crossword).
- Encourage person to keep own records if possible (e.g., intake and output).
- Provide tasks to perform (addressing envelopes, occupational therapy).

Refer to Risk for Injury for Strategies for Assessing and Manipulating the Environment for Hazards.

👫 Pediatric Interventions

For Children With Thought Disturbance, Assess for Signs of Dissociative Disorder:

Abusive history (physical, sexual)
Amnesic periods
Switching between alter personalities
Affect disturbances
Abrupt behavioral changes

Refer for Multidisciplinary Evaluation.

▶ Memory, Impaired

DEFINITION

The state in which an individual experiences a temporary or permanent inability to remember or recall bits of information or behavioral skills.

■■■■ **AUTHOR'S NOTE**
This diagnosis is useful when the person can be helped to function better because of improved memory. If the person's memory cannot be improved because of cerebral degeneration, this diagnosis is not appropriate. Instead the nurse should evaluate the effects of impaired memory on functioning as *Self-Care Deficits* or *Risk for Injury*. The focus of interventions would be on improving self-care or protection, not on improving memory.

DEFINING CHARACTERISTICS
Major (Must Be Present, One or More)

Observed or reported experiences of forgetting
Inability to determine if a behavior was performed
Inability to learn or retain new skills or information
Inability to perform a previously learned skill
Inability to recall factual information
Inability to recall recent or past events

RELATED FACTORS

Pathophysiologic

Related to central nervous system changes secondary to:

Degenerative brain disease	Lesion
Head injury	Cerebrovascular accident

Related to reduced quantity and quality of information processed secondary to:

Visual deficits	Poor physical fitness
Learning habits	Educational level
Hearing deficits	Fatigue
Intellectual skills	

Related to nutritional deficiencies (e.g., vitamins C, B12, folate, niacin, thiamine)

Treatment-Related

Related to effects of medication (specify) on memory storage

Situational (Personal, Environmental)

Related to self-fulfilling expectations

Related to excessive self-focusing and worrying secondary to grieving, depression, or anxiety

Related to alcohol consumption

Related to lack of motivation

Related to lack of stimulation

Related to difficulty concentrating secondary to:

Stress	Sleep disturbances
Lack of intellectual stimulation	Distractions
	Pain

NOC

Cognitive Orientation, Memory

Goals

The person will report increased satisfaction with memory.

Indicators

- Identify three techniques to improve memory.
- Relate factors that deter memory.

NIC

Reality Orientation, Memory Training, Environmental Management

Generic Interventions

Discuss the Person's Beliefs About Memory Deficits.

Correct misinformation.

Explain that negative expectations can result in memory deficits.

If a person is older, provide accurate information about age-related changes.

Explain that If One Wants to Improve Memory, the Intent to Remember and the Knowledge About Techniques for Remembering Are Needed (Miller, 2009).

If the Person Has Difficulty Concentrating, Explain the Favorable Effects of Relaxation and Imagery.

Teach the Person Two or Three Methods for Improving Memory Skills (Maier-Lorentz, 2000; Miller, 2009):

Write things down (e.g., use lists, calendars, and notebooks).

Use auditory cues (e.g., timers, alarm clocks) in conjunction with written cues.

Have specific places for specific items, and keep the items in their proper place (e.g., keep keys on a hook near the door).

Put reminders in appropriate places (e.g., place shoes to be repaired near the door).

Use active observation—pay attention to details of what's going on around you, and be alert to the environment.

Make associations between names and mental images (e.g., Carol and Christmas carol).

Rehearse items you want to remember by repeating them aloud or writing the information on paper.

Divide information into small "chunks" that can be remembered easily (e.g., to remember an address or a zip code, divide it into groups ["seven hundred sixty, fifty five"]).

Search the alphabet while focusing on what you are trying to remember (e.g., to remember that someone's name is Martin, start with names that begin with "A" and continue naming names through the alphabet until your memory is jogged for the correct one).

Explain that When One Is Trying to Learn or Remember Something:

Minimize distractions.
Do not rush.
Maintain some form of organization of routine tasks.
Carry a note pad or calendar or use written cues.

When Teaching (Miller, 2009; Stanley & Beare, 2000):

Eliminate distractions.
Present information as concretely as possible.
Use practical examples.
Allow learner to pace the learning.
Use visual, auditory aids.
Provide advance organizers: outlines, written cues.
Encourage use of aids.
Make sure glasses are clean and lights are soft-white.
Correct wrong answers immediately.
Encourage verbal responses.

Ⓒ Geriatric Interventions

Encourage Client to Share Concerns About Memory Problems.

Explain that Short-Term Memory May Decline With Aging.

Explain that Memory Aids Can Improve Memory. Refer to Generic Interventions.

TISSUE PERFUSION, INEFFECTIVE

Tissue Perfusion, Ineffective
Cardiac Tissue Perfusion, Risk for Decreased
Cerebral Tissue Perfusion, Risk for Ineffective
Peripheral Tissue Perfusion, Ineffective
Renal Perfusion, Risk for Ineffective

DEFINITION

The state in which an individual experiences, or is at risk of experiencing, a decrease at the capillary level in oxygenation.

■■■■ AUTHOR'S NOTE

This nursing diagnosis is restricted to represent only diminished peripheral tissue perfusion situations in which nurses prescribe definitive treatment to reduce, eliminate, or prevent the problem.

In the other situations of diminished cardiopulmonary, cerebral, renal, or gastrointestinal tissue perfusion, the nurse should focus on the functional abilities of the individual that are or may be compromised because of the decreased tissue perfusion. The nurse should also monitor to detect physiologic complications of decreased tissue perfusion and label these situations as collaborative problems. The following illustrates examples of a compromised functional health problem (nursing diagnosis) and a potential complication (collaborative problem) for an individual with compromised cerebral tissue perfusion:

Risk for Injury related to vertigo secondary to recent head injury
(nursing diagnosis)
Risk for Complications of Increased Intracranial Pressure (collaborative problem)

Refer to Section 3 of Carpenito, L. J. (2010). *Nursing Diagnosis: Application to Clinical Practice* (13th ed.), Philadelphia: Lippincott Williams & Wilkins, for additional information on collaborative problems. For additional examples of nursing diagnoses and collaborative problems grouped under medical conditions, refer to Section 3 of this handbook.

▶ Risk for Decreased Cardiac Tissue Perfusion

DEFINITION (NANDA)

The state in which an individual is at risk for a decrease in cardiac tissue perfusion.

RISK FACTORS (NANDA)

Birth Control Pills (medication side effect of combination pills)

Cardiac Surgery (treatment with multiple complications and associated nursing diagnoses)

Cardiac Tamponade (clinical emergency)

Coronary artery spasm (clinical emergency)

Diabetes mellitus (medical diagnosis with multiple complications and associated nursing diagnoses)

Drug abuse (clinical situations with multiple complications)

Elevated C-reactive protein (positive laboratory test)

Family history of coronary artery disease (These relate to nursing diagnoses of Risk Prone Health Behavior and/or Ineffective Self-Health Management)

Hyperlipidemia (medical diagnosis with multiple complications and associated nursing diagnoses)

Hypertension (medical diagnosis with multiple complications with associated modifiable risk lifestyles)

Hypoxemia (collaborative problem refer to Section 3)

Hypovolemia (collaborative problem refer to Section 3)

Hypoxia (collaborative problem refer to Section 3)

Lack of knowledge of modifiable risk factors (e.g., smoking, sedentary lifestyle, obesity)

(These relate to nursing diagnoses of Risk Prone Health Behavior and/or Ineffective Self-Health Management)

▪▪▪▪ **AUTHOR'S NOTE**

This new NANDA-I nursing diagnosis represents a collection of risk factors that have very different clinical implications. Some are single complications as RC of Hypovolemia and RC of Hypoxia and are discussed in Section 3. Some are medical emergencies as cardiac tamponade, coronary artery spasm or occlusion, which will have protocols for medical interventions.

Birth control pills can have side effects of nausea, breast discomforts, elevated blood pressure and adverse events as cardiovascular or cerebral thrombus; using a nursing diagnosis as Risk for Decreased Cardiac Perfusion to describe one adverse event is not clinically usefully. If a diagnosis is needed for this clinical situation, use Risk for Complications of Medication Therapy Adverse Effects, specifically Risk for Complications of Oral Combination Contraception Therapy.

Some have a collection of physiological complications that are related to the situation and can be labeled as Risk for Complications of Cardiac Surgery, RC of Acute Coronary

(continued)

■■■■ **AUTHOR'S NOTE** *(Continued)*

Syndrome, or RC of Diabetes Mellitus. For example, Risk for Complications of Alcohol Abuse would have the following collaborative problems:*

Risk for Complications of Delirium Tremors

Risk for Complications of Seizures

Risk for Complications of Autonomic Hyperactivity

Risk for Complications of Hypovolemia

Risk for Complications of Hypoglycemia

Risk for Complications of Alcohol Hallucinosis

Risk for Complications of Cardio/Vascular Shock.

Nursing Diagnoses associated with alcohol abuse:

Anxiety related to loss of control, memory loss, and fear of withdrawal.

Ineffective Coping or Ineffective Denial related to inability to constructively manage stressors without alcohol.

Imbalanced Nutrition: Less than Body Requirements related to inadequate intake of balanced diet and water-soluble vitamins

Ineffective Self-Health Management related to insufficient knowledge of condition, treatments available, high-risk situations and community recovery programs

Interventions/Outcomes

Refer to Section 3 Risk for Complications of Cardiovascular Dysfunction for specific interventions for cardiovascular complications. If the focus is on modifying one's lifestyle, refer to Sedentary Lifestyle, Risk-Prone Health Behavior or Ineffective Self-Health Management in Section 1.

▶ Risk for Ineffective Cerebral Tissue Perfusion

DEFINITION (NANDA)

The state in which an individual is at risk for a decrease in cerebral tissue circulation.

---

*For more specific care plans with nursing interventions and outcomes for clinical situations (Medical Diagnoses, e.g., stroke, seizures; Surgeries, e.g., cranial surgery; Treatments/Therapies, e.g., mechanical ventilation, chemotherapy, and 70 other clinical situations) refer to Carpenito-Moyet, L.J. (2009) *Nursing Care Plans and Documentation*, 5th ed., Lippincott Williams & Wilkins.

RISK FACTORS (NANDA)

Abnormal partial thromboplastin time
Abnormal Prothrombin time
Akinetic left ventricular segment
Aortic atherosclerosis
Arterial dissection
Atrial fibrillation
Atrial myxoma
Brain Tumor
Carotid stenosis
Cerebral aneurysm
Coagulopathies (e.g., sickle cell anemia)
Dilated Cardiomyopathy
Disseminated intravascular coagulation
Embolism
Head trauma
Hypercholesterolemia
Hypertension
Endocardiitis
Left atrial appendage thrombosis
Mechanical prosthetic valve
Mitral stenosis
Neoplasm of the brain
Recent myocardial infarction
Sick sinus syndrome
Substance abuse
Thrombolytic therapy
Treatment-related side effects (cardiopulmonary bypass,
    medications)

■■■■ **AUTHOR'S NOTE**

This newly accepted NANDA-I nursing diagnosis represents
a collection of risk factors that have very different clinical
implications. Some are physiological complications that
are related to a medical diagnosis or treatment and can be
labeled as Risk for Complications of Head Trauma, RC of
Brain Tumor, or RC of Thrombolytic Therapy. These clinical situations have both nursing diagnoses and collaborative
problems that require interventions.

For example Risk for Complications of Cranial Surgery
would have the following collaborative problems:

Risk for Complications of Increased Intracranial Pressure
Risk for Complications of Bleeding, Hypovolemia/shock

(continued)

■■■■ **AUTHOR'S NOTE** *(Continued)*
Risk for Complications of Thromboembolism
Risk for Complications of Cranial Nerve Dysfunction
Risk for Complications of Cardiac Dysrhythmias
Risk for Complications of Seizures
Risk for Complications of Sensory/Motor Alterations

and nursing diagnoses associated with this clinical situation:*
Anxiety to impending surgery and fear of outcomes
Acute Pain related to compression/displacement of brain
tissue and increased intracranial pressure
Risk for Ineffective Self-Health Management related to
insufficient knowledge of wound care signs and symptoms
of complications, restrictions and follow-up care.

Interventions/Goals

Refer to Section 3 for specific collaborative problems under Risk
for Complications of Neurologic Dysfunction

▶ Ineffective Peripheral Tissue Perfusion

DEFINITION

The state in which an individual experiences, or is at risk for experiencing, a decrease in nutrition and respiration at the peripheral cellular level because of a decrease in capillary blood supply.

DEFINING CHARACTERISTICS

Major (Must Be Present, One or More)

Presence of One of the Following Types:
Claudication (arterial)   Aching pain (arterial)
Rest pain (arterial)

Diminished or Absent Arterial Pulses

---

*For more specific care plans with nursing interventions and outcomes for
clinical situations (Medical Diagnoses, e.g., stroke, seizures; Surgeries, e.g.,
cranial surgery; Treatments/Therapies, e.g., mechanical ventilation, chemotherapy, and 70 other clinical situations) refer to Carpenito-Moyet, L.J.
(2009) *Nursing Care Plans and Documentation*, 5th ed., Lippincott Williams
& Wilkins.

Skin Color Changes

Pallor (arterial)   Reactive hyperemia (arterial)
Cyanosis (venous)

Skin Temperature Changes

Cooler (arterial)   Warmer (venous)

Decreased Blood Pressure (Arterial)

Capillary Refill Greater than 3 Seconds (Arterial)

Minor (May Be Present)

Edema (venous)
Change in sensory function (arterial)
Change in motor function (arterial)
Trophic tissue changes (arterial):
  • Hard, thick nails
  • Loss of hair
  • Nonhealing wound

RELATED FACTORS

Pathophysiologic

Related to compromised blood flow secondary to:

Vascular disorders

Arteriosclerosis   Raynaud's disease/syndrome
Hypertension   Aneurysm
Varicosities   Arterial thrombosis
Buerger's disease   Deep vein thrombosis
Sickle cell crisis   Collagen vascular disease
Cirrhosis   Rheumatoid arthritis
Alcoholism   Leriche's syndrome
Diabetes mellitus
Hypotension
Blood dyscrasias (platelet disorders)
Renal failure
Cancer/tumor

Treatment-Related

Related to immobilization
Related to invasive lines
Related to pressure sites/constriction (Ace bandages, stockings)
Related to blood vessel trauma or compression

Situational (Personal, Environmental)

*Related to pressure of enlarging uterus on peripheral
circulation*

*Related to pressure of enlarged abdomen on pelvic and
peripheral circulation*
Related to dependent venous pooling
Related to hypothermia
Related to vasoconstricting effects of tobacco
*Related to decreased circulating volume secondary to
dehydration*
Related to pressure of muscle mass secondary to weightlifting

NOC

Sensory Function: Cutaneous, Tissue Integrity, Tissue
Perfusion: Peripheral

Goals

The individual will report a decrease in pain.

Indicators

- Define peripheral vascular problem in own words.
- Identify factors that improve peripheral circulation.
- Identify necessary lifestyle changes.
- Identify medical regimen, diet, medications, activities that pro-
  mote vasodilatation.
- Identify factors that inhibit peripheral circulation.
- State when to contact physician or health care professional.

NIC

Peripheral Sensation Management, Circulatory
Care: Venous Insufficiency, Circulatory Care: Arterial
Insufficiency, Positioning, Exercise Promotion

Generic Interventions

Teach Person to

Keep extremity in a dependent position.
Keep extremity warm. (Do not use heating pad or hot water
    bottle, because the individual with a peripheral vascular
    disease may have a disturbance in sensation and will not be
    able to determine if the temperature is hot enough to damage
    tissue; the use of external heat may also increase the metabolic
    demands of the tissue beyond its capacity.)

Reduce Risk for Trauma.

Change positions at least every hour.
Avoid leg crossing.

Reduce external pressure points (inspect shoes daily for rough lining).

Avoid sheepskin heel protectors (they increase heel pressure and pressure across dorsum of foot).

Encourage range-of-motion exercises.

Plan a Daily Walking Program.

Instruct individual in reasons for program.

Teach individual to avoid fatigue.

Instruct to avoid increase in exercise until assessed by physician for cardiac problems.

Reassure individual that walking does not harm the blood vessels or the muscles; "walking into the pain," resting, and resuming walking assists in developing collateral circulation.

Teach Factors that Improve Venous Blood Flow.

Elevate extremity above the level of the heart (may be contraindicated if severe cardiac or respiratory disease is present).

Avoid standing or sitting with legs dependent for long periods.

Consider the use of Ace bandages or below-knee elastic stockings to prevent venous stasis.

Reduce or remove external venous compression that impedes venous flow:
- Avoid pillows behind the knees or Gatch bed that is elevated at the knees.
- Avoid leg crossing.
- Change positions; move extremities or wiggle fingers and toes every hour.
- Avoid garters and tight elastic stockings above the knees.

Measure Baseline Circumference of Calves and Thighs If Individual Is at Risk for Deep Venous Thrombosis or If It Is Suspected.

Teach Person to:

Avoid long car or plane rides (get up and walk around at least every hour).

Keep dry skin lubricated (cracked skin eliminates the physical barrier to infection).

Wear warm clothing during cold weather.

Wear cotton or wool socks.

Avoid dehydration in warm weather.

Give special attention to feet and toes:
- Wash feet and dry well daily.
- Do not soak feet.

- Avoid harsh soaps or chemicals (including iodine) on feet.
- Keep nails trimmed and filed smooth.

Inspect feet and legs daily for injuries and pressure points:

- Wear clean socks.
- Wear shoes that offer support and fit comfortably.
- Inspect the inside of shoes daily for rough lining.

Teach Risk-Factor Modification.

Diet:

- Avoid foods high in cholesterol.
- Modify sodium intake to control hypertension.
- Refer to dietitian.

Relaxation techniques to reduce effects of stress

Smoking cessation

Exercise program

👥 Maternal Interventions

Explain that Uterine Pressure Can Cause Pooling of Venous Blood in Lower Extremities.

Teach to Report Immediately Signs and Symptoms of Thrombosis:

Pain in leg, groin

Unilateral leg swelling

Pale skin

Refer to Generic Interventions for Specific Techniques to Reduce Edema.

▶ Risk for Ineffective Renal Perfusion

DEFINITION (NANDA)

The state in which the individual is at risk for a decrease in blood circulation to the kidney that may compromise health.

RISK FACTORS (NANDA)

Abdominal compartment syndrome

Advanced age

Bilateral cortical necrosis

Burns

Cardiac surgery

Cardiopulmonary bypass
Diabetes mellitus
Exposure to toxins
Female glomerulonephritis
Hyperlipidemia
Hypertension
Hypovolemia
Hypoxemia
Hypoxia
Infection
Malignancy
Malignant Hypertension
Metabolic acidosis
Multitrauma
Polynephritis
Renal artery stenosis
Renal disease (polycystic kidney)
Smoking
Systemic inflammatory response syndrome
Treatment-related side effects (e.g., medications)
Vascular embolism vasculitis

■■■■ AUTHOR'S NOTE

This NANDA-I diagnosis represents a potential complication which is a collaborative problem, Risk for Complications of Renal Insufficiency

If the situation is a medical diagnosis of Acute Kidney Failure or Chronic Renal Disease, using Risk for Complications of Acute Kidney Failure would include the following collaborative problems:*

Risk for Complications of Fluid Overload
Risk for Complications of Metabolic Acidosis
Risk for Complications of Acute Albuminemia
Risk for Complications of Hypertension
Risk for Complications of Pulmonary Edema
Risk for Complications of Dysrhythmias
Risk for Complications of Gastrointestinal Bleeding

(continued)

*For more specific care plans with nursing interventions/rationales and outcomes for clinical situations (medical diagnoses such as Chronic Renal Disease or Acute Kidney Failure; surgical procedures such as nephrectomy; treatments/procedures such as hemodialysis, peritoneal dialysis, and 70 other clinical situations), refer to Carpenito-Moyet, L.J.. (2009) *Nursing Care Plans and Documentation*, 5th ed., Lippincott Williams & Wilkins.

Related nursing diagnoses include:

Risk for Infection Related to Invasive Procedures
Imbalanced Nutrition
Risk for Impaired Tissue Integrity

Interventions/Goals

Refer to Section 3 for interventions/goals for Risk for
   Complications of Renal Insufficiency
Refer to Section 1 for interventions and goals for specific related
   nursing diagnoses.

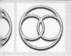

UNILATERAL NEGLECT

DEFINITION

The state in which a person cannot attend to or ignores the hemi-
plegic side of the body and/or, on the affected side, objects, persons, or sounds in the environment.

DEFINING CHARACTERISTICS

Major (Must Be Present, One or More)

Neglect of involved body parts and/or extrapersonal space
   (hemispatial neglect) *and/or*
Denial of the existence of the affected limb or side of the body
   (anosognosia)

Minor (May Be Present)

Difficulty with spatial–perceptual tasks
Hemiplegia (usually of the left side)

RELATED FACTORS

Pathophysiologic

Related to impaired perceptual abilities secondary to:
Cerebrovascular accident   Cerebral tumors
Brain injury/trauma   Cerebral aneurysms

NOC

Body Image, Body Positioning: Self-Initiated, Self-Care Status

Goals

The person will demonstrate an ability to scan the visual field to compensate for loss of function/sensation in affected limbs.

Indicators
• Identify safety hazards in the environment.
• Describe the deficit and the rationale for treatment.

NIC

Unilateral Neglect Management, Self-Care Assistance

Generic Interventions

Initially Adapt the Environment to the Deficit.

Position bed, call light, bedside stand, television, telephone, and personal items on the unaffected side.

Approach and speak to person from unaffected side.

If you must approach from affected side, announce your presence as soon as you enter the room to avoid startling the person.

Gradually Change the Environment As You Teach Person to Compensate and Learn to Recognize the Forgotten Field; Move Furniture and Personal Items out of Visual Field.

For a Person in a Wheelchair, Obtain a Lapboard (Preferably Plexiglas), and Position Affected Arm on Lapboard With Fingertips at Midline; Encourage Person to Look for Arm on Board.

For an Ambulatory Person, Obtain an Arm Sling to Prevent the Arm from Dangling and Causing Shoulder Subluxation.

Constantly Cue Person to the Environment.

Encourage Person to Wear Prescribed Corrective Lenses or Hearing Aids.

For Bathing, Dressing, and Toileting:

Instruct person to attend to affected extremity/side first when performing activities of daily living.

Encourage person to integrate affected extremity during bathing; encourage person to feel extremity by rubbing and massage.

For Eating:

Instruct person to eat in small amounts; place food on unaffected side of mouth.

Instruct person to use tongue to sweep out pockets of food from affected side after every bite.

Check oral cavity for pocketed food/medication after meals/ medications.

Provide oral care three times per day and as needed.

Initially place food in visual field; gradually move food out of field and teach person to scan entire visual field.

Retrain Person to Scan Entire Environment.

Have Person Stroke Involved Side With Uninvolved Hand; the Person Should Watch Arm or Leg As He or She Strokes It.

Evaluate that Both Person and Family Understand the Purpose and Rationale of All Interventions.

IMPAIRED URINARY ELIMINATION

Impaired Urinary Elimination
Maturational Enuresis*
Functional Incontinence
Reflex Incontinence
Stress Incontinence
Continuous Incontinence
Urge Incontinence
Urge Incontinence, Risk for
Overflow Incontinence*

AUTHOR'S NOTE

All of these diagnoses pertain to urine elimination, not urine formulation. Anuria, oliguria, and renal failure should be

(continued)

---

*This diagnosis is not currently on the NANDA list, but has been included for clarity or usefulness.

■■■■ **AUTHOR'S NOTE** *(Continued)*
labeled collaborative problems, such as Risk for Complications of Anuria.

Impaired Urinary Elimination represents a broad diagnosis, probably too broad for clinical use. It is recommended that a more specific diagnosis such as *Stress Incontinence* be used instead. When the etiologic or contributing factors have not been identified for incontinence, the diagnosis can temporarily be written *Urinary Incontinence related to unknown etiology*.

DEFINITION

The state in which an individual experiences, or is at risk of experiencing, urinary elimination dysfunction.

DEFINING CHARACTERISTICS

Major (Must Be Present, One or More)

Reports or experiences a urinary elimination problem, such as:

Urgency	Dribbling
Frequency	Bladder distention
Hesitancy	Incontinence
Nocturia	Large residual urine volumes
Enuresis	

RELATED FACTORS

Pathophysiologic

Related to incompetent bladder outlet secondary to congenital urinary tract anomalies

Related to decreased bladder capacity or irritation to bladder secondary to infection, trauma, urethritis, glucosuria, or carcinoma

Related to diminished bladder cues or impaired ability to recognize bladder cues secondary to:

Cord injury/tumor/infection	Diabetic neuropathy
Brain injury/tumor/infection	Alcoholic neuropathy
Cerebrovascular accident	Tabes dorsalis
Demyelinating diseases	Parkinsonism
Multiple sclerosis	Alpha adrenergic agents

Treatment-Related

Related to effects of surgery on bladder sphincter secondary to prostatectomy or extensive pelvic dissection
Related to diagnostic instrumentation

Related to decreased bladder muscle tone secondary to:
General or spinal anesthesia
Drug therapy (iatrogenic)

Antihistamines	Immunosuppressant therapy
Epinephrine	Diuretics
Anticholinergics	Tranquilizers
Sedatives	Muscle relaxants

Post-indwelling catheters

Situational (Personal, Environmental)

Related to weak pelvic floor muscles secondary to:

Obesity	Aging
Recent substantial weight loss	Childbirth

Related to inability to communicate needs
Related to bladder outlet obstruction secondary to fecal impaction or chronic constipation
Related to decreased bladder muscle tone secondary to dehydration

Related to decreased attention to bladder cues secondary to:

Depression	Confusion
Intentional suppression	Delirium

Related to environmental barriers to bathroom:

Distant toilets	Poor lighting
Unfamiliar surroundings	Bed too high, or side rails

Related to inability to access bathroom on time secondary to:

Impaired mobility	Caffeine/alcohol use

Maturational

Child
Related to small bladder capacity
Related to lack of motivation

Goals

The person will be continent (specify during day, night, 24 hours).

Indicators
- Be able to identify the cause of incontinence.
- Provide rationale for treatments.

Generic Interventions

Determine If There Is Acute Cause of Problem.

Infection (e.g., urinary tract, sexually transmitted disease, gonorrhea)
Renal disease
Renal calculi
Medication effects
Anesthesia effects

Refer to a Urologist If Acute Cause Is Determined.

If Incontinence Is the Problem, Determine Type. Assess:

History of continence
Onset and duration (day, night, just certain times)
Factors that increase incidence:
- Coughing
- Laughing
- Standing
- Turning in bed
- Delay in getting to bathroom
- When excited
- Leaving bathroom
- Running

Perception of need to void: present, absent, diminished
Ability to delay urination after urge
Relief after voiding:
- Complete
- Continued desire to void after bladder is emptied

Using Data from Assessment, Refer to Specific Type of Incontinence.

▶ Maturational Enuresis

DEFINITION

The state in which a child experiences involuntary voiding during sleep, which is not pathophysiologic in origin.

■■■■ **AUTHOR'S NOTE**
This diagnosis would represent enuresis that is not caused by pathophysiologic or structural deficits, such as strictures.

DEFINING CHARACTERISTICS

Major (Must Be Present)

Reports or demonstrates episodes of involuntary voiding during sleep

RELATED FACTORS

Situational (Personal, Environmental)

Related to stressors (school, siblings)
Related to inattention to bladder cues
Related to unfamiliar surroundings

Maturational

Child
Related to small bladder capacity
Related to lack of motivation
Related to attention-seeking behavior

NOC

Urinary Continence, Knowledge: Enuresis, Family Functioning

Goals

The child will remain dry during the sleep cycle.

Indicator

The child and family will be able to list factors that decrease enuresis.

NIC

Urinary Incontinence Care: Enuresis, Urinary Habit Training, Anticipatory Guidance, Family Support

👫 Pediatric Interventions

Explain the Nature of Enuresis, the Physiologic Development of Bladder Control and Its High Rate of Spontaneous Remission to Parents and Child.

Explain to Parents that Disapproval (Shaming, Punishing) Is Useless in Stopping Enuresis but Can Make Child Shy, Ashamed, and Afraid.

Offer Reassurance to Child that Other Children Wet the Bed at Night and Child Is Not Bad.

Teach:

After child drinks fluids, encourage him or her to postpone voiding to help stretch the bladder.

Have child void before retiring.

Restrict fluids at bedtime.

If child is awakened later (about 11 P.M.) to void, attempt to awaken child fully for positive reinforcement.

Teach child awareness of sensations that occur when it is time to void.

Teach child ability to control urination (have child start and stop the stream; have child "hold" the urine during the day, even if only for a short time).

Have Child Keep a Record of Progress; Emphasize Dry Days or Nights (e.g., Stars on a Calendar).

Explain How Nocturnal Enuresis Alarm Works.

Teach Child and Family Techniques to Control the Embarrassing Effects of Enuresis (e.g., Use of Plastic Mattress Covers, Use of Child's Own Sleeping Bag [Machine Washable] When Staying Overnight Away from Home).

With School Age Children, Assess If the Child Is Using the Bathroom at School. Do They Get Sufficient Bathroom Breaks?

Seek Opportunities to Teach the Public About Enuresis and Incontinence (e.g., School and Parent Organizations, Self-Help Groups).

▶ Functional Incontinence

DEFINITION

The state in which an individual experiences incontinence because of a difficulty or inability to reach the toilet in time.

DEFINING CHARACTERISTICS

Major (Must Be Present)

Incontinence before or during an attempt to reach the toilet

RELATED FACTORS

Pathophysiologic

Related to diminished bladder cues and impaired ability to recognize bladder cues secondary to:

Brain injury/tumor/infection	Alcoholic neuropathy
Cerebrovascular accident	Parkinsonism
Demyelinating diseases	Progressive dementia
Multiple sclerosis	

Treatment-Related

Related to decreased bladder tone secondary to:

Antihistamines	Immunosuppressant therapy
Epinephrine	Diuretics
Anticholinergics	Tranquilizers
Sedatives	Muscle relaxants

Situational (Personal, Environmental)

Related to impaired mobility

Related to decreased attention to bladder cues

Depression	Intentional suppression
Confusion	(self-induced reconditioning)

Related to environmental barriers to bathroom:

Distant toilets	Poor lighting
Unfamiliar surroundings	Bed too high, side rails

Maturational

Older Adult

Related to motor and sensory losses

NOC

Tissue Integrity, Urinary Continence, Urinary Elimination

Goals

The person will report no or fewer episodes of incontinence.

Indicators
- Remove or minimize environmental barriers from home.
- Use proper adaptive equipment to assist with voiding, transfers, and dressing.
- Describe causative factors for incontinence.

NIC

Perineal Care, Urinary Incontinence Care, Prompted Voiding, Urinary Habit Training, Urinary Elimination Management, Teaching: Procedure/Treatment

Generic Interventions

Determine If There Is Another Cause Contributing to Incontinence (e.g., Stress, Urge, or Reflex Incontinence, Urinary Retention, Infection).

Assess for Sensory/Cognitive Deficits.

Assess for Motor/Mobility Deficits.

Reduce Environmental Barriers:

Obstacles, lighting, and distance
Adequacy of toilet height and need for grab-bars

Provide a Commode Between Bathroom and Bed, If Needed.

For an Individual with Cognitive Deficits, Offer Toileting Reminders Every 2 Hours, After Meals, and Before Bedtime.

For Persons with Limited Hand Function:

Assess person's ability to remove and replace clothing. Clothing that is loose is easier to manipulate.

Provide dressing aids as necessary: Velcro closures in seams for wheelchair patients, zipper pulls; all garments with fasteners may be adapted with Velcro closures.

Initiate Referral to Visiting Nurse (Occupational Therapy Department) for Assessment of Bathroom Facilities at Home.

Ⓒ Geriatric Interventions

Emphasize that Incontinence Is Not an Inevitable Age-Related Event.

Explain Not to Restrict Fluid Intake for Fear of Incontinence.

Explain Not to Rely on Thirst As a Signal to Drink Fluids.

Teach the Need to Have Easy Access to Bathroom at Night. If Needed, Consider Commode Chair or Urinal.

▶ Reflex Incontinence

DEFINITION

The state in which an individual experiences predictable, involuntary loss of urine with no sensation of urge, voiding, or bladder fullness.

DEFINING CHARACTERISTICS

Major (Must Be Present, One or More)

Uninhibited bladder contractions
Involuntary reflexes that produce spontaneous voiding
Partial or complete loss of sensation of bladder fullness or urge to void

RELATED FACTORS

Pathophysiologic

Related to impaired conduction of impulses above the reflex arc level secondary to:

Cord injury   Tumor
Infection

NOC

See *Functional Incontinence*

Goals

The person will report a state of dryness that is personally satisfactory.

Indicators
- Have a residual urine volume of less than 50 mL.
- Use triggering mechanisms to initiate reflex voiding.

NIC

See *Functional Incontinence*

Generic Interventions

Explain to Person Rationale for Treatment.

Teach Cutaneous Triggering Mechanisms:

Repeated deep, sharp suprapubic tapping (most effective)
Instruct individual to:
- Position self in a half-sitting position.
- Tapping is aimed directly at bladder wall.
- Rate is seven or eight times for 5 seconds (40 single blows).
- Use only one hand.
- Shift site of stimulation over bladder to find most successful site.
- Continue stimulation until a good stream starts.
- Wait approximately 1 minute, then repeat stimulation until bladder is empty.
- One or two series of stimulations without response signifies that nothing more will be expelled.

If the Above Is Ineffective, Perform Each of the Following for 2 to 3 Minutes Each. Wait 1 Minute Between Facilitation Attempts:

Stroking glans penis
Punching abdomen above inguinal ligaments (lightly)
Stroking inner thigh

Encourage Person to Void or Trigger at Least Every 3 Hours.

Persons with Abdominal Muscle Control Should Use Valsalva's Maneuver During Triggered Voiding.

Indicate on Intake and Output Sheet Which Mechanism Was Used to Induce Voiding.

Teach Person that if Fluid Intake Is Increased, He or She Also Needs to Increase the Frequency of Triggering to Prevent Overdistention.

If Needed, Schedule Intermittent Catheterization Program.

Instruct Person in Signs and Symptoms of Dysreflexia:

Elevated blood pressure, decreasing pulse
Flushing and sweating above the level of the lesion
Cool and clammy below the level of the lesion
Pounding headache
Nasal stuffiness
Anxiety, feeling of impending doom
Goose pimples
Blurred vision

Instruct Person in Measures to Reduce or Eliminate Symptoms:

Elevate head.
Check blood pressure.
Rule out bladder distention; empty bladder by catheter (do not trigger); use lidocaine lubricant for catheter.

If Condition Persists After Emptying Bladder, Check for Bowel Distention. If Stool Is Present in the Rectum, Use a Dibucaine (Nupercainal) Suppository to Desensitize the Area Before Removing Stool.

If Condition Persists or Person Has Not Been Able to Identify Cause, Notify Physician Immediately or Seek Help in an Emergency Room.

Instruct Person to Carry an Identification Card that States Signs, Symptoms, and Management in the Event that He or She Cannot Direct Others.

▶ Stress Incontinence

DEFINITION

The state in which an individual experiences an immediate involuntary loss of urine during an increase in intra-abdominal pressure.

DEFINING CHARACTERISTICS

Major (Must Be Present)

The individual reports loss of urine (usually less than 50 mL) occurring with increased abdominal pressure from standing, sneezing, coughing, running, or lifting heavy objects.

RELATED FACTORS

Pathophysiologic

Related to incompetent bladder outlet secondary to congenital urinary tract anomalies

Related to degenerative changes in pelvic muscles and structural supports secondary to estrogen deficiency

Situational (Personal, Environmental)

Related to high intra-abdominal pressure and weak pelvic muscles secondary to:

Obesity	Pregnancy
Sex	Poor personal hygiene
Smoking	

Related to weak pelvic muscles and sphincter incompetence secondary to:

Recent substantial weight loss	Childbirth

Maturational

Older Adult
Related to loss of muscle tone

NOC

See *Functional Incontinence*

Goals

The person will report a reduction or elimination of stress incontinence.

Indicator

Be able to explain the cause of incontinence and rationale for treatment.

NIC

See also *Functional Incontinence*, Pelvic Muscle Exercise, Weight Management

Generic Interventions

Assess Pattern of Voiding/ Incontinence and Fluid Intake.

Explain the Effect of Incompetent Floor Muscles on Continence.

Teach Person to Identify Pelvic Floor Muscles and Strengthen Them With Exercise (Kegel Exercises). (Wilkinson & Van Leuven, 2007)

- Tighening muscles as if you were trying to stop urination, this includes tightening the rectal muscles.
- Hold the contraction for 5-10 seconds and release. Relax between contractions taking care to keep contraction and relaxation times equal. If you contract for 10 seconds, relax for 10 seconds before next contraction.
- Perform 40 to 60 contractions divided in 2-4 sessions each time. These should be spread out through the day and incorporate different positions: sitting, standing and lying.
- A good way to remember to do your exercises is to incorporate them into your daily routine, such as stopping at a traffic light or washing dishes.

Explain the Relationship of Obesity and Stress Incontinence.

Refer to community programs if weight loss is desired.
Instruct to void every 2 hours and avoid prolonged periods of standing.

Explain the Relationship of Decreased Estrogen Production and Stress Incontinence.

Suggest Vaginal Estrogen Cream.

If There Is No Improvement, Refer to a Urologist for Evaluation of Possible Detrusor Instability or Atony, Mechanical Obstruction, or Neuron Injury.

👫 Maternal Interventions

Teach Woman to Decrease Abdominal Pressure During Pregnancy.

Avoid prolonged periods of standing.
Void at least every 2 hours.
Practice Kegel exercises. (Refer to Generic Interventions.)

▶ **Continuous Incontinence**

DEFINITION

The state in which an individual experiences continuous unpredictable loss of urine without distention or awareness of bladder fullness.

◼◼◼ **AUTHOR'S NOTE**

This diagnosis was accepted in 2008. Previously this author had developed Total Incontinence. Total Incontinence has been changed to Continuous Incontinence. This diagnosis should be used only after the other types of incontinence have been ruled out.

DEFINING CHARACTERISTICS

Major (Must Be Present)

Constant flow of urine without distention
Nocturia more than two times during sleep
Incontinence refractory to other treatments

Minor (May Be Present)

Unaware of bladder cues to void
Unaware of incontinence

RELATED FACTORS

Pathophysiologic

Refer to *Impaired Urinary Elimination*.

NOC

See *Functional Incontinence*

Goals

The person will be continent (specify during day, night, 24 hours).

Indicators

- Identify the cause of incontinence and rationale for treatment.
- Identify daily goal for fluid intake.

NIC

See also *Functional Incontinence*, Environmental Management, Urinary Catheterization, Teaching: Procedural Treatment, Tube Care: Urinary, Urinary Bladder Training

Generic Interventions

Maintain Optimal Hydration.

Increase fluid intake to 2 to 3 L/day, unless contraindicated.

Space fluids every 2 hours.

Decrease fluid intake after 7 p.m., and provide only minimal fluids during the night.

Reduce intake of coffee, tea, dark colas, alcohol, and grapefruit juice because of their diuretic effect.

Avoid large amounts of tomato and orange juice because they tend to make the urine more alkaline.

Maintain Adequate Nutrition to Ensure Bowel Elimination at Least Once Every 3 Days.

Promote Micturition.

Ensure privacy and comfort.

Use toilet facilities, if possible, instead of bedpans.

Provide male with opportunity to stand, if possible.

Assist person on bedpan to flex knees and support back.

Teach postural evacuation (bend forward while sitting on toilet).

Promote Personal Integrity and Provide Motivation to Increase Bladder Control.

Convey to Person that Incontinence Can Be Cured or at Least Controlled to Maintain Dignity.

Expect Person to Be Continent, Not Incontinent (e.g., Encourage Street Clothes, Discourage Use of Bedpans, Protective Pads).

Promote Skin Integrity.

Identify individuals at risk for developing pressure ulcers.

Wash area, rinse, and dry gently after incontinent episode.

Avoid harsh soaps, alcohol products.

Use a no-rinse perineal cleanser.

Select a moisturizer that is occlusive (e.g., lanolin, petroleum).

Assess the Person's Potential for Participation in a Bladder-Retraining Program (Cognition, Willingness to Participate, Desire to Change Behavior).

Provide Individual with Rationale for Plan, and Acquire Informed Consent.

Encourage Individual to Continue Program by Providing Accurate Information Concerning Reasons for Success or Failure.

Assess Voiding Pattern:

Time and amount of fluid intake
Type of fluid
Amount of incontinence
Amount of void, whether it was voluntary or involuntary
Presence of sensation of need to void
Amount of retention
Amount of residual urine
Amount of triggered urine
Identify certain activities that precede voiding (e.g., restlessness, yelling, exercise)

Schedule Fluid Intake and Voiding Times.

Schedule Intermittent Catheterization Program, If Indicated.

Teach Intermittent Catheterization to Person and Family for Long-Term Management of Bladder.

Explain the reasons for the catheterization program.
Explain the relationship of fluid intake and the frequency of catheterization.
Explain the importance of emptying the bladder at the prescribed time regardless of circumstances because of the hazards of an overdistended bladder (e.g., circulation contributes to infection, and stasis of urine contributes to bacterial growth).

Teach Prevention of Urinary Tract Infections.

Encourage regular, complete emptying of the bladder.
Ensure adequate fluid intake.
Keep urine acidic; avoid citrus juices, dark colas, and coffee.
Monitor urine pH.

Teach Individual to Monitor for Signs and Symptoms of Urinary Tract Infections:

Increase in mucus and sediment
Blood in urine (hematuria)
Change in color (from normal straw-colored) or odor
Elevated temperature, chills, and shaking
Changes in urine properties
Suprapubic pain
Painful urination
Urgency
Frequent, small voids or frequent, small incontinences
Increased spasticity in spinal cord–injured individuals
Increase in urine pH
Nausea/vomiting
Lower back or flank pain

Refer to Community Nurse for Assistance in Bladder Reconditioning If Indicated.

▶ Urge Incontinence

DEFINITION

The state in which an individual experiences an involuntary loss of urine associated with a strong sudden desire to void.

DEFINING CHARACTERISTICS

Major (Must Be Present)

Urgency followed by incontinence

RELATED FACTORS

Pathophysiologic

Related to decreased bladder capacity secondary to:

Infection	Cerebrovascular accident
Trauma	Demyelinating diseases
Urethritis	Diabetic neuropathy
Neurogenic disorders or injury	Alcoholic neuropathy
Parkinsonism	Brain injury/tumor/infection

Treatment-Related

Related to decreased bladder capacity secondary to:
Abdominal surgery
Post-indwelling catheters

Situational (Personal, Environmental)

Related to irritation of bladder stretch receptors secondary to:

Alcohol   Excess fluid intake
Caffeine

Related to decreased bladder capacity secondary to frequent voiding

Maturational

Child
Related to small bladder capacity

Older Adult
Related to decreased bladder capacity

NOC

Refer to *Functional Incontinence*

Goals

The person will report an absence or decreased episodes of incontinence (specify).

Indicators
- Explain causes of incontinence.
- Describe bladder irritants.

NIC

Refer to *Functional Incontinence*

Generic Interventions

Explain the Causative or Contributing Factors:

Bladder irritants:
- Infection
- Inflammation
- Alcohol, caffeine, or dark cola ingestion
- Concentrated urine

Diminished bladder capacity:
- Self-induced deconditioning (frequent, small voids)
- Post-indwelling catheter

Overdistended bladder:
- Increased urine production (diabetes mellitus, diuretics)
- Intake of alcohol or large quantities of fluids

Uninhibited bladder contractions:
- Neurologic disorders (cerebrovascular accident, brain tumor/trauma/infection, Parkinson's disease)

Explain the Risk of Insufficient Fluid Intake and Its Relation to Infection and Concentrated Urine.

Explain the Relationship Between Incontinence and Intake of Alcohol, Caffeine, and Dark Colas (Irritants).

Determine Amount of Time Between Urge to Void and Need to Void (Record How Long Person Can Hold off Urination).

For a Person with Difficulty Prolonging Waiting Time, Communicate to Personnel the Need to Respond Rapidly to Request for Assistance for Toileting (Note on Care Plan).

Teach Person to Increase Waiting Time by Increasing Bladder Capacity.

Determine volume of each void.
Ask person to "hold off" urinating as long as possible.
Give positive reinforcement.
Discourage frequent voiding that is result of habit not need.
Develop bladder reconditioning program.

For Uninhibited Bladder Contractions, Provide an Opportunity to Void on Awakening, After Meals, Physical Exercise, Bathing, Drinking Coffee or Tea, and Before Going to Sleep.

▶ Urge Incontinence, Risk for

DEFINITION

The state in which an individual is at risk to experience an involuntary loss of urine associated with a strong, sudden desire to void.

RISK FACTORS

Refer to Related Factors in *Urge Incontinence*.

NOC

Refer to *Functional Incontinence*

Goals

The person will report continued continence.

Indicators

- Explain causes of incontinence.
- Explain strategies to maintain continence.

NIC

Refer to *Functional Incontinence*

Interventions

Refer to *Urge Incontinence*.

▶ Overflow Incontinence

DEFINITION

The state in which an individual experiences a chronic inability to void followed by involuntary voiding (overflow incontinence).

AUTHOR'S NOTE

This diagnosis is not recommended for use with individuals with acute episodes of urinary retention (e.g., fecal impaction, post anesthesia, post delivery); in these patients, catheterization, treatment of the cause, or surgery (prostatic hypertrophy) cures urinary retention. These situations are collaborative problems: Risk for Complications of Acute Urinary Retention.

DEFINING CHARACTERISTICS

Major (Must Be Present, One or More)

Bladder distention (not related to acute, reversible etiology)
Bladder distention with small, frequent voids or dribbling (overflow incontinence)
100 mL or more residual urine

Minor (May Be Present)

The individual states that it feels as though the bladder is not empty after voiding.

RELATED FACTORS

Pathophysiologic

Related to sphincter blockage secondary to:

Strictures

Prostate enlargement

Perineal swelling

Ureterocele

Bladder neck contractures

Related to impaired afferent pathways or inadequacy secondary to:

Cord injury/tumor/infection

Brain injury/tumor/infection

Cerebrovascular accident

Demyelinating diseases

Multiple sclerosis

Diabetic neuropathy

Alcoholic neuropathy

Tabes dorsalis

Treatment-Related

Related to bladder outlet obstruction or impaired afferent pathways secondary to drug therapy (iatrogenic):

Antihistamines

Epinephrine

Anticholinergics

Theophylline

Isoproterenol

Situational (Personal, Environmental)

Related to bladder outlet obstruction secondary to fecal impaction

Related to detrusor inadequacy secondary to deconditioned voiding associated with stress or discomfort

NOC

See *Functional Incontinence*

Goals

The person will achieve a state of dryness that is personally satisfactory.

Indicators

- Empty the bladder using Credé's and/or Valsalva's maneuvers with residual urine of less than 50 mL if indicated.
- Void voluntarily.

NIC

See also *Functional Incontinence*, Urinary Retention
Care, Urinary Bladder Training

Generic Interventions

Develop a Bladder Retraining or Reconditioning Program (See **Continuous Incontinence** for Generic Interventions).

Teach Abdominal Strain and Valsalva's Maneuver, If Indicated.

Lean forward on thighs.
Contract abdominal muscles if possible, and strain or "bear
   down"; hold breath while straining (Valsalva's maneuver).
Hold strain or breath until urine flow stops; wait 1 minute, and
   strain again as long as possible.
Continue until no more urine is expelled.

Teach Credé's Maneuver, If Indicated.

Place hands flat (or place fist) just below umbilical area.
Place one hand on top of the other.
Press firmly down and in toward the pelvic arch.
Repeat six or seven times until no more urine can be expelled.
Wait a few minutes and repeat to ensure complete emptying.

Teach Anal Stretch Maneuver, If Indicated.

Sit on commode or toilet.
Lean forward on thighs.
Place one gloved hand behind buttocks.
Insert one or two lubricated fingers into the anus to the anal
   sphincter.
Spread fingers apart, or pull to posterior direction.
Gently stretch the anal sphincter and hold it distended.
Bear down and void.
Take a deep breath and hold it while straining (Valsalva's
   maneuver).
Relax and repeat the procedure until the bladder is empty.

Instruct Individual to Try All Three Techniques or a Combination of Techniques to Determine Which Is Most Effective in Emptying the Bladder.

Indicate on the Intake and Output Record Which Technique Was Used to Induce Voiding.

**Obtain Postvoid Residuals After Attempts
at Emptying Bladder; If Residual Urine
Volumes Are Greater Than 100 mL, Schedule
Intermittent Catheterization Program.**

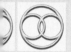

VIOLENCE, RISK FOR OTHER-DIRECTED

DEFINITION

The state in which an individual has been, or is at risk to be, assaultive toward others or the environment.

RISK FACTORS

Presence of risk factors (see also Related Factors)

RELATED FACTORS

Pathophysiologic

*Related to history of aggressive acts and perception of
environment as threatening secondary to: or*

*Related to history of aggressive acts and delusional thinking
secondary to: or*

*Related to history of aggressive acts and manic excitement
secondary to: or*

*Related to history of aggressive acts and inability to verbalize
feelings secondary to: or*

*Related to history of aggressive acts and psychic overload
secondary to:*

Temporal lobe epilepsy	Hormonal imbalance
Progressive CNS deterioration	Viral encephalopathy
(brain tumor)	Mental retardation
Head injury	
Minimal brain dysfunction	

Related to toxic response to alcohol or drugs
Related to organic brain syndrome

Treatment-Related

Related to toxic reaction to medication

Situational (Personal, Environmental)

Related to history of overt aggressive acts

Related to increase in stressors within a short period

Related to acute agitation

Related to suspiciousness

Related to persecutory delusions

Related to verbal threats of physical assault

Related to low frustration tolerance

Related to poor impulse control

Related to fear of the unknown

Related to response to catastrophic event

Related to response to dysfunctional family throughout developmental stages

Related to dysfunctional communication patterns

Related to drug or alcohol abuse

NOC

Abuse Cessation, Abusive Behavior Self-Control, Aggression Control, Impulse Self Control

Goals

The person will have no or fewer violent responses.

Indicators (Varcarolis, 2007)

- Seeks assistance when emotions are escalating
- Refrains from threatening. Loud language toward others
- Responds to external controls when at high risk for loss of control
- Explain rationale for interventions.

NIC

Abuse Protection Support, Anger Control Assistance, Environmental Management: Violence Prevention, Impulse Control Training, Crisis Intervention, Seclusion, Physical Restraint

Generic Interventions

Acknowledge the Individual's Feelings; Be Genuine and Empathetic.

Tell Individual that You Will Help Control Behavior and Not Let Him or Her Do Anything Destructive.

Set Limits When Individual Presents a Risk to Others. Refer to Anxiety for Further Interventions on Limit Setting.

Offer Choices and Options. At Times, It Is Necessary to Give in to Some Demands to Avoid a Power Struggle.

Encourage Individual to Express Anger and Hostility Verbally Instead of "Acting Out."

Remain Calm. If You Are Becoming Upset, Leave the Situation in the Hands of Others, If Possible.

Allow the Acutely Agitated Individual Space that Is Five Times Greater Than that for an Individual Who Is in Control. Do Not Touch the Person Unless You Have a Trusting Relationship. Avoid Physical Entrapment of Individual or Staff.

When interpersonal and pharmacological interventions fail to control the angry, aggressive person, physical interventions (restraints, seclusion) are the final resort. Always follow agency protocols (Varcarolis, 2007).

Do Not Approach a Violent Individual Alone. Often the Presence of Four or Five Staff Members Will Be Enough to Reassure the Individual that You Will Not Let Him or Her Lose Control.

When Assault Is Imminent, Quick, Coordinated Action Is Essential.

Approach Individual in a Calm, Self-Assured Manner to Avoid Communicating Your Anxiety or Fear.

Establish an Environment that Reduces Agitation.

Decrease noise level.
Give short, concise explanations.
Control the number of persons present at one time.
Provide single or semiprivate room.

Establish the Expectation that Person Can Control Behavior, and Continue to Reinforce the Expectation.

Provide Positive Feedback When Person Is Able to Exercise Restraint.

Allow Appropriate Verbal Expressions of Anger. Give Positive Feedback.

Set Limits on Verbal Abuse. Do Not Take Insults Personally. Support Others (Clients, Staff) Who May Be Targets of Abuse.

Plan for Unpredictable Violence.

Assess person's potential for violence and history.
Ensure availability of staff before potential violent behavior (never try to assist person alone when physical restraint is necessary).
Determine who will be in charge of directing personnel to intervene in violent behavior if it occurs.
Ensure protection for oneself (door nearby for withdrawal, pillow to protect face).

Use Seclusion or Restraint, According to Policy.

Remove Individual from Situation If Environment Is Contributing to Aggressive Behavior, Using the Least Amount of Control Needed (e.g., Ask Others to Leave and Take Individual to Quiet Room).

Reinforce that You Are Going to Help Person Control Self.

Repeatedly Tell the Person What Is Going to Happen Before External Control Is Begun.

When Using Seclusion, Institutional Policy Will Provide Specific Guidelines; the Following Are General.

Observe individual at least every 15 minutes.
Search the individual before secluding to remove harmful objects.
Check seclusion room to see that safety is maintained.
Offer fluids and food periodically (in nonbreakable containers).
Have sufficient staff present when approaching an individual to be secluded.
Explain concisely what is going to happen ("You will be placed in a room by yourself until you can better control your behavior."), and give person a chance to cooperate.
Assist person in toileting and personal hygiene (assess ability to be out of seclusion; a urinal or commode may need to be used).

If person is taken out of seclusion, someone must be present continually.

Maintain verbal interaction during seclusion (provides information necessary to assess person's degree of control).

When person is allowed out of seclusion, a staff member needs to be in constant attendance to determine whether person can handle additional stimulation.

Assist Individual in Developing Alternative Coping Strategies When Crisis Has Passed and Learning Can Occur.

Teach Negotiation Skills With Significant Others and Persons in Authority.

Encourage an Increase in Recreational Activities.

Use Group Therapy to Decrease Sense of Aloneness and Increase Communication Skills.

Consult With Person's Therapist or Your Supervisor If Third Parties Need to Be Warned of Danger from the Client (e.g., Police, Potential Victim).

VIOLENCE, RISK FOR SELF-DIRECTED

DEFINITION

The state in which an individual is at risk for behaviors that can be physically, emotionally and/or sexually harmful to self.

RISK FACTORS

Age 15–19
Age over 45
Engagement in autoerotic sexual acts

■■■■ **AUTHOR'S NOTE**
The remaining risk factors are risk factors for suicide, e.g., suicidal ideation or history of multiple suicide attempts. *Risk for Self-Directed Violence* should be replaced with *Risk for Suicide*. Refer to this diagnosis for additional content.

WANDERING

DEFINITION

A state in which an individual with dementia has meandering, aimless, or repetitive locomotion that exposes him or her to harm.

DEFINING CHARACTERISTICS

Person with dementia who (Algase, 1999; Edgerly & Donovick, 1998):

- Ambulates in an aimless, endless manner
- Has repetitive locomotion in a circular pattern
- Paces repetitively
- Exceeds or transgresses environmental limits into hazardous or unauthorized locations
- Has spatial disorientation or navigational deficits
- Is unable to find what he or she is seeking

RELATED FACTORS

Pathophysiologic

Related to impaired cerebral function secondary to:*

Cerebrovascular accident

Mental retardation

Alzheimer's dementia

Related to physiologic urge (e.g., hunger, thirst, pain, urination, constipation)

Situational (Personal, Environmental)

Related to increased frustration, anxiety, boredom, depression, or agitation

Related to over/understimulating environment

Related to separation from familiar people and places

---

*This related factor must be present. Other related factors can also be present concurrently.

Maturational

Older Adult
Related to faulty judgments secondary to motor and sensory deficits, medications

NOC
Risk Detection, Safe Wandering

Goals

The person will not elope or get lost.

Indicators (Person, Family)
- Ambulate safely.
- Identify factors that contribute to wandering behaviors.
- Anticipate wandering behaviors.

NIC
Surveillance: Safety, Environmental Management: Safety, Support Groups, Family Mobilization

Generic Interventions

Assess for Contributing Factors:

Anxiety
Confusion
Frustration
Boredom
Agitation
Separation from familiar people and places
Faulty judgment
Physiologic urge (hunger, thirst, pain, urination, constipation)

Reduce or Eliminate Factors, If Possible.

Physiologic Urges
Anticipate need for toileting with a schedule.
Schedule times for fluids and food.
Evaluate presence of pain.

Anxiety/Agitation
Refer to *Anxiety* for interventions.

Unfamiliar Environment
Select a familiar picture to exhibit on person's door.
Redirect if lost.

Provide a safe route for walking.

Encourage activities that increase exercise (e.g., sweeping, raking).

Create nature scenes in hallways (Cohen-Mansfield & Werner, 1998).

Mark exit door with big signs.

Make horizontal stripes on exit door or use a cloth panel across the width of door.

Promote a Safe Environment.

Install locks on doors and windows.

Install electronic devices with buzzers on door, property boundaries.

Use pressure-sensitive alarms (doormats, bed sensor, chair sensor).

Provide regular opportunities to walk with a companion or in a safe area.

Notify others about person's wandering behaviors:
- Neighbors
- Police
- Other patients in residence
- Staff
- Community resources

Explain the use of electronic devices.

Instruct them to notify if person is seen wandering.

Have recent photograph and current identification information (age, height, weight, hair color, description of clothes, identifying characteristics).

Contact local Alzheimer's Association for safety programs.

SECTION 2

Health Promotion/ Wellness Nursing Diagnoses

This section organizes all the Health Promotion/Wellness Diagnoses for individuals. All these diagnoses are organized under *Health-Seeking Behaviors*. *Health–Seeking Behaviors* is a broad nursing diagnosis that can be useful if a specific wellness diagnosis does not address the targeted health topic.

Wellness nursing diagnoses are "a clinical judgment about an individual, group or community in transition from a specific level of wellness to a higher level of wellness" (NANDA, 2007, p. 10). A valid wellness nursing diagnosis has two requirements: (1) the person has a desire for increased wellness in a particular area and (2) the person is currently functioning effectively in a particular area.

Wellness nursing diagnoses are one-part statements with no related factors. The goals established by the person or group will direct their actions to enhance their health.

There is still confusion about the clinical usefulness of this type of diagnosis. This author takes the position that some of these diagnoses can be strengthened and are clinically useful, such as *Readiness for Enhanced Parenting* or *Readiness for Enhanced Community Coping*. The clinical usefulness of others, for example, *Readiness for Enhanced Power*, *Readiness for Enhanced Urinary Elimination*, and other similar diagnoses, is questionable. Under each diagnosis, Author's Notes will elaborate on the clinical usefulness of the diagnosis.

Clinically, data that represent strengths can be important for nurses to know. These strengths can assist the nurse in selecting interventions to reduce or prevent a problem in another health pattern. If nurses want to designate strength, it should be documented as a strength on the assessment form or care plan. If the client desires assistance in promoting a higher level of function, *Readiness for Enhanced (specify)* would be useful in certain settings e.g., schools, community centers, older-assisted living facilities. Interested clinicians can utilize these health-promotion/wellness diagnoses and are invited to share their work with NANDA and this author.

HEALTH-SEEKING BEHAVIORS

DEFINITION

State in which a person in stable health actively seeks ways to alter personal health habits and/or the environment to move toward a higher level of wellness.*

DEFINING CHARACTERISTICS

Major (Must Be Present)

Expressed or observed desire to seek information for health promotion.

Minor (May Be Present)

Expressed or observed desire for increased control of health.
Expression of concern about current environmental conditions on health status.
Stated or observed unfamiliarity with wellness community resources.
Demonstrated or observed lack of knowledge of health-promotion behaviors.

■■■ AUTHOR'S NOTE

This diagnosis can be used to focus on a personal or life-style change in a specific area that is effective and can be enhanced. If the specific wellness diagnoses do not target the specific area of wellness, this diagnosis can be used— for example, *Health-Seeking Behaviors: Cross-Training Exercise Program.*

---

*Stable health status is defined as the following: age-appropriate illness prevention measures are achieved; client reports good or excellent health; and signs and symptoms of disease, if present, are controlled.

HEALTH PROMOTION/WELLNESS ASSESSMENT (ADAPTED FROM GORDON, 1994; EDELMAN & MANDLE, 2006)

Subjective Data

Health Perception–Health Management Pattern

Ask the person to place a check in front of a category that they observe regularly; place two checks if they are perfect in the category (Breslow, 2004).

- Three meals a day at regular times and no snacking
- Breakfast every day
- Moderate exercise two or three times a week
- 7 to 8 hours of sleep, not more or less
- No smoking
- Moderate weight
- No alcohol or in moderation

What is the Person/Family's Perception of Their Overall Health?

- What personal practices maintain their health?
- What sources does the person or family access to maintain or improve their healthy lifestyle?

Nutrition–Metabolic Pattern

- What is the person's body mass index (BMI)?
- Typical daily fluid intake
- Supplements (vitamins, types of snacks)
- Daily intake of whole grain or enriched breads, cereals, rice or pasta.
- Two pieces of fruit daily
- Unlimited raw, non-starch vegetables daily
- Skim or low-fat dairy products
- Meats and poultry trimmed of fat and skin
- No fried foods/snacks
- Do you see a relationship among stress and tension, emotional upsets, and your diet or eating habits?

Elimination Pattern

Bowel elimination pattern? (Describe)
  - Frequency, character
Urinary elimination? (Describe)
  - Character (amber, yellow, straw-colored)

Activity–Exercise Pattern

Exercise pattern? Type, frequency
Leisure activities? Frequency
Energy level? (High, moderate, adequate, low)

Are there barriers to exercising?
What are five things that you do to play?
What things do you do that make you feel good?

Sleep–Rest Pattern

Satisfied and rested?
Average hours of sleep per night
Relaxation periods? How often, how long?

Cognitive–Perceptual Pattern

Satisfied with:
- Decision-making?
- Memory?
- Ability to learn?

Describe briefly your educational background.

Self-Perception–Self-Concept Pattern

Describe how you feel about:
- Yourself?
- Your body? Changes?

Do you have trouble expressing anger, sadness, happiness, love, and/or sexuality?
What are your major strengths or personal qualities?
What are your weaknesses or negative aspects?
In your life right now, what is your most meaningful activity?
How many more years do you expect to live, and how do you think you will die?
How do you imagine your future?
What would you like to accomplish in your future? Are there changes you need to make to accomplish this?

List the Most Important Events, Crises, Transitions, and/or Changes (Positive or Negative) in Your Life.

Take time to reflect on how they affected you. Place an asterisk in front of one or two that were especially important.

Roles–Relationships Pattern

- Satisfied with job? Need a change?
- Satisfied with role responsibilities?
- Describe your relationship with your family/partner.
- Describe your friendships (close, casual).
- List the most important people in your life right now and why they are important.

Sexuality–Reproductive Pattern

- Is sex an important aspect of your life?
- Are you currently in a sexual relationship?

- What would you want to change about your current sexual relationship?

Coping–Stress Tolerance Pattern

- List the most regular sources of stress in your life. How could you make them less stressful?
- How do you usually respond to stressful situations? (get angry, withdraw, take it out on others, get sick, drink, eat?)
- What situations make you feel calm or relaxed?
- What situations make you feel anxious or upset? What can you do to make yourself feel better?

Values–Beliefs Pattern

- Write ten things you most value in life.
- Would you describe yourself as a religious or spiritual person?
- How do your beliefs help you?

NOC
Adherence Behavior, Health Beliefs, Health Promoting Behaviors, Well-Being

Generic Goals

The person will express a desire to move from wellness to a higher level of wellness in (specify), for example, nutrition, decision-making.

Indicators
Identify two new strategies (specify) to enhance well-being.

Generic Interventions

The following interventions are appropriate for any health promotion/wellness nursing diagnosis that focuses on lifestyle changes and choices, for example, *Readiness for Enhanced Nutrition*, *Parenting*, *Sleep*, *Breastfeeding*, *Family Coping* and *Family Processes*. These areas of wellness and health promotion can be found readily in the self-help literature and on the Internet. Some of the interventions for the wellness diagnoses, such as *Readiness for Enhanced Grieving*, *Readiness for Enhanced Coping*, or *Readiness for Enhanced Decision-Making* can be found in Section One under the individual nursing diagnoses. For example, in *Decisional Conflict* there are interventions that can promote better decision-making even for someone already making good decisions.

Complete Assessment of One or More or All Patterns as the Individual Desires.

Renew Data with Person or Group.

- Does the person/group report good or excellent health?
- Does the person desire to learn a behavior to maximize health in a specific pattern?

Encourage the Person/Group to Select Only One Wellness Focus at a Time.

Refer to Educational Resources on a Particular Focus (Printed, Web Sites). Examples of Generic Data Bases/Web Sites Include:

- www.seekwellness.com/wellness/
- www.cdc.gov/—Centers for Disease Control and Prevention
- www.agingblueprint.org—focuses on aging well
- www.wellness-community.org—education, support for people and families with cancer
- www.nhlbi.nih.gov—U.S. Department of Health and Human Services
- www.ahrq.gov—U.S. Preventive Services Task Force
- www.health.gov—various health topics
- www.nih.gov—National Institutes of Health
- www.fda.gov—Food and Drug Administration
- www.mbmi.org—Mind-Body Medical Institute
- www.ahha.org—American Holistic Health Association

Advise the Person to Contact the Nurse to Discuss the Outcome of Resource Review via Phone or e-Mail.

Discuss the Strategies or Targeted Behavior Changes. Have the Person Record Realistic Goals and Time Frames that Are Highly Specific:

- For example, Goal—I will reduce my daily intake of CHO.
  - Indicators—Reduce cookie intake from five to two each day.
  - Change pasta to multigrain pasta.
  - Reduce potato intake by 50% and replace the 50% with root vegetables.

Ask the Person If You Can Contact Him or Her at Designated Intervals (Every Month, at 4 to 6 Months, at 1 Year); Call or E-Mail Person to Discuss Progress.

Advise the Person that This Process Can Be Repeated as They Desire in Other Functional Health Patterns.

EFFECTIVE BREASTFEEDING

DEFINITION

The state in which a mother–infant dyad exhibits adequate proficiency and satisfaction with the breastfeeding process.

DEFINING CHARACTERISTICS

Major (Must Be Present)

Mother's ability to position infant at breast to promote a
  successful latch-on response
Infant content after feeding
Regular and sustained suckling/swallowing at the breast
Infant weight patterns appropriate for age
Effective mother–infant communication patterns (infant cues,
  maternal interpretation and response)

Minor (May Be Present)

Signs or symptoms of oxytocin release (let-down or milk ejection
  reflex)
Adequate infant elimination patterns for age
Eagerness of infant to nurse
Maternal verbalization of satisfaction with breastfeeding

■■■■ **AUTHOR'S NOTE**
  This diagnosis reportedly represents a newly proposed
  NANDA wellness diagnosis, defined as "a clinical judgment
  about an individual, family, or community in transition from
  a specific level of wellness to a higher level of wellness." The
  definition does not describe a mother–infant dyad seeking
  higher-level breastfeeding, but "adequate proficiency and
  satisfaction with the breastfeeding process." *This diagnosis
  Effective Breastfeeding should be changed to Readiness for Enhanced Breastfeeding for terminology that is consistent for wellness
  diagnoses.*

(continued)

■■■■ **AUTHOR'S NOTE** *(Continued)*

In the management of breastfeeding, nurses will encounter three situations covered by the following nursing diagnoses:

- *Ineffective Breastfeeding*
- *Risk for Ineffective Breastfeeding*
- *Readiness for Enhanced Breastfeeding*

The nurse would use *Ineffective Breastfeeding* to describe an evaluation judgment of a mother's and infant's breastfeeding session for both ineffective and potentially ineffective breastfeeding. This evaluation results from the nurse observing or the mother reporting those signs and symptoms listed as defining characteristics. These signs and symptoms do not describe higher-level breastfeeding.

If the nurse cares for a mother reporting proficiency and satisfaction with breastfeeding and desiring additional teaching to achieve even greater proficiency and satisfaction, *Readiness for Enhanced Breastfeeding* would be appropriate. The focus of this teaching and continued support would not be on preventing ineffective breastfeeding or maintaining adequate proficiency and satisfaction, but on promoting higher-quality breastfeeding.

This diagnosis is not useful in its present form; instead, the nurse should use *Ineffective Breastfeeding* or *Risk for Ineffective Breastfeeding*. Nurses desiring to use a wellness nursing diagnosis could use *Readiness for Enhanced Breastfeeding*. Because this diagnosis is not on the NANDA list, nurses using it should send their experiences to NANDA.

READINESS FOR ENHANCED BREASTFEEDING*

DEFINITION

The state in which a mother-infant dyad exhibits adequate proficiency and satisfaction with the breastfeeding process.

*This diagnosis is not on the NANDA-I list but has been added for usefulness and clarity.

DEFINING CHARACTERISTICS
Major (Must Be Present)

Mother's ability to position infant at breast to promote a
  successful latch-on response
Infant content after feeding
Regular and sustained suckling/swallowing at the breast
Infant weight patterns appropriate for age
Effective mother-infant communication patterns (infant cues,
  maternal interpretation and response)

Minor (May Be Present)

Signs or symptoms of oxytocin release (let-down or milk ejection
  reflex)
Adequate infant elimination patterns for age
Eagerness of infant to nurse
Maternal verbalization of satisfaction with breastfeeding

NOC
Knowledge: Breastfeeding

Goals

The mother will report an increase in confidence and satisfaction
with breastfeeding.

Indicators
Identify two new strategies (specify) to enhance breastfeeding.

NIC
Refer to Health-Seeking Behaviors

Interventions

Refer to the Internet for sites for resources and information on
breastfeeding.

*Refer to Ineffective Breastfeeding for interventions to enhanced breast-
  feeding*

READINESS FOR ENHANCED CHILDBEARING PROCESS

DEFINITION (NANDA)

A pattern of preparing for, maintaining and strengthening a healthy pregnancy and child birth process and care of newborn.

DEFINING CHARACTERISTICS (NANDA)

During Pregnancy

Reports appropriate prenatal lifestyle (e.g., diet, elimination, sleep, bodily movement, exercise, personal hygiene
Reports appropriate physical preparations
Reports managing unpleasant symptoms in pregnancy
Demonstrates respect for unborn baby
Reports a realistic birth plan
Prepares necessary newborn care items
Seeks necessary newborn care items
Seeks necessary knowledge (e.g., of labor and delivery, newborn care
Reports available support systems
Has regular prenatal health visits

During Labor and Delivery

Reports lifestyle (e.g., diet, elimination, sleep, bodily movement, personal hygiene) that is appropriate for the stage of labor
Responds appropriately to the onset of labor
Is proactive in labor and delivery
Uses relaxation techniques appropriate for the stage of labor
Demonstrates attachment behavior to the newborn baby
Utilizes support systems appropriately

After Birth

Demonstrates appropriate baby feeding techniques
Demonstrates appropriate breast care
Demonstrates attachment behavior to the baby
Demonstrates basic baby care techniques
Provides safe environment for the baby
Reports appropriate postpartum lifestyle (e.g., diet, elimination, sleep, bodily movement, exercise, personal hygiene)
Utilizes support system appropriately

■■■ **AUTHOR'S NOTE**
This new NANDA-I nursing diagnosis represents the comprehensive care that is needed to promote a healthy pregnancy, childbirth and postpartum process, enhanced relationships (mother, father, infant siblings) and optimal care of the newborn. This care is beyond the scope possible in this text. Refer to a text on maternal-child health for the specific interventions for this diagnosis.

READINESS FOR ENHANCED COMFORT

DEFINITION (NANDA)

A pattern of ease, relief, and transcendence in physical, psycho-spiritual, environmental, and/or social dimensions that can be strengthened.

DEFINING CHARACTERISTICS (NANDA)

Expresses desire to enhance comfort
Expresses desire to enhance feeling of contentment
Expresses desire to enhance relaxation
Expresses desire to enhance resolution of complaints

■■■ **AUTHOR'S NOTE**
This diagnosis is very general and therefore does not direct specific interventions. It encompasses physical, psychological, spiritual, environmental, and social dimensions. It would be more clinically useful to focus on a particular dimension, such as *Readiness for Enhanced Spiritual Well-Being*.

READINESS FOR ENHANCED COMMUNICATION

DEFINITION (NANDA)

A pattern of exchanging information and ideas with others that is sufficient for meeting one's needs and life's goals, and can be enhanced.

DEFINING CHARACTERISTICS (NANDA)

Able to speak a language
Able to write a language
Expresses feelings
Expresses satisfaction with ability to share ideas with others
Expresses satisfaction with ability to share information with others
Expresses willingness to enhance communication
Forms phrases
Forms sentences
Forms words
Interprets nonverbal cues appropriately
Uses nonverbal cues appropriately

AUTHOR'S NOTE

This diagnosis represents a person with good communications skills. Interventions to enhance communication skills can be found in Section 1 in *Impaired Communication* and *Impaired Verbal Communication*.

READINESS FOR ENHANCED COPING

DEFINITION (NANDA)

A pattern of cognitive and behavioral efforts to manage demands that is sufficient for well-being and can be strengthened.

DEFINING CHARACTERISTICS (NANDA)

Acknowledges power
Aware of possible environmental changes
Defines stressors as manageable
Seeks knowledge of new strategies
Seeks social support
Uses a broad range of emotion-oriented strategies
Uses a broad range of problem-oriented strategies
Uses spiritual resources

Goals

The individual/group will report increased satisfaction with coping with stressors.

Indicators

Identify two new strategies (specify) to enhance coping with stressors

Interventions

If anxiety diminishes one's effective coping, teach:

- Abdominal relaxation breathing
- Abdominal breathing with imagining a peaceful scene, e.g., ocean, woods, mountains

  Imagine the feel of the warm sand on your feet, sun on your face, the sound of water

Explain reframing (Varcarolis, 2007 p.153)

- Reassess the situation, ask yourself:
  What positive thing came out of the situation?
  What did I learn?
  What would I do differently next time?
  What might be going on with your (boss, partner, sister, friend) that would cause him/her to say or do that?
  Is she or he stressed out or having problems?

Acknowledge stress reducing tips for living (Varcarolis, 2007 p. 154)

Exercise regularly, at least 3 times weekly
Reduce caffeine intake
Engage in meaningful, satisfying work
Don't let work dominate your life
Guard your personal freedom
Choose your friends. Associate with gentle people
Live with and love who you choose
Structure your time as you see fit
Set your own life goals
Refer to the Internet for sites for resources and information on
    stress reduction techniques.

READINESS FOR ENHANCED DECISION-MAKING

DEFINITION (NANDA)

A pattern of choosing courses of action that is sufficient for meeting short- and long-term health-related goals and can be strengthened.

DEFINING CHARACTERISTICS (NANDA)

Expresses desire to enhance decision-making
Expresses desire to enhance congruency of decisions with
    personal and/or sociocultural values and goals
Expresses desire to enhance risk-benefit analysis of decisions
Expresses desire to enhance understanding of choices and the
    meaning of the choices
Expresses desire to enhance use of reliable evidence for decisions

KEY CONCEPTS
Refer to *Decisional Conflict* for principles of effective
decision-making.

Focus Assessment

Refer to Health Promotion/Wellness Assessment under Cognitive–Perceptual Pattern.

NOC
Decision-Making, Information Processing

Goals
The individual/group will report increased satisfaction with decision-making.

Indicators
Identify two new strategies (specify) to enhance decision-making.

NIC
Decision-Making Support, Mutual Goal Setting

Interventions
Refer to the Internet for sites for resources and information on decision-making.

Refer to Interventions for *Health-Seeking Behaviors* and *Decisional Conflict*.

READINESS FOR ENHANCED FAMILY COPING

DEFINITION (NANDA)
Effective management of adaptive tasks by a family member involved with the individual's health challenge and who is now exhibiting the desire and readiness for enhanced health and growth in regard to self and in relation to the client.

AUTHOR'S NOTE
This diagnosis describes a family that seeks the opportunity to adapt together to changes and to have a sense of control over outcomes.

DEFINING CHARACTERISTICS (NANDA)
Family member attempts to describe the growth impact of a crisis on his or her own values, priorities, goals, or relationships.

Family member moves in the direction of a health-promoting and enriching lifestyle that supports and monitors maturational processes, audits and negotiates treatment programs, and generally chooses experiences that optimize wellness.

Individual expresses interest in making contact on a one-to-one basis or in a mutual-aid group with another person who has experienced a similar situation.

RELATED FACTORS

See *Health-Seeking Behaviors* and *Interrupted Family Processes*.

Generic Interventions

See also *Interrupted Family Processes*.

READINESS FOR ENHANCED FAMILY PROCESSES

DEFINITION (NANDA)

A pattern of family functioning that is sufficient to support the well-being of family members and can be strengthened.

DEFINING CHARACTERISTICS (NANDA)

- Expresses willingness to enhance family dynamics
- Family functioning meets physical, social, and psychological needs of family members
- Activities support the safety and growth of family members
- Communication is adequate
- Relationships are generally positive; interdependent with community; family tasks are accomplished
- Family roles are flexible and appropriate for developmental stages
- Respect for family members is evident
- Family adapts to change
- Boundaries of family members are maintained
- Energy level of family supports activities of daily living
- Family resilience is evident
- Balance exists between autonomy and cohesiveness

READINESS FOR ENHANCED FLUID BALANCE

DEFINITION

A pattern of equilibrium between fluid volume and chemical composition of body fluids that is sufficient for meeting physical needs and can be strengthened.

DEFINING CHARACTERISTICS

- Expresses willingness to enhance fluid balance
- Stable weight
- Moist mucous membranes
- Food and fluid intake adequate for daily needs
- Straw-colored urine with specific gravity within normal limits
- Good tissue turgor
- No excessive thirst
- Urine output appropriate for intake
- No evidence of edema or dehydration

■■■ **AUTHOR'S NOTE**
If a person has a pattern of equilibrium between fluid volume and the chemical composition of body fluids that is sufficient for meeting physical needs, how can this be strengthened? Would it be more useful to focus on education under the diagnosis *Risk for Deficient Fluid Volume*?

Refer to *Imbalanced Nutrition* and *Deficient Fluid Volume* for Key Concepts on balanced nutrition and fluid volume.

NOC
Fluid Balance, Hydration, Electrolyte Balance

Goals
The individual will report increased satisfaction with fluid balance.

Indicators

NIC
Fluid/Electrolyte Management; See also Health-Seeking Behaviors

Identify two new strategies (specify) to enhance fluid balance.

Interventions
Refer to the Internet for sites for resources and information on nutrition.

Refer to Interventions for *Health-Seeking Behavior* and *Deficient Fluid Balance*.

READINESS FOR ENHANCED HOPE

DEFINITION (NANDA)
A pattern of expectations and desires that is sufficient for mobilizing energy on one's own behalf and can be strengthened.

DEFINING CHARACTERISTICS (NANDA)
- Expresses expectations congruent with desires
- Sets achievable goals
- Conducts problem-solving to meet goals
- Expresses belief in possibilities
- Expresses a sense of spirituality and meaning to life
- Interconnected with others
- Expresses desire or agrees to enhanced hope

NOC
See *Hopelessness*

Goals

The individual/group will report increased hope.

Indicators

Identify two new strategies (specify) to enhance hope.

NIC

Refer to Internet Sites for Resources and Information on Hope, Refer to *Hopelessness* for Interventions to Promote Hope, Refer to *Health-Seeking Behaviors* for Generic Interventions

READINESS FOR ENHANCED IMMUNIZATION STATUS

DEFINITION (NANDA)

A pattern of conforming to local, national, and/or international standards of immunization to prevent infectious disease(s) that is sufficient to protect a person, family, or community and that can be strengthened.

DEFINING CHARACTERISTICS (NANDA)

- Obtains immunizations appropriate for age and health status
- Expresses knowledge of immunization standards
- Exhibits behavior to prevent infectious diseases
- Keeps records of immunizations
- Values immunizations as a health priority; describes possible problems associated with immunizations

■■■ AUTHOR'S NOTE

This diagnosis would apply to an individual or group that needs an immunization according to a national/international standard. All individuals qualify for immunization depending on their age or risk factors. An individual either is a candidate for immunizations or is not. The diagnosis *Risk for Altered Health Maintenance* would be more useful to describe an individual who needs immunizations and/or age-related screening such as mammograms. Thus, *Readiness for Enhanced Immunization* is not clinically useful.

READINESS FOR ENHANCED ORGANIZED INFANT BEHAVIOR

DEFINITION (NANDA)

A pattern of modulation of the physiologic and behavioral systems of functioning of an infant (i.e., autonomic, motor, state, organizational, self-regulatory, and attentional-interactional) that is satisfactory but that can be improved, resulting in higher levels of integration in response to environmental stimuli.

DEFINING CHARACTERISTICS (BLACKBURN & VANDENBERG, 1993)

Autonomic System

- Regulated color and respiration
- Reduced visceral signals (e.g., smooth)
- Reduces tremors, twitches
- Digestive functioning, feeding tolerance

Motor System

Smooth, well-modulated posture and tone
Synchronous smooth movements with:

- Hand/foot clasping
- Suck/suck searching
- Grasping
- Hand holding
- Hand-to-mouth activity
- Tucking

State System

Well-differentiated range of states
Clear, robust sleep states
Focused, shiny-eyed alertness with intent or animated facial expressions
Active self-quieting/consoling "Ooh" face
Attentional smiling
Cooing

■■■ **AUTHOR'S NOTE**
This diagnosis describes an infant who is responding to the
environment with stable and predictable autonomic, motor,
and state cues. The focus of interventions is to promote
continued stable development and to reduce excess environmental stimuli that may stress the infant. Because this is a
wellness diagnosis, the use of related factors is not needed.
The nurse can write the diagnostic statement as *Readiness
for Enhanced Organized Infant Behavior as evidenced by ability
to regulate autonomic, motor, and state systems to environmental
stimuli.*

NOC

Child Development: Specify Age, Sleep, Comfort Level

Goals

The infant will continue age-appropriate growth and development and not experience excessive environmental stimuli.

The parent(s) will demonstrate handling that promotes
stability.

Indicators

- Describe developmental needs of infant.
- Describe early signs of stress or exhaustion.
- Demonstrate:
  - Gentle, soothing touch
  - Melodic tone of voice, coos
  - Mutual gazing
  - Rhythmic movements
  - Acknowledgment of all baby's vocalizations
  - Recognition of soothing qualities of actions

NIC

Developmental Care, Infant Care, Sleep Enhancement,
Environmental Management: Comfort, Parent
Education: Infant Attachment Promotion, Caregiver
Support, Calming Technique

General Interventions

Explain to Parents the Effects of Excess Environmental Stress on the Infant.

Provide a List of Signs of Stress for Their Infant. Refer to Disorganized Infant Behavior for a List of Signs.

Teach Them to Terminate Stimulation If Infant Shows Signs of Stress.

Role-Model Developmental Interventions.

- Offer only when the infant is alert (if possible, show parents examples of alert and not alert).
- Begin with one stimulus at a time (touch, voice).
- Provide intervention for a short time.
- Increase interventions according to infant's cues.
- Provide frequent, short interventions instead of infrequent, long-term ones.
- Stimulation (visual, auditory, vestibular, tactile, olfactory, gustatory)
- Periods of alertness
- Sleep requirements

Explain, Role-Model, and Observe Parents Engaging in Developmental Interventions.

Visual

Eye-to-eye contact

Face-to-face experiences

High-contrast colors, geometric shapes (e.g., black and white shapes on paper mobile); up to 4 weeks, simple mobiles of four dessert-size paper plates with stripes, four-square checkerboards, a black dot, and a simple bull's eye, hung 10 to 13 inches from baby's eyes.

Auditory

Use high-pitched vocalizations.

Play classical music softly.

Use a variety of voice inflections.

Avoid loud talking.

Call infant by name.

Avoid monotone speech patterns.

Vestibular (Movement)

Rock baby in chair.

Place infant in sling and rock.

Close infant's fist around a soft toy.

Slowly change position during handling.
Provide head support.

Tactile
Use firm, gentle touch as initial approach.
Use skin-to-skin contact in a warm room.
Provide alternative textures (e.g., sheepskin, velvet, satin).
Avoid stroking if responses are disorganized.

Olfactory
Wear a light perfume.

Gustatory
Allow non-nutritive sucking (e.g., pacifier, hand in mouth).

Promote Adjustment and Stability in Caregiving Activities (Blackburn & Vandenberg, 1993; Merenstein & Gardner, 1998).

Waking
Enter room slowly.
Turn on light and open curtains slowly.
Avoid waking baby if he or she is asleep.

Changing
Keep room warm.
Gently change position; contain limbs during movement.
Stop changing if infant is irritable.

Feeding
Time feedings with alert states.
Hold infant close and, if needed, swaddle in a blanket.

Bathing
Ventral openness may be stressful. Cover body parts not being bathed.
Proceed slowly; allow for rest.
Offer a pacifier or hand to suck.
Eliminate unnecessary noise.
Use a soft, soothing voice.

Explain the Need to Reduce Environmental Stimuli When Taking the Infant Outside.
Shelter the eyes from light.
Swaddle the infant so his or her hands can reach the mouth.
Protect from loud noises.

Praise Parent(s) on Interaction Patterns; Point Out Infant's Engaging Responses.

Initiate Health Teaching and Referrals If Needed.

Explain that developmental interventions will change with
maturity. Refer to *Delayed Growth and Development* for specific
age-related developmental needs.

Provide parent (s) with resources for assistance at home (e.g.,
community resources).

Refer to the Internet for sites for resources and information on
preterm newborns.

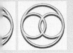

READINESS FOR ENHANCED KNOWLEDGE (SPECIFY)

DEFINITION (NANDA)

The presence of acquisition of cognitive information related to a
specific topic is sufficient for meeting health-related goals and can
be strengthened.

DEFINING CHARACTERISTICS (NANDA)

- Expresses an interest in learning
- Explains knowledge of the topic
- Behaviors congruent with expressed knowledge
- Describes previous experiences pertaining to the topic

AUTHOR'S NOTE

Readiness for Enhanced Knowledge is very broad. All nursing diagnoses—actual, risk, and wellness—seek to enhance
knowledge. Once the specific area of enhanced knowledge
is identified, refer to that specific diagnosis, for example,
*Readiness for Enhanced Nutrition, Grieving, Risk for Ineffec-
tive Parenting, Risk-Prone Health Behavior,* or *Ineffective Self
Health Management. Readiness for Enhanced Knowledge* is not
needed because it lacks the reason for the desired or needed
knowledge.

READINESS FOR ENHANCED NUTRITION

DEFINITION (NANDA)

A pattern of nutrient intake that is sufficient for meeting metabolic needs and can be strengthened.

DEFINING CHARACTERISTICS (NANDA)

- Expresses willingness to enhance nutrition
- Eats regularly
- Consumes adequate food and fluid
- Expresses knowledge of healthy food and fluid choices
- Follows an appropriate standard for intake (e.g., the food pyramid or American Diabetic Association guidelines)
- Safe preparation and storage for food and fluids
- Attitude toward eating and drinking is congruent with health goals

■■■ KEY CONCEPTS

Refer to *Imbalanced Nutrition* for principles of balanced nutrition.

NOC

Nutritional Status, Teaching Nutrition

Indicators

Identify two new strategies (specify) to enhance nutrition

NIC

Nutrition Management, Nutrition Monitoring

Generic Interventions

Refer to Internet sites for resources and information on nutrition:

- www.mypyramid.gov
- www.health.gov/dietaryguidelines
- www.lifestyleadvantage.org

Refer to *Health-Seeking Behaviors* for generic interventions.

DEFINITION (NANDA)

A pattern of participating knowingly in change that is sufficient for well-being and can be strengthened.

DEFINING CHARACTERISTICS (NANDA)

Expresses readiness to enhance awareness of possible changes to be made

Expresses readiness to enhance freedom to perform actions for change

Expresses readiness to enhance identification of choices that can be made for change

Expresses readiness to enhance involvement in creating change

Expresses readiness to enhance knowledge for participation in change

Expresses readiness to enhance participation in choices for daily living and health

Expresses readiness to enhance power

NOC

Health Beliefs: Perceived Control, Participation: Health Care Decisions

Goals

The individual/group will report increased power.

Indicators

Identify two new strategies (specify) to enhance power.

NIC

Decision-Making Support, Self-Responsibility Facilitation, Teaching: Individual

Interventions

Refer to *Powerlessness* for strategies to increase power and to *Health-Seeking Behaviors* for generic interventions.

READINESS FOR ENHANCED RELATIONSHIP

DEFINITION (NANDA)

A pattern of mutual partnership that is sufficient to provide each other's needs and can be strengthened.

DEFINING CHARACTERISTICS (NANDA)

Expresses desire to enhance communication between partners
Expresses satisfaction with sharing of informatioon and ideas between partners
Expresses satisfaction with fulfilling physical and emotional needs by one's partner
Demonstrates mutual respect between partners
Meets developmental goals appropriate for family life-cycle stage
Demonstrates well-balanced autonomy and collaboration between partners
Demonstrates mutual support in daily activities between partners
Identifies each other as a key person
Demonstrates understanding of partner's insufficient (physical, social, psychological) function
Expresses satisfaction with complementary relation between partners

Goals

The individual will report increased satisfaction with partnership.

Indicators
Identify two new strategies (specify) to enhance partnership

Interventions

Teach client to: (Murray, Zentner, Yakimo, 2009 p. 563)
- Talk daily about feelings
- Elicit feelings of partner
- Explore " what if… conversations.

Vary family responsibilities, schedule, chores and roles.

Engage partner to discuss individual problems, validate solutions or ask for partner's opinion on the problem.

Establish a support system that can help when needed. Provide such support to other families or individuals in need.

During times of high stress or crisis, share feelings of guilt, anger, helplessness.

Engage in activities together as partners, family

Refer to the internet for sites for resources for coping with difficult family situations, e.g., death of member, ill family member.

READINESS FOR ENHANCED RELIGIOSITY

DEFINITION (NANDA)

Ability to increase reliance on religious beliefs and/or participate in rituals of a particular faith tradition.

DEFINING CHARACTERISTICS (NANDA)

Expresses a desire to strengthen religious belief patterns:
- Comfort of religion in the past
- Questions belief patterns that are harmful
- Rejects belief patterns that are harmful
- Requests assistance expanding religious options
- Requests assistance to increase participation in prescribed religious beliefs
- Requests forgiveness
- Requests reconciliation
- Requests meeting with religious leaders/facilitators
- Requests religious materials and/or experiences

AUTHOR'S NOTE
This diagnosis represents a variety of foci. Request for forgiveness may be related to an actual nursing diagnosis such as *Grieving, Ineffective Individual Coping*, or *Compromised Family Coping*. Further assessment is needed for interventions. Refer to *Impaired Religiosity* in Section 2, Part 1 for additional information.

READINESS FOR ENHANCED RESILIENCE

DEFINITION (NANDA)

A pattern of positive responses to an adverse situation or crisis that can be strengthened to optimize human potential.

DEFINING CHARACTERISTICS (NANDA)

Access to resources
Demonstrates positive outlook
Effective use of conflict management strategies
Enhances personal coping skills
Expresses desire to enhance resilience
Identifies available resources
Identifies support systems
Increases positive relationships with others
Involvement in activities
Makes progress towards goals
Presence of a crisis
Safe environment is maintained
Sets goals
Takes responsibilities for actions
Use of effective communication skills
Verbalizes an enhanced sense of control
Verbalizes self control

RELATED FACTORS (NANDA)

Demographics that increase chance of maladjustment
Drug use
Gender
Inconsistent parenting
Low intelligence
Low maternal education
Large family size
Minority status
Parental mental illness
Poor impulse control
Poverty
Psychological disorders
Vulnerability factors that encompass indices that exacerbate the
    negative effects of the risk
Condition
Violence

AUTHOR'S NOTE

This new NANDA-I diagnosis focuses on the concept of resilience. Resilience is a strength that one has, which allows one to persist and overcome difficulties. When faced with a crisis or problem resilient people respond constructively with solutions or effective adaption. Resilience is not a nursing diagnosis. It is an important and vital characteristic that can be nurtured and taught to children to assist them to cope with problematic life events.

The defining characteristics listed describe enhanced or effective coping. In contrast the related factors are contributing factors for ineffective coping.

This author recommends:

- Using *Risk for Ineffective Coping* related to the related factors listed above to assist someone to prevent ineffective coping
- Using *Ineffective Coping* related to the above related factors if Defining characteristics if *Ineffective Coping* exists. (refer to Section 2 under *Ineffective Coping* for specific defining characteristics)
- Referring to the interventions for promoting resiliency in children and adults (refer to index under resiliency for specific pages)

READINESS FOR ENHANCED SELF-CARE

DEFINITION (NANDA)

A pattern of performing activities for oneself that helps to meet health-related goals and can be strengthened.

DEFINING CHARACTERISTICS (NANDA)

Expresses a desire to enhance independence in maintaining life
Expresses desire to enhance independence in maintaining health
Expresses desire to enhance knowledge of strategies of self-care
Expresses a desire to enhance responsibility for self-care
Expresses desire to enhance self-care

■■■■ **AUTHOR'S NOTE**
This diagnosis focuses more on improving self-care activities. Refer to *Self-Care Deficits* for interventions to improve self-care.

READINESS FOR ENHANCED SELF-CONCEPT

DEFINITION (NANDA)

A pattern of perceptions or ideas about the self that is sufficient for well-being and can be strengthened

DEFINING CHARACTERISTICS (NANDA)

- Expresses willingness to enhance self-concept.
- Expresses satisfaction with thoughts about self, sense of worthiness, role performance, body image, and personal identity.
- Actions are congruent with expressed feelings and thoughts.
- Expresses confidence in abilities.

NOC
Quality of Life, Self-Esteem, Coping

Goals

The individual will report increased self-concept in (specify situation).

Indicators
Identify two new strategies (specify) to enhance self-concept.

NIC
Hope Instillation, Values Clarification, Coping Enhancement

Interventions

Refer to *Disturbed Self-Concept* for interventions to improve
self-concept.

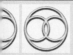

READINESS FOR ENHANCED SELF-HEALTH MANAGEMENT*

DEFINITION (NANDA)

A pattern of integrating a program(s) for treatment of illness and
its sequelae that is sufficient for meeting health-related goals and
can be strengthened.

DEFINING CHARACTERISTICS (NANDA)

- Expresses desire to manage the treatment of illness and prevention of sequelae.
- Choices of daily living are appropriate for meeting the goals of treatment or prevention.
- Expresses little to no difficulty with regulation/integration of one or more prescribed regimens for treatment of illness or prevention of complications.
- Describes reduction of risk factors for progression of illness and sequelae.
- No unexpected acceleration of illness symptoms.

AUTHOR'S NOTE

This diagnosis describes a person who is managing an illness
or a condition successfully. The concept of "enhanced" is appropriate: the nurse can assist the person to enhance his or
her management. The focus is anticipatory guidance (e.g.,
teaching what events could negatively affect the person's
management and how to reduce them).

NOC

Knowledge: Treatment Regimen, Participation: Health
Care Decisions

---

*This diagnostic label was changed from Readiness for Enhanced Therapeutic
Regimen Management by NANDA-I in 2008.

Goal

The person will describe strategies to address progression or complications of condition should they arise.

Indicators
- Discuss situations that can challenge continued successful management.
- Describe or demonstrate self-care techniques needed.

NIC

Decision-Making Support, Teaching: Individual

General Interventions

Discuss Possible Changes in Client's Condition that May Affect Illness and Usual Management.

Exacerbation   Complications   Side effects of medication

Advise Early Contact With Care Provider to Discuss Possible Changes in Management Regimen.

Discuss How Increased Stress Can Negatively Affect Previous Successful Management and Possibly Decrease Resistance to Colds or Influenza.

Explore With Client His or Her Usual Level of Stress.
Usual level of stress   Signs of overload

Emphasize That Stress Accompanies Favorable and Unfavorable Life Events (e.g., Marriage, Divorce, Birth, Death, Vacations, Work).
Refer to *Stress Overload* for additional interventions.
Refer to the Internet for resources and information on specific topics (e.g., amputation, diabetes mellitus).

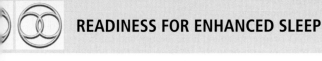

READINESS FOR ENHANCED SLEEP

DEFINITION (NANDA)

A pattern of natural, periodic suspension of consciousness that provides adequate rest, sustains a desired lifestyle and can be enhanced.

DEFINING CHARACTERISTICS (NANDA)

Amount of sleep is congruent with developmental needs
Expresses a feeling of being rested after sleep
Expresses willingness to enhance sleep
Follows sleep routines that promote sleep habits
Occasional use of medications to induce sleep

Goals

The individual will report satisfactory sleep pattern.

Indicators

Identify two new strategies (specify) to enhance sleep

Interventions

Refer to Disturbed Sleep patterns for strategies to promote sleep

READINESS FOR ENHANCED SPIRITUAL WELL-BEING

DEFINITION

A person who experiences affirmation of life in a relationship with a higher power (as defined by the person), self, community, and environment that nurtures and celebrates wholeness.

DEFINING CHARACTERISTICS (CARSON, 1989)

- Inner strength that nurtures:
  - Sense of awareness
  - Inner peace
  - Sacred source
  - Unifying force
  - Trust relationships
- Intangible motivation and commitment directed toward ultimate values of love, meaning, hope, beauty, and truth.
- Trusts relations with or in the transcendent that provide bases for meaning and hope in life's experiences and love in one's relationships.
- Has meaning and purpose to existence.

NOC

Hope, Spiritual Well-Being

Goals

The person will express enhanced spiritual harmony and wholeness.

Indicators

- Maintain previous relationship with higher being.
- Continue spiritual practices not detrimental to health.

NIC

Spiritual Growth Facilitation, Spiritual Support, Hope

Interventions

Refer to the Internet for resources and information on spiritual health.

Refer to *Health-Seeking Behaviors* for additional generic interventions.

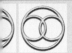

READINESS FOR ENHANCED URINARY ELIMINATION

DEFINITION (NANDA)

A pattern of urinary function that is sufficient for meeting eliminatory needs and can be strengthened.

DEFINING CHARACTERISTICS (NANDA)

- Expresses willingness to enhance urinary elimination.
- Urine is straw colored with no odor.
- Specific gravity is within normal limits.
- Amount of output is within normal limits for age and other factors.
- Positions self for emptying of bladder.
- Fluid intake is adequate for daily needs.

Goals

The individual will report an increased balance in urinary elimination.

Indicators

Identify two new strategies (specify) to enhance urinary elimination.

Interventions

Refer to the Internet for resources and information on fluid balance:

- www.health.gov/dietaryguidelines
- www.seekwellness.com/wellness

See also *Health-Seeking Behaviors* for generic interventions.

SECTION 3

Collaborative Problems

This new section, Collaborative Problems, presents 22 specific collaborative problems grouped under eight generic body system categories. These problems have been selected because of their high incidence and as alternatives to nursing diagnoses in Section 1 that require medical and nursing interventions.

New to this edition is a terminology change for collaborative problems. *Potential Complication: (specify)* has been replaced with *Risk for Complications of (specify)*. This statement change will provide more clarity for clinical situations that are actual complications such as *Increased Intracranial Pressure* or when a person is at risk for *Increased Intracranial Pressure*.

A statement in parentheses and italics with interventions gives the scientific explanation for why an intervention produces the desired response. Keep in mind that for many of the collaborative problems in Section 3, there are associated nursing diagnoses that can be predicted to be present. For example, a client with diabetes mellitus would receive care under the collaborative problem *Risk of Complications of Hypo/Hyperglycemia* along with the nursing diagnosis *Risk for Ineffective Self-Health Management related to Insufficient Knowledge of (specify)*.

CARDIAC/VASCULAR SYSTEM

Cardiac/Vascular System
Risk for Complications of Cardiac/Vascular Dysfunction
Risk for Complications of Decreased Cardiac Ouput
Risk for Complications of Bleeding
Risk for Complications of Dysrhythmias
Risk for Complications of Deep Vein Thrombosis
Risk for Complications of Hypovolemia

▶ Risk for Complications of Cardiac/Vascular Dysfunction

DEFINITION

Describes a person experiencing or at high risk to experience various cardiac and/or vascular dysfunctions.

The nurse can use this generic collaborative problem to describe a person at risk for several types of cardiovascular problems. For example, for a client in a critical care unit vulnerable to cardiovascular dysfunction, using *Risk for Complications of Cardiac/Vascular Dysfunction* would direct nurses to monitor cardiovascular status for various problems, based on focus assessment findings. Nursing interventions for this client would focus on detecting and diagnosing abnormal functioning.

▶ Risk for Complications of Decreased Cardiac Output

DEFINITION

Describes a person experiencing or at high risk to experience inadequate blood supply for tissue & organ needs because of insufficient blood pumping by the heart.

HIGH-RISK POPULATIONS

Coronary artery disease (CAD) and its antecedents, including angina or the more preferred term acute coronary syndrome (ACS)

- Acute myocardial infarction
- Aortic or mitral valve disease with a murmur and/or history of rheumatic fever
- Cardiomyopathy
- Cardiac tamponade
- Hypothermia
- Septic shock
- Coarctation of the aorta
- Chronic obstructive pulmonary disease (COPD)
- Congenital heart disease
- Hypovolemia (e.g., due to severe bleeding or burns)
- Bradycardia
- Tachycardia
- Congestive heart failure
- Cardiogenic shock
- Hypertension

Nursing Goals

The nurse will monitor and manage episodes of decreased cardiac output

Indicators

Calm, alert, oriented
Oxygen saturation >95%
Normal sinus rhythm
No chest pain
No life-threatening dysrhythmias
Skin warm and dry
Usual skin color (appropriate for race)
Pulse: regular rhythm, rate 60–100 beats/min.
Respirations 16–20 breaths/min
Blood pressure >90/60, <140/90mm Hg, MAP >70, or CVP >11
Urine output >5 mL/kg/h
Serum ph.7.35–7.45
Serum PCO_2 35–45 mm Hg
SaO_2 goals >95% for those without history of lung disease
Breath sounds without evidence of new, abnormal sounds (rales)
No presence of distended neck veins (JVD)

General Interventions and Rationales

- Monitor for signs and symptoms of decreased cardiac output/index:
  - Increased, decreased, and/or irregular pulse rate
  - Increased respiratory rate
  - Decreased blood pressure, increased blood pressure
  - Abnormal heart sounds
  - Abnormal lung sounds (crackles) (rales)
  - Decreased urine output (<5 mL/kg/hr)
  - Changes in mentation
  - Cool, moist, cyanotic, mottled skin
  - Delayed capillary refill time
  - Neck vein distention
  - Weak peripheral pulses
  - Abnormal pulmonary artery pressures
  - Abnormal renal artery pressures
  - Decreased mixed venous oxygen saturation
  - Electrocardiogram (ECG) changes
  - Dysrhythmias, decreased SaO_2, decreased ($ScvO_2$)
  (Decreased cardiac output/index leads to insufficient oxygenated blood to meet the metabolic needs of tissues. Decreased circulating volume

can result in hypoperfusion of the kidneys and decreased tissue perfusion with a compensatory response of decreased circulation to extremities and increased pulse and respiratory rates. Changes in mentation may result from cerebral hypoperfusion. Vasoconstriction and venous congestion in dependent areas [e.g., limbs] produce changes in skin and pulses.)

- Initiate appropriate protocols or standing orders, depending on the underlying etiology of the problem affecting ventricular function. *(Nursing management differs based on etiology [e.g., measures to help increase preload for hypovolemia and to decrease preload for impaired ventricular contractility].)*
- During acute episodes, maintain absolute bed rest and minimize all controllable stressors. Administer intravenous (IV) morphine PRN according to protocol. (Morphine is the preferred agent in most cases.) Use with caution if client is hypotensive. *(These measures decrease metabolic demands.)*
- Assist client with measures to conserve strength, such as resting before and after activities (e.g., meals, baths). *(Adequate rest reduces oxygen consumption and decreases the risk of hypoxia.)*
- Monitor intake and output and weight. *(Changes can indicate fluid retention.)*
- In a client with impaired ventricular function, cautiously administer IV fluids. Consult with physician or advanced practice nurse if ordered rate exceeds 125 mL/h. Be sure to include any additional IV fluids (e.g., antibiotics) when calculating hourly allocation. *(A client with poorly functioning ventricles may not tolerate increased blood volumes.)*
- If decreased cardiac output results from hypovolemia, septic shock, or dysrhythmia, refer to the specific collaborative problem in this section.
- Administer inotropic and vasoactive agents (e.g., digoxin, dopamine, dobutamine) as prescribed to improve contractility.
- Assist with insertion and/or maintenance of mechanical cardiac assist devices as indicated (e.g., intraaortic balloon pumps, hemapump, ventricular assist devices).

▶ Risk for Complications of Bleeding

DEFINITION

Describes a person experiencing or at high risk to experience a decrease in blood volume.

HIGH-RISK POPULATIONS

- Intraoperative status
- Postoperative status
  Post-procedural cannulation of any arterial vessel but particularly those at risk for retro-peritoneal bleed due to cannulation of femoral vessel
- Anaphylactic shock
- Trauma
- A history of bleeding disease or dysfunction
- Anticoagulant use, including over-the-counter use of aspirin or NSAIDs (nonsteroidal anti-inflammatory drugs)
- Chronic steroid use
- Acetaminophen use with associated liver dysfunction
- Anemia
- Liver disease
- Disseminated intravascular coagulation (DIC)
- Rupture of esophageal varices
- Dissecting aneurysms
- Trauma in pregnancy
- Pregnancy-related complications (placenta previa, molar pregnancy, abruptio placentae)

Nursing Goals

The nurse will manage and minimize bleeding episodes.

Indicators
Refer to *Decreased Cardiac Output* for indicators.

General Interventions and Rationales

- Monitor fluid status; evaluate
  - Intake (parenteral and oral)
  - Output and other losses (urine, drainage, and vomiting), nasogastric tube
  (Early detection of fluid deficit enables interventions to prevent shock.)
- Monitor the surgical site for bleeding, dehiscence, and evisceration. *(Careful monitoring allows early detection of complications.)*
- Teach client to splint the surgical wound with a pillow when coughing, sneezing, or vomiting. *(Splinting reduces stress on suture line by equalizing pressure across the wound.)*
- Monitor for bleeding from esophageal varices
  Hematemesis (vomiting blood)
  Melena (black, sticky stools)

(Varices are dilated tortuous veins in the lower esophagus. Portal hypertension caused by obstruction of the portal venous system from cirrhosis results in increased pressure on the vessels in the esophagus, making them fragile and at risk to bleed. [Porth, 2007])

- Test stools daily for occult blood if indicated. (Signs of gastrointestinal bleeding may be dected early.)
- If anticoagulant therapy, monitor for:
    Bruises, nosebleeds
    Bleeding gums
    Hematuria
    Severe headaches
    Red or black stools
  (The prolonged clotting time of anticoagulants by anticoagulant therapy can cause spontaneous bleeding anywhere in the body. Hematuria is a common early sign.)
- Monitor for signs of bleeding with venous access devices e.g., IVs, long term venous access devices
    Hematoma at site
    Bleeding at site (Bleeding can occur several hours after insertion after blood pressure returns to normal and puts increased pressure on newly formed clot at the insertion site. It can also develop later, secondary to vascular erosion due to infection)
- Monitor for bleeding during pregnancy and post-partum (refer to specific collaborative problems as *Risk for Complications of Placenta Previa*)
- Monitor for signs and symptoms of shock:
    - Increased pulse rate with normal or slightly decreased blood pressure, narrowing pulse pressure, decrease in mean or mean arterial pressure (MAP)
    - Urine output <5 mL/kg/h
    - Restlessness, agitation, decreased mentation
    - Increased respiratory rate, thirst
    - Diminished peripheral pulses
    - Cool, pale, moist, or cyanotic skin
    - Decreased oxygenation saturation (SaO_2, SvO_2), pulmonary artery pressures
    - Decreased hemoglobin/hematocrit, decreased cardiac output/index
    - Decreased central venous pressure
    - Decreased right atrial pressure
    - Decreased wedge pressure
    (The compensatory response to decreased circulatory volume aims to increase oxygen delivery through increased heart and respiratory

rates and decreased peripheral circulation [manifested by diminished peripheral pulses and cool skin]. Decreased oxygen to the brain alters mentation. Decreased circulation to the kidneys leads to decreased urine output. Hemoglobin and hematocrit values decline if bleeding is significant.)

- If shock occurs, place client in the supine position unless contraindicated (e.g., head injury). *(This position increases blood return [preload] to the heart.)*
- Insert an IV line; use a large-bore catheter if blood replacement is anticipated. Initiate appropriate protocols for shock (e.g., vasopressor therapy). Refer also to *Risk for Complications of Acidosis* or *Risk for Complications of Alkalosis*, if indicated, for more information. *(Protocols aim to increase peripheral resistance and elevate blood pressure.)*
- Contact physician or advanced practice nurse with assessment data that may indicate bleeding. Replace fluid losses at a rate sufficient to maintain urine output >0.5 mL/kg/h (e.g., saline or Ringer's lactate). *(This measure promotes optimal renal tissue perfusion.)*
- Restrict client's movement and activity. *(This helps decrease tissue demands for oxygen.)*
- Provide reassurance, simple explanations, and emotional support to help reduce anxiety. *(High anxiety increases metabolic demands for oxygen.)*
- Administer oxygen as ordered (Diminished blood volume causes decreased circulating oxygen levels.)

▶ Risk for Complications of Dysrhythmias

DEFINITION

Describes a person experiencing or at high risk to experience a disorder of the heart's conduction system that results in an abnormal heart rate, abnormal rhythm, or a combination of both.

HIGH-RISK POPULATIONS

A-type coronary artery disease (CAD)
- Angina
- Myocardial infarction (acute coronary syndrome [ACS])
- Congestive heart failure
- Hypoendocrine or hyperendocrine states
- Sepsis or severe sepsis/septic shock
- Increased intracranial pressure

- Electrolyte imbalances (calcium, potassium, magnesium, phosphorus)
- Atherosclerotic heart disease
- Medication side effects (e.g., aminophylline, dopamine, stimulants, digoxin, beta blockers, dobutamine, lidocaine, procainamide, quinidine, diuretics)
- COPD
- Cardiomyopathy, valvular heart disease
- Anemia
- Postoperative cardiac surgery
- Postoperative after any major anesthesia
- Trauma
- Sleep apnea

Nursing Goals

The nurse will manage and minimize dysrhythmic episodes.

Indicators
Refer to *Decreased Cardiac Output* indicators

General Interventions and Rationales

- Monitor for signs and symptoms of dysrhythmias.
  - Abnormal rate, rhythm
  - Palpitations, chest pain, syncope, fatigue
  - Decreased SaO_2
  - ECG changes
  - Hypotension
  - Change in level of consciousness
  (*Ischemic tissue is electrically unstable, causing dysrhythmias. Certain congenital cardiac conditions, electrolyte imbalances, and medications also can cause disturbances in cardiac conduction.*)
- Initiate appropriate protocols depending on the type of dysrhythmia; this may include:
- Administer supplemental oxygen (*It increases circulating oxygen levels and decreases cardiac workload.*)
- Monitor oxygen saturation (SaO_2) with pulse oximetry and ABGs as necessary.
- Monitor serum electrolyte levels (e.g., sodium, potassium, calcium, magnesium). (*High or low electrolyte levels may exacerbate a dysrhythmia.*)
- Monitor pacemaker and automatic implantable cardioverter (cardiac) defibrillator (AICD) therapy.

▶ Risk for Complications of Deep Vein Thrombosis

DEFINITION

Describes a person experiencing venous clot formation because of blood stasis, vessel wall injury, or altered coagulation.

HIGH-RISK POPULATIONS (FETTERMAN & LEMBURG, 2004)

- Immobility >72 h
- Fractures (especially hip, pelvis, and leg)
- Chemical irritation of vein
- Blood dyscrasias
- All major surgeries that involve general anesthesia and immobility in the operative course (pre-op, peri-op, and post-op combined), especially surgeries involving abdomen, pelvis & lower extremities.
- Orthopedic, urologic, or gynecologic surgery
- History of venous insufficiency
- Obesity
- Estrogen use (high dose)
- Cancer
- Heart failure
- Varicose veins
- Inflammatory bowel disease
- Pregnancy
- Severe COPD
- History of deep vein thrombosis (DVT) or pulmonary embolism
- Surgery greater than 30 min
- Over 40 years of age
- CVA
- MI
- Critical illness
- Indwelling central venous catheters
- Nephrotic syndrome

Nursing Goals

The nurse will manage and minimize complications of DVT.

Indicators

No leg pain
No leg edema

No pain with dorsiflexion of feet (Homans' sign)
No change in skin temperature or color

General Interventions and Rationales

- Monitor the status of venous thrombosis, noting:
  - Diminished or absent peripheral pulses (*Insufficient circulation causes pain and diminished peripheral pulses.*)
  - Unusual warmth and redness or coolness and cyanosis, increased leg swelling (*Unusual warmth and redness point to inflammation; coolness and cyanosis indicate vascular obstruction.*)
  - Increasing leg pain (*Leg pain results from tissue hypoxia.*)
  - Sudden, severe chest pain, increased dyspnea, tachypnea (*These findings may indicate mobilization of thrombi to the lungs.*)
  - Positive Homans' sign (*In a positive Homans' sign, dorsiflexion of the foot causes pain because of insufficient circulation.*)
  - Consult physician for use of below-knee antiembolic stockings or sequential pressure devices, low-dose dextran, or anticoagulant therapy for high-risk clients. (*These assist to reduce venous stasis.*)
- Refer to High-Risk Populations.
- Evaluate hydration status based on urine specific gravity, intake/output, weights, and serum osmolality. Take steps to ensure adequate hydration. (*Increased blood viscosity and coagulability and decreased cardiac output may contribute to thrombus formation.*)
- Encourage client to perform isotonic leg exercises. (*They promote venous return.*)
- Ambulate as soon as possible with at least 5 min of walking each waking hour. Avoid prolonged chair sitting with legs dependent. (*Walking contracts leg muscles, stimulates the venous pump, and reduces stasis.*)
- Elevate the affected extremity above the level of the heart. (*This positioning can help reduce interstitial swelling by promoting venous return.*)
- Discourage smoking. (*Nicotine can cause vasospasms.*)
- Administer anticoagulant therapy as the physician or advanced practice nurse prescribes, and monitor blood coagulation results daily. (*Anticoagulant therapy prevents extension of a thrombosis by delaying the clotting time of blood.*)
- For a client receiving anticoagulant therapy, monitor for early signs of abnormal bleeding (e.g., hematuria, bleeding gums, ecchymoses, petechiae, epistaxis). (*Prolonged clotting time can increase the risk of bleeding.*)
- Administer analgesics for leg pain as prescribed.
- Explain the importance of external compression devices (graded compression below-knee elastic stockings, sequential compres-

sion/decompression stockings [SCDs], intermittent external pneumatic compression [IEPC] impulse boots). *(Venous return is increased; pooling is decreased. IPC and impulse boots increase the rate and velocity of venous flow and decrease hypercoagulability [Morton et al., 2005].)*

▶ Risk for Complications of Hypovolemia

DEFINITION

Describes a person experiencing or at high risk to experience inadequate cellular oxygenation and inability to excrete waste products of metabolism secondary to decreased fluid volume (e.g., from bleeding, plasma loss, prolonged vomiting, or diarrhea).

HIGH-RISK POPULATIONS

- Intraoperative status
- Postoperative status
  Post-procedural cannulation of any arterial vessel but particularly those at risk for retro-peritoneal bleed due to cannulation of femoral vessel
- Anaphylactic shock
- Trauma
- Bleeding
  A history of bleeding disease or dysfunction
  Anticoagulant use, including over-the-counter use of aspirin or NSAIDs (nonsteroidal anti-inflammatory drugs)
  Chronic steroid use
  Acetaminophen with associated liver dysfunction
  Anemia
  Liver disease
- Diabetic ketoacidosis (DKA) or Hyperosmolar Hyperglycemic State (HHS)
- Prolonged vomiting or diarrhea
- Infants, children, elderly
- Acute pancreatitis
- Major burns
- Disseminated intravascular coagulation (DIC)
- Rupture of esophageal varices
- Dissecting aneurysms
- Prolonged pregnancy
- Trauma in pregnancy
- Diabetes insipidus

- Ascites
- Peritonitis
- Intestinal obstruction
- Sepsis (Bridges & Dukes, 2005)

Nursing Goals

The nurse will manage and minimize hypovolemic episodes.

Indicators
Refer to *Decreased Cardiac Output* for indicators

General Interventions and Rationales

- Monitor fluid status; evaluate: intake (parenteral and oral), output and other losses (urine, drainage, and vomiting), nasogastric tube *(Early detection of fluid deficit enables interventions to prevent shock.)*
- Monitor the surgical site for bleeding, dehiscence, and evisceration. *(Careful monitoring allows early detection of complications.)*
- Teach client to splint the surgical wound with a pillow when coughing, sneezing, or vomiting. *(Splinting reduces stress on suture line by equalizing pressure across the wound.)*
- Monitor for signs and symptoms of shock:
  - Increased pulse rate with normal or slightly decreased blood pressure, narrowing pulse pressure, decrease in mean or mean arterial pressure (MAP)
  - Urine output <5 mL/kg/h
  - Restlessness, agitation, decreased mentation
  - Increased respiratory rate, thirst
  - Diminished peripheral pulses
  - Cool, pale, moist, or cyanotic skin
  - Decreased oxygenation saturation (SaO_2, SvO_2), pulmonary artery pressures
  - Decreased hemoglobin/hematocrit, decreased cardiac output/index
  - Decreased central venous pressure
  - Decreased right atrial pressure
  - Decreased wedge pressure

  (The compensatory response to decreased circulatory volume aims to increase oxygen delivery through increased heart and respiratory rates and decreased peripheral circulation [manifested by diminished peripheral pulses and cool skin]. Decreased oxygen to the brain alters mentation. Decreased circulation to the kidneys leads to decreased urine output. Hemoglobin and hematocrit values decline if bleeding is significant.)

- If shock occurs, place client in the supine position unless contraindicated (e.g., head injury). *(This position increases blood return [preload] to the heart.)*
- Collaborate with physician or advanced practice nurse to replace fluid losses at a rate sufficient to maintain urine output >0.5 mL/kg/h (e.g., saline or Ringer's lactate). *(This measure promotes optimal renal tissue perfusion.)*
- Restrict client's movement and activity. *(This helps decrease tissue demands for oxygen.)*
- Provide reassurance, simple explanations, and emotional support to help reduce anxiety. *(High anxiety increases metabolic demands for oxygen.)*
- Administer oxygen as ordered.

RESPIRATORY SYSTEM

Respiratory System
Risk for Complications of Respiratory Dysfunction
Risk for Complications of Hypoxemia

▶ Risk for Complications of Respiratory Dysfunction

DEFINITION

Describes a person experiencing or at high risk to experience various respiratory problems.

AUTHOR'S NOTE

The nurse uses the generic collaborative problem *Risk for Complications of Respiratory Dysfunction* to describe a person at risk for several types of respiratory problems and to identify the nursing focus—monitoring respiratory status for detection and diagnosis of abnormal functioning. Nursing management of a specific respiratory complication is then described under the appropriate collaborative problem for that complication. For example, a nurse using *Risk for*

(continued)

■■■■ **AUTHOR'S NOTE** *(Continued)*
Complications of Respiratory Dysfunction for a client in whom hypoxemia later develops would then add *Risk for Complications of Hypoxemia* to the client's problem list. If the risk factors or etiology were not related directly to the primary medical diagnosis, the nurse would add this information to the diagnostic statement (e.g., *Risk for Complications of Hypoxemia related to COPD* in a client with chronic obstructive pulmonary disease [COPD] who experiences respiratory problems after gastric surgery).

For a person vulnerable to respiratory problems because of immobility or excessive tenacious secretions, the nurse should apply the nursing diagnosis *Risk for Ineffective Respiratory Function related to immobility* rather than *Risk for Complications of Respiratory Dysfunction*.

▶ Risk for Complications of Hypoxemia

DEFINITION

Describes a person experiencing or at high risk to experience insufficient plasma oxygen saturation (PO_2 less than normal for age) because of alveolar hypoventilation, pulmonary shunting, or ventilation–perfusion inequality.

HIGH-RISK POPULATIONS

- COPD
- Pneumonia
- Atelectasis
- Pulmonary edema
- Adult respiratory distress syndrome
- Central nervous system depression
- Medulla or spinal cord disorders
- Guillain-Barré syndrome
- Myasthenia gravis
- Muscular dystrophy
- Obesity
- Compromised chest wall movement (e.g., trauma)
- Drug overdose
- Head injury
- Near-drowning

- Multiple trauma
- Anemia and/or hypovolemia
- Pulmonary embolism

Nursing Goals

The nurse will manage and minimize complications of hypoxemia.

Indicators
Serum pH 7.35–7.45
$PaCO_2$ 35-45
PaO_2 80-100
Pulse: regular rhythm, rate 60–100 beats/min
Respirations 16–20 breaths/min.
Blood pressure <140/90, >90/60 mmHg (MAP [mean arterial pressure] >70) (CVP >11)
Urine output >30 mL/h (use of a standardized volume that is weight based, i.e., >5 mL/kg/h)

General Interventions and Rationales
- Monitor for signs of acid–base imbalance:
  - ABG analysis: pH < 7.35, $PaCO_2$ > 48 mm Hg *(ABG analysis helps evaluate gas exchange in the lungs. In mild to moderate COPD, the client may have a normal $PaCO_2$ level as chemoreceptors in the medulla respond to increased $PaCO_2$ by increasing ventilation. In severe COPD, however, the client cannot sustain this increased ventilation, and the $PaCO_2$ value gradually increases.)*
  - Increased and irregular pulse, and increased respiratory rate initially, followed by decreased rate. *(Respiratory acidosis develops as a result of excessive CO_2 retention. A client with respiratory acidosis from chronic disease at first experiences increased heart rate and respirations in an attempt to compensate for decreased oxygenation. After a while, the client breathes more slowly and with prolonged expiration. Eventually, the respiratory center may stop responding to the higher CO_2 levels, and breathing may stop abruptly.)*
  - Changes in mentation (somnolence, confusion, irritability, anxiety). *(Changes in mentation result from cerebral tissue hypoxia.)*
  - Decreased urine output (<5 mL/kg/h); cool, pale, or cyanotic skin. *(The compensatory response to decreased circulatory oxygen aims to increase blood oxygen by increasing heart and respiratory rates and to decrease circulation to the kidneys and extremities [marked by decreased pulses and skin changes].)*
- Administer low-flow (2 L/min) oxygen as needed through nasal cannula, if indicated. *(Oxygen therapy increases circulating oxygen*

levels. High flow rates increase CO$_2$ retention in people with COPD. Using a cannula rather than a mask may help reduce the client's fears of suffocation.)

- Evaluate the effects of positioning on oxygenation, using ABG values as a guide. Change client's position every 2 h, avoiding positions that compromise oxygenation. *(This measure promotes optimal ventilation.)*
- Ensure adequate hydration. Teach client to avoid dehydrating beverages (e.g., caffeinated drinks, grapefruit juice). *(Optimal hydration helps liquefy secretions. Avoid milk-based products.)*
- Teach client effective coughing technique. *(Effective coughing moves mucus from the lower airways to the trachea for expectoration.)*
- If client cannot expectorate secretions, use coughing, chest physiotherapy, or both to move secretions up from the trachea for suctioning. *(Suctioning is effective only at the tracheal level.)*
- Administer supplemental oxygen before and after suctioning. *(This measure helps prevent decreased PO$_2$ as a result of suctioning.)*
- Obtain a sputum sample for culture and sensitivity and Gram stain testing. *(Sputum culture and sensitivity determine whether an infection is contributing to symptoms.)*
- Eliminate smoke and strong odors from the client's room. *(Irritation of the respiratory tract can exacerbate symptoms.)*
- Monitor the electrocardiogram for dysrhythmias secondary to altered oxygenation. *(Hypoxemia may precipitate cardiac dysrhythmias.)*
- Monitor for signs of right-sided congestive heart failure:
  - Elevated diastolic pressure
  - Distended neck veins
  - Edema
  - Elevated central venous pressure

  (The combination of arterial hypoxemia and respiratory acidosis acts locally as a strong vasoconstrictor of pulmonary vessels. This leads to pulmonary arterial hypertension, increased right ventricular systolic pressure, and, eventually, right ventricular hypertrophy and failure.)
- Refer to the nursing diagnosis *Activity Intolerance* in Section 2 for specific adaptive techniques to teach a client with chronic pulmonary insufficiency.

METABOLIC/IMMUNE/ HEMATOPOIETIC SYSTEMS

Risk for Complications of Metabolic/Immune/Hematopoietic
    Dysfunction
Risk for Complications of Electrolyte Imbalances
Risk for Complications of Hypo/Hyperglycemia

DEFINITION

Describes a person experiencing or at high risk to experience various endocrine, immune, or metabolic dysfunctions.

AUTHOR'S NOTE

The nurse can use this generic collaborative problem to describe a person at risk for several types of metabolic and immune system problems. For example, for a client with pituitary dysfunction who is at risk for various metabolic problems, using *Risk for Complications of Metabolic/Immune/ Hematopoietic Dysfunction* directs nurses to monitor endocrine system function for specific problems, based on focus assessment findings. Under this collaborative problem, nursing interventions would focus on monitoring metabolic status to detect and diagnose abnormal functioning. If the client developed a specific complication, the nurse would add the appropriate specific collaborative problem, along with nursing management information, to the client's problem list.

▶ Risk for Complications of Electrolyte Imbalances*

- Risk for Complications of Hypokalemia
- Risk for Complications of Hyperkalemia
- Risk for Complications of Hyponatremia
- Risk for Complications of Hypernatremia
- Risk for Complications of Hypocalcemia
- Risk for Complications of Hypercalcemia

---

*For a person experiencing or at high risk for experiencing a deficit or excess in a single electrolyte, use *Risk for Complications of Hypokalemia related to diuretic therapy.*

- Risk for Complications of Hypophosphatemia
- Risk for Complications of Hyperphosphatemia
- Risk for Complications of Hypomagnesemia
- Risk for Complications of Hypermagnesemia
- Risk for Complications of Hypochloremia
- Risk for Complications of Hyperchloremia

DEFINITION

Describes a person experiencing or at risk to experience a deficit or excess of one or more electrolytes

HIGH-RISK POPULATIONS

For Hypokalemia

- Crash dieting
- Diabetic ketoacidosis
- Metabolic or respiratory alkalosis
- Excessive intake of licorice
- Diuretic therapy
- Loss of gastrointestinal (GI) fluids (through excessive nasogastric suctioning, nausea, vomiting, or diarrhea)
- Steroid use
- Estrogen use
- Hyperaldosteronism
- Severe burns
- Decreased potassium intake
- Liver disease with ascites
- Renal tubular acidosis
- Malabsorption
- Severe catabolism
- Salt depletion
- Hemolysis
- Hypoaldosteronism
- Rhabdomyolysis
- Laxative abuse
- Villous adenoma
- Hyperglycemia
- Severe magnesium depletion

For Hyperkalemia

- Renal failure
- Excessive potassium intake (oral or IV)
- Cell damage (e.g., from burns, trauma, surgery)
- Crushing injuries
- Potassium-sparing diuretic use
- Adrenal insufficiency

- Lupus
- Sickle cell disease
- Post-transplant
- Chemotherapy
- Metabolic acidosis
- Transfusion of old blood
- Internal hemorrhage
- Hypoaldosteronism
- Acidosis
- Rhabdomyolysis

For Hyponatremia

- Water intoxication (oral or IV)
- Renal failure
- Gastric suctioning
- Vomiting, diarrhea
- Burns
- Potent diuretic use
- Excessive diaphoresis
- Excessive wound drainage
- Congestive heart failure
- Hyperglycemia
- Malabsorption syndrome
- Cystic fibrosis
- Addison's disease
- Psychogenic polydipsia
- Oxytocin administration
- Syndrome of inappropriate antidiuretic hormone (SIADH) (resulting from central nervous system [CNS] disorders, major trauma, malignancies, or endocrine disorders)
- Adrenal gland insufficiency
- Chronic illness (e.g., cirrhosis)
- Hypothyroidism (moderate, severe)

For Hypernatremia

- Elderly, infants
- Inadequate fluid intake
- Heat stroke
- Diarrhea
- Severe insensible fluid loss (e.g., through hyperventilation or sweating)
- Diabetes insipidus
- Excessive sodium intake (oral, IV, medications)
- Hypertonic tube feeding
- Coma
- High protein feeding with inadequate H_2O intake

For Hypocalcemia

- Renal failure (increased phosphorus)
- Protein malnutrition (e.g., due to malabsorption)
- Inadequate calcium intake
- Diarrhea
- Burns
- Malignancy
- Hypoparathyroidism
- Vitamin D deficiency
- Osteoblastic tumors

For Hypercalcemia

- Chronic renal failure
- Sarcoidosis and granulomatous disease
- Excessive vitamin D intake
- Hyperparathyroidism
- Decreased hypophosphatemia
- Bone tumors
- Cancers (Hodgkin's disease, myeloma, leukemia, neoplastic bone disease)
- Prolonged use of thiazide diuretics
- Paget's disease
- Parathyroid hormone-secreting tumors (e.g., lung, kidney)
- Hemodialysis
- Multiple fractures
- Prolonged immobilization
- Excessive calcium-containing antacids

For Hypophosphatemia

- Diabetic ketoacidosis
- Prolonged use of IV dextrose solutions
- Malabsorption disorders
- Renal wasting of phosphorus
- Low-phosphate diet (oral, total parenteral nutrition)
- Rickets
- Excessive use of phosphate binders
- Osteomalacia
- Alcoholism

For Hyperphosphatemia

- Excessive vitamin D intake
- Renal failure
- Healing fractures
- Bone tumors
- Hypoparathyroidism

- Hypocalcemia
- Phosphate laxatives
- Excessive IV or PO phosphate
- Chemotherapy
- Catabolism
- Lactic acidosis

For Hypomagnesemia

- Malnutrition
- Prolonged diuretic use
- Chronic alcoholism
- Excessive lactation
- Severe diarrhea, nasogastric suctioning
- Cirrhosis
- Severe dehydration
- Ulcerative colitis
- Toxemia
- Burns
- Cisplatinum use
- Hyperthyroidism/Cushing's disease
- Prolonged IV therapy without magnesium

For Hypermagnesemia

- Addison's disease
- Renal failure
- Severe dehydration with oliguria
- Excessive intake of magnesium-containing antacids, laxatives
- Thiazide use

For Hypochloremia

- Loss of GI fluids (e.g., through vomiting, diarrhea, suctioning)
- Metabolic alkalosis
- Diabetic acidosis
- Prolonged use of IV dextrose
- Excessive diaphoresis
- Excessive diuretic use
- Ulcerative colitis
- Fever
- Acute infections
- Severe burns

For Hyperchloremia

- Metabolic acidosis
- Severe diarrhea
- Excessive parenteral isotonic saline solution infusion
- Urinary diversion

- Renal failure
- Cushing's syndrome
- Hyperventilation
- Eclampsia
- Anemia
- Cardiac decompensation

Nursing Goals

The nurse will manage and minimize episodes of electrolyte imbalances using laboratory values and norms from organization.

Indicators
Serum magnesium 1.3–2.4 mEq/L
Serum sodium 135–145 mEq/L
Serum potassium 3.8–5 mEq/L
Serum calcium 8.5–10.5 mg/dL
Serum phosphates 125–300 mg/dL
Serum chloride 98–108 mEq/L

General Interventions

Identify the electrolyte imbalances for which the client is vulnerable, and intervene as follows. (Refer to High-Risk Populations under the specific imbalance.)

Risk for Complications of Hypo/Hyperkalemia

- Monitor for signs and symptoms of hyperkalemia:
    - Weakness to flaccid paralysis
    - Muscle irritability
    - Paresthesias
    - Nausea, abdominal cramping, or diarrhea
    - Oliguria
    - Electrocardiogram (ECG) changes: tall, tented T waves, ST segment depression, prolonged PR interval (>0.2 s), first-degree heart block, bradycardia, broadening of the QRS complex, eventual ventricular fibrillation, and cardiac standstill (Porth, 2002)

    (Hyperkalemia can result from the kidney's decreased ability to excrete potassium or from excessive potassium intake. Acidosis increases the release of potassium from cells. Fluctuations in potassium level affect neuromuscular transmission, producing cardiac dysrhythmias, and reducing action of GI smooth muscle. There is an increase in cardiac irritability and cardiac monitoring may show early changes as premature ventricular beats.)

- For a client with hyperkalemia

- Restrict potassium-rich foods, fluids, and IV solutions with potassium. *(High potassium levels necessitate a reduction in potassium intake.)*
- Provide range-of-motion (ROM) exercises to extremities. *(ROM improves muscle tone and reduces cramps.)*
- Per orders or protocols, give medications to reduce serum potassium levels, such as:
  - IV calcium *(To block effects on the heart muscle temporarily)*
  - Sodium bicarbonate, glucose, insulin *(To force potassium back into cells)*
  - Cation-exchange resins (e.g., Kayexalate, hemodialysis; *to force excretion of potassium*)
- Monitor for signs and symptoms of hypokalemia:
  - Weakness or flaccid paralysis
  - Decreased or absent deep tendon reflexes
  - Hypoventilation, change in consciousness
  - Polyuria
  - Hypotension
  - Paralytic ileus
  - ECG changes: U wave, low-voltage or inverted T wave, dysrhythmias, and prolonged QT interval
  - Nausea, vomiting, anorexia

  (Hypokalemia results from losses associated with vomiting, diarrhea, or diuretic therapy, or from insufficient potassium intake. Hypokalemia impairs neuromuscular transmission and reduces the efficiency of respiratory muscles. Kidneys are less sensitive to antidiuretic hormone and thus excrete large quantities of dilute urine. GI smooth muscle action also is reduced. Abnormally low potassium levels also impair electrical conduction of the heart [Porth, 2007].)
- For a client with hypokalemia:
  - Encourage increased intake of potassium-rich foods. *(An increase in dietary potassium intake helps ensure potassium replacement.)*
  - If parenteral potassium replacement (always diluted) is instituted, do not exceed 10 mEq/h in adults. Monitor serum potassium levels during replacement. *(Excessive levels can cause cardiac dysrhythmias.)*
  - Observe the IV site for infiltration. *(Potassium is very caustic to tissues.)*
  - Monitor for discomfort at peripheral infusion site, consider lidocaine additive to reduce/prevent discomfort

Risk for Complications of Hypo/Hypernatremia

- Monitor for signs and symptoms of hyponatremia:
  - CNS effects ranging from lethargy to coma, headache
  - Weakness

- Abdominal pain
- Muscle twitching or convulsions
- Nausea, vomiting, diarrhea
- Apprehension

(Hyponatremia results from sodium loss through vomiting, diarrhea, or diuretic therapy; excessive fluid intake; or insufficient dietary sodium intake. Cellular edema, caused by osmosis, produces cerebral edema, weakness, and muscle cramps.)

- For a client with hyponatremia, initiate IV sodium chloride solutions and discontinue diuretic therapy, as ordered. *(These interventions prevent further sodium losses.)*
- Monitor for signs and symptoms of hypernatremia with fluid overload:
  - Thirst, decreased urine output
  - CNS effects ranging from agitation to convulsions
  - Elevated serum osmolality
  - Weight gain, edema
  - Elevated blood pressure
  - Tachycardia

(Hypernatremia results from excessive sodium intake or increased aldosterone output. Water is pulled from the cells, causing cellular dehydration and producing CNS symptoms. Thirst is a compensatory response to dilute sodium.)

- For a client with hypernatremia:
  - Initiate fluid replacement in response to serum osmolality levels, as ordered. *(Rapid reduction in serum osmolality can cause cerebral edema and seizures.)*
  - Monitor for seizures. *(Sodium excess causes cerebral edema.)*
  - Monitor intake and output, weight. *(This evaluates fluid balance.)*

Risk for Complications of Hypo/Hypercalcemia

- Monitor for signs and symptoms of hypocalcemia:
  - Altered mental status
  - Numbness or tingling in fingers and toes
  - Muscle cramps
  - Seizures
  - ECG changes: prolonged QT interval, prolonged ST segment, and dysrhythmias
  - Chvostek's or Trousseau's sign
  - Tetany

(Hypocalcemia can result from the kidney's inability to metabolize vitamin D [needed for calcium absorption]. Retention of phosphorus causes a reciprocal drop in serum calcium level. A low serum calcium level produces increased neural excitability, resulting in muscle spasms *[cardiac, facial, extremities] and CNS irritability [seizures]. It also causes cardiac muscle hyperactivity, as evidenced by ECG changes.)*

- For a client with hypocalcemia:
  - Per orders for acute hypocalcemia, administer calcium by way of IV bolus infusion.
  - Consult with the dietitian for a high-calcium, low-phosphorus diet. *(Lower serum calcium level necessitates dietary replacement.)*
  - Assess for hyperphosphatemia or hypomagnesemia. *(Hyperphosphatemia inhibits calcium absorption; in hypomagnesemia, the kidneys excrete calcium to retain magnesium.)*
  - Monitor for ECG changes: prolonged QT interval, irritable dysrhythmias, and atrioventricular conduction defects. *(Calcium imbalances can cause cardiac muscle hyperactivity.)*
- Monitor for signs and symptoms of hypercalcemia:
  - Altered mental status
  - Anorexia, nausea, vomiting, constipation
  - Numbness or tingling in fingers and toes
  - Muscle cramps, hypotoxicity
  - Deep bone pain
  - AV blocks (ECG)

  (Insufficient calcium level reduces neuromuscular excitability, resulting in decreased muscle tone, numbness, anorexia, and mental lethargy.)
- For a client with hypercalcemia:
  - Initiate normal saline IV therapy and loop diuretics, as ordered; avoid thiazide diuretics. *(IV fluids dilute serum calcium. Loop diuretics enhance calcium excretion; thiazide diuretics inhibit calcium excretion.)*
  - Per order, administer phosphorus preparations and mithramycin (contraindicated in clients with renal failure). *(These increase bone deposition of calcium.)*
  - Monitor for renal calculi (see *RC of Renal Calculi*).

Risk for Complications of Hypo/Hyperphosphatemia

- Monitor for signs and symptoms of hypophosphatemia:
  - Muscle weakness, pain
  - Bleeding
  - Depressed white cell function
  - Confusion
  - Anorexia

  (Phosphorus deficiency impairs cellular energy resources and oxygen delivery to tissues and also causes decreased platelet aggregation.)
- For a client with hypophosphatemia, per order, replace phosphorus stores slowly by oral supplements, and discontinue phosphate binders. *(This helps prevent precipitation with calcium.)*

- Monitor for signs and symptoms of hyperphosphatemia:
  - Tetany
  - Numbness or tingling in fingers and toes
  - Soft tissue calcification
  - Chvostek's and Trousseau's signs
  - Coarse, dry skin

  (Hyperphosphatemia can result from the kidneys' decreased ability to excrete phosphorus. Elevated phosphorus does not cause symptoms in itself, but contributes to tetany and other neuromuscular symptoms in the short term and to soft tissue calcification in the long term.)

- For a client with hyperphosphatemia, administer phosphorus-binding antacids, calcium supplements, or vitamin D, and restrict phosphorus-rich foods. *(Supplements are needed to overcome vitamin D deficiency and to compensate for a calcium-poor diet. High phosphate decreases calcium, which increases parathyroid hormone [PTH]. PTH is ineffective in removing phosphates due to renal failure, but causes calcium reabsorption from bone and decreases tubular reabsorption of phosphate.)*

Risk for Complications of Hypo/Hypermagnesemia

- Monitor for hypomagnesemia:
  - Dysphagia, nausea, anorexia
  - Muscle weakness
  - Facial tics
  - Athetoid movements (slow, involuntary twisting movements)
  - Cardiac dysrhythmias, flat or inverted T waves, prolonged QT intervals, tachycardia, depressed ST segment. Torsades, a specific type of ventricular dysrhythmia, is associated with hypomagnesemia
  - Confusion

  (Magnesium deficit causes neuromuscular changes and hyperexcitability.)

- For a client with hypomagnesemia, initiate magnesium sulfate replacement (dietary for mild deficiency, parenteral for severe deficiency), as ordered.
- Initiate seizure precautions. *(This protects from injury.)*
- Monitor for hypermagnesemia:
  - Decreased blood pressure, bradycardia, decreased respirations
  - Flushing
  - Lethargy, muscle weakness
  - Peaked T waves

  (Magnesium excess causes depression of central and peripheral neuromuscular function, producing vasodilation.)

- If respiratory depression occurs, consult with the physician for possible hemodialysis. *(Magnesium-free dialysate causes excretion.)*

Risk for Complications of Hypo/Hyperchloremia

- Monitor for hypochloremia:
  - Hyperirritability
  - Slow respirations
  - Decreased blood pressure
  (Hypochloremia occurs with metabolic alkalosis, resulting in loss of calcium and potassium, which produces the symptoms.)
- For a client with hypochloremia, see *RC of Alkalosis* for interventions.
- Monitor for hyperchloremia:
  - Weakness
  - Lethargy
  - Deep, rapid breathing
  (Metabolic acidosis causes loss of chloride ions.)
- For a client with hyperchloremia, see *Risk for Complications of Acidosis* for interventions.

▶ Risk for Complications of Hypo/Hyperglycemia

DEFINITION

Describes a person experiencing or at high risk to experience a blood glucose level that is too low or too high for metabolic function.

▦ AUTHOR'S NOTE

In 2006, NANDA approved the nursing diagnosis, *Risk for Unstable Blood Sugar*. This author defines this condition as a collaborative problem. The nurse can choose which terminology is preferred. The student should consult with the instructor for direction. If the client is only high risk for hyperglycemia as with corticosteroid therapy, use only *Risk for Complications of Hyperglycemia*.

HIGH-RISK POPULATIONS

- Diabetes mellitus
- Parenteral nutrition
- Sepsis
- Enteral feedings
- Corticosteroid therapy
- Neonate of diabetic mother

- Small-for-gestational-age neonate
- Neonate of narcotic-addicted mother
- Thermal injuries (severe)
- Pancreatitis (hyperglycemia), cancer of pancreas
- Addison's disease (hypoglycemia)
- Adrenal gland hyperfunction
- Liver disease (hypoglycemia)

Nursing Goals

The nurse will manage and minimize episodes of hypoglycemia or hyperglycemia.

Indicators
Alert, calm, oriented
No complaints of dizziness
Warm, dry skin
No complaints of fatigue, nausea, abdominal pain, diaphoresis
Pulse: no significant increase
Respirations: no significant increase

General Interventions and Rationales

Many labs and institutions require a repeat of or a second method of validation for treatment of "Critical Lab Values." The organizations define them and require them even for Point of Care (POC) testing for blood glucose values.

For Hypoglycemia

- Monitor serum glucose level at the bedside before administering hypoglycemic agents and/or before meals and hour of sleep. (*Serum glucose is a more accurate parameter than urine glucose, which is affected by renal threshold and renal function.*)
- Monitor for signs and symptoms of hypoglycemia:
  - Blood glucose level below institutional guide, commonly 50–60 mg/dL
  - Pale, moist, cool skin
  - Tachycardia, diaphoresis
  - Jitteriness, irritability, nervousness
  - Hypoglycemia unawareness
  - Incoordination, difficulty speaking
  - Drowsiness, confusion, lightheadedness
  - Hunger
  - Weakness

  (*Hypoglycemia [insufficient glucose levels] can result from excessive insulin, insufficient food intake, excessive physical activity, excessive*) *alcohol intake, medications, diseases, hormone or enzyme deficiencies, or tumors. A rapid drop in blood glucose level stimulates the sympathetic system to produce adrenaline, which causes diaphoresis, cool skin, tachycardia, and jitteriness.*

- Check standard for hypoglycemia oral treatment. If client can swallow, give him or her ½ cup of fruit juice or non-diet soda; 1 cup of milk; 5-6 pieces of hard candy; 2-3 glucose tablets; or 1-2 teaspoons of sugar or honey, every 15 min until blood glucose level exceeds 69 mg/dL. Check glucose level prior to administering more glucose. (*Simple carbohydrates are metabolized quickly.*)

- If client cannot swallow, administer glucagon hydrochloride subcutaneously or 50 mL of 50% glucose in water intravenously (IV), according to protocol. (*Glucagon causes glycogenolysis in the liver when glycogen stores are adequate. In a client in critical condition who has been in a coma for some time, glycogen stores likely have already been used up, and IV glucose is the only effective treatment.*)

- Recheck blood glucose level 1 h after an initial blood glucose reading of greater than 69 mg/dL. (*Regular monitoring detects early signs of high or low levels.*)

- If indicated, consult with a dietitian to provide a complex carbohydrate snack at bedtime. (*This measure can help prevent hypoglycemia during the night.*)

For Hyperglycemia

- Monitor for signs and symptoms of diabetic ketoacidosis:
  - Anion gap
  - Blood glucose level >300 mg/dL
  - Positive plasma ketone, acetone breath
  - Headache
  - Kussmaul's respirations
  - Anorexia, nausea, vomiting
  - Tachycardia
  - Decreased blood pressure
  - Polyuria, polydipsia
  - Decreased serum sodium, potassium, and phosphate levels

  (*When insulin is unavailable, blood glucose levels rise and the body metabolizes fat for energy-producing ketone bodies. Excessive ketone bodies cause headaches, nausea, vomiting, and abdominal pain. Respiratory rate and depth increase to help increase CO_2 excretion and reduce acidosis. Glucose inhibits water reabsorption in the renal glomerulus, leading to osmotic diuresis with severe loss of water, sodium, potassium, and phosphates. Diabetic ketoacidosis occurs in type I diabetes.*)

- If ketoacidosis occurs, initiate appropriate protocols to reverse dehydration, restore the insulin–glucagon ratio, and treat circulatory collapse, ketoacidosis, and electrolyte imbalances.
- Continue to monitor hydration status every 30 min; assess skin moisture and turgor, urine output and specific gravity, and fluid intake. *(Accurate assessments are needed during the acute stage [first 10–12 h] to prevent overhydration or underhydration.)*
- Continue to monitor blood glucose levels according to protocol. *(Careful monitoring enables early detection of medication-induced hypoglycemia or continued hyperglycemia.)*
- Monitor serum potassium, sodium, and phosphate levels. *(Acidosis causes hyperkalemia and hyponatremia. Insulin therapy promotes potassium and phosphate return to the cells, causing serum hypokalemia and hypophosphatemia.)*
- Monitor neurologic status every hour. *(Fluctuating glucose levels, acidosis, and fluid shifts can affect neurologic functioning.)*
- Carefully protect client's skin from microorganism invasion, injury, and shearing force; reposition every 1 to 2 h. *(Dehydration and tissue hypoxia increase the skin's vulnerability to injury.)*
- Do not allow a recovering client to drink large quantities of water. Give a conscious client ice chips to quench thirst. *(Excessive fluid intake can cause abdominal distention and vomiting.)*
- Monitor for signs and symptoms of hyperosmolar hyperglycemic nonketotic (HHNK) coma:
  - Blood glucose 600–2000 mg/dL
  - Serum sodium, potassium normal or elevated
  - Elevated hematocrit, blood urea nitrogen (BUN)
  - Nausea, vomiting
  - Hypotension, tachycardia
  - Dehydration, weight loss, poor skin turgor
  - Lethargy, stupor, coma
  - Elevated urine glucose (>2$^+$)
  - Urine ketones negative or <2$^+$
  - Polyuria

  (HHNK results from relative insulin deficiency. Hyperglycemia and hyperosmolality are present, but there is an absence of significant ketones. HHNK coma can be a response to acute stress [e.g., from myocardial infarction, burns, severe infection, dialysis, or hyperalimentation]. People with type II insulin-resistant diabetes who experience marked dehydration are especially at risk. Glucose inhibits water reabsorption in the renal glomerulus, leading to osmotic diuresis with loss of water, sodium, potassium, and phosphates. Cerebral impairment results from intracellular dehydration in the brain [Porth, 2007; Morton et al., 2005].)

- Monitor cardiac function and circulatory status; evaluate:

- Rate, rhythm (cardiac, respiratory)
- Skin color
- Capillary refill time, central venous pressure
- Peripheral pulses
- Serum potassium

(Severe dehydration can cause reduced cardiac output and compensatory vasoconstriction. Cardiac dysrhythmias can result from potassium imbalances.)
- Follow protocols for ketoacidosis, as indicated.
- Investigate for causes of ketoacidosis or hypoglycemia, and teach prevention and early management, using the nursing diagnosis *Risk for Ineffective Self-Health Management related to insufficient knowledge of (specify)* (see Section 2).

RENAL/URINARY SYSTEMS

Renal/Urinary Systems
Risk for Complications of Renal/Urinary Dysfunction
Risk for Complications of Acute Urinary Retention
Risk for Complications of Renal Insufficiency

▶ Risk for Complications of Renal/Urinary Dysfunction

DEFINITION

Describes a person experiencing or at high risk to experience various renal or urinary tract dysfunctions.

AUTHOR'S NOTE

The nurse can use this generic collaborative problem to describe a person at risk for several types of renal or urinary problems. For such a client (e.g., a client in a critical care unit, who is vulnerable to various renal/urinary problems), using *Risk for Complications of Renal/Urinary Dysfunction* directs nurses to monitor renal and urinary status, based on the focus assessment, to detect and diagnose abnormal functioning. Nursing management of a specific renal or urinary

(continued)

complication would be addressed under the collaborative problem applying to the specific complication. For example, a standard of care for a client recovering from coronary bypass surgery could contain the collaborative problem *Risk for Complications of Renal/Urinary Dysfunction*, directing the nurse to monitor renal and urinary status. If urinary retention developed in this client, the nurse would add *Risk for Complications of Urinary Retention* to the problem list, along with specific nursing interventions to manage this problem. If the risk factors or etiology were not directly related to the primary medical diagnosis, the nurse still would specify them in the diagnostic statement (e.g., *RC of Renal Insufficiency related to chronic renal failure* in a client who has sustained a myocardial infarction). For a person vulnerable to respiratory problems because of immobility or excessive tenacious secretions, the nurse should apply the nursing diagnosis *Risk for Ineffective Respiratory Function related to immobility* rather than *Risk for Complications of Respiratory Dysfunction*.

▶ Risk for Complications of Acute Urinary Retention

DEFINITION

Describes a person experiencing or at high risk to experience an acute abnormal accumulation of urine in the bladder and the inability to void due to a temporary situation (e.g., postoperative status) or to a condition reversible with surgery (e.g., prostatectomy) or medications.

HIGH-RISK POPULATIONS

- Postoperative status (e.g., surgery of the perineal area, lower abdomen)
- Postpartum status
- Anxiety
- Prostate enlargement, prostatitis
- Medication side effects (e.g., atropine, antidepressants, antihistamines)
- Postarteriography status
- Bladder outlet obstruction (infection, tumor)
- Impaired detrusor contractility

Nursing Goals

The nurse will manage and minimize acute urinary retention episodes.

Indicators

Urinary output >5mL/kg/h

Can verbalize bladder fullness

No complaints of lower abdominal pressure

General Interventions and Rationales

- Monitor a postoperative client for urinary retention. *(Trauma to the detrusor muscle and injury to the pelvic nerves during surgery can inhibit bladder function. Anxiety and pain can cause spasms of the reflex sphincters. Bladder neck edema also can cause retention. Sedatives and narcotics can affect the CNS and effectiveness of smooth muscles [Porth, 2007].)*

- Monitor for urinary retention by palpating and percussing the suprapubic area for signs of bladder distention (overdistention, etc.). Instruct client to report bladder discomfort or inability to void. *(These problems may be early signs of urinary retention.)*

- Monitor for urinary retention in postpartum women. *(Labor and delivery can slacken the tone of the bladder wall temporarily, causing urinary retention.)*

- Encourage client to void within 6 to 8 hours after delivery. *(Desire to void may be diminished because of increased bladder capacity related to reduced intraabdominal pressure after delivery.)*

- In a postpartum client, differentiate between bladder distention and uterine enlargement:
  - A distended bladder protrudes above the symphysis pubis.
  - When the nurse massages the uterus to return it to its midline position, the bladder protrudes further.
  - Percussion and palpation can distinguish between a rebounding bladder (from fluid) and a firm uterus.

  (A distended bladder can push the uterus up and to the side and cause uterine relaxation.)

- If client does not void within 8 to 10 h after surgery or complains of bladder discomfort, take the following steps:
  - Warm the bedpan.
  - Encourage client to get out of bed to use the bathroom, if possible.
  - Instruct a man to stand when urinating, if possible. If unable to stand, even sitting at the side of the bed helps.
  - Run water in the sink as client attempts to void.
  - Pour warm water over client's perineum.

(These measures help promote relaxation of the urinary sphincter and facilitate voiding.)

- After the first voiding postdelivery or postsurgery, continue to monitor and to encourage client to void again in 1 hour or so. *(The first voiding usually does not empty the bladder completely.)*
- If the client still cannot void after 10 h, follow protocols for straight catheterization, as ordered by physician/advanced practice nurse. *(Straight catheterization is preferable to indwelling catheterization because it carries less risk of urinary tract infection from ascending pathogens.)*
- For a client with chronic urinary retention, refer to the nursing diagnosis *Urinary Retention* in Section I.
- If person is voiding small amounts, use straight catheterization; if postvoid residual is >200 mL, leave catheter indwelling. Notify physician or advanced practice nurse.

▶ Risk for Complications of Renal Insufficiency

DEFINITION

Describes a person experiencing or at high risk to experience a decrease in glomerular filtration rate that results in oliguria or anuria.

HIGH-RISK POPULATIONS

- Renal tubular necrosis from ischemic causes
  - Excessive diuretic use
  - Pulmonary embolism
  - Burns
  - Intrarenal thrombosis
  - Rhabdomyolysis
  - Renal infections
  - Renal artery stenosis/thrombosis
  - Peritonitis
  - Sepsis
  - Hypovolemia
  - Hypotension
  - Congestive heart failure
  - Myocardial infarction
  - Aneurysm
  - Aneurysm repair
- Renal tubular necrosis from toxicity
  - Nonsteroidal anti-inflammatory drugs

- Gout (hyperuricemia)
- Hypercalcemia
- Certain street drugs (e.g., PCP)
- Gram-negative infection
- Radiocontrast media
- Aminoglycoside antibiotics
- Antineoplastic agents
- Methanol, carbon tetrachloride
- Snake venom, poison mushroom
- Phenacetin-type analgesics
- Heavy metals
- Insecticides, fungicides
- Aminoglycosides
- Diabetes mellitus
- Primary hypertensive disease
- Hemolysis (e.g., from transfusion reaction)

Nursing Goals

The nurse will manage and minimize complications of renal insufficiency.

Indicators

Urine specific gravity 1.005–1030
Urine output >5 mL/kg/h
Urine sodium 130–200 mEq/24 h
Blood urea nitrogen 10–20 mg/dL
Serum potassium 3.8–5 mEq/L
Serum sodium 135–145 mEq/L
Phosphorus 2.5–4.5 mg/dL
Creatinine clearance 100–150 mL of blood cleared/mm

General Interventions and Rationales

- Monitor for early signs and symptoms of renal insufficiency:
  - Sustained elevated urine specific gravity, elevated urine sodium levels
  - Sustained insufficient urine output (<5 mL/kg/h), elevated blood pressure
  - Elevated BUN, serum creatinine, potassium, phosphorus, and ammonia; decreased creatinine clearance
  - Dependent edema (periorbital, pedal, pretibial, sacral)
  - Nocturia
  - Lethargy
  - Itching
  - Nausea/vomiting

(Hypovolemia and hypotension activate the renin–angiotensin system, increasing renal vasculature resistance, which decreases renal plasma flow and glomerular filtration rate. Decreased glomerular filtration rate eventually causes insufficient urine output and stimulates renin production, elevating the blood pressure in an attempt to increase blood flow to the kidney. Decreased excretion of urea and creatinine in the urine elevates BUN and creatinine levels. Dependent edema results from increased plasma hydrostatic pressure, salt and water retention, and/or decreased colloid osmotic pressure from plasma protein losses [Porth, 2007].)

- Weigh the client daily at a minimum; more often, if indicated. Ensure accurate findings by weighing at the same time each day, on the same scale, and with the client wearing the same amount of clothing. *(Daily weights and intake and output records help evaluate fluid balance and guide fluid intake recommendations.)*

- Maintain strict intake and output records; determine the net fluid balance and compare with daily weight loss or gain for correlation. (A 1-kg [2.2-lb] weight gain correlates with excess intake of 1 L.)

- Explain prescribed fluid management goals. *(Client and family understanding may enhance cooperation.)*

- Adjust client's daily fluid intake so it approximates fluid loss plus 300–500 mL/day. *(Careful replacement therapy is necessary to prevent fluid overload.)*

- Distribute fluid intake fairly evenly throughout the entire day and night. It may be necessary to match fluid intake with loss every 8 h or even every hour if the client is critically imbalanced. *(Maintaining a constant fluid balance, without major fluctuations, is essential. Allowing toxins to accumulate because of poor hydration can cause complications such as nausea and sensorium changes.)*

- Consult with a dietitian regarding the fluid and diet plan. *(Important considerations in fluid management, requiring a specialist's attention, include the fluid content of nonliquid food, appropriate amount and type of liquids, liquid preferences, and sodium content.)*

- Administer oral medications with meals whenever possible. If medications must be administered between meals, give with the smallest amount of fluid necessary. *(This measure avoids using parts of the fluid allowance unnecessarily.)*

- Avoid continuous IV fluid infusion whenever possible. Dilute all necessary IV drugs in the smallest amount of fluid that is safe for IV administration. Use small IV bags and an IV controller or pump, if possible, to prevent accidental infusion of a large volume of fluid. *(Extremely accurate fluid infusion is necessary to prevent fluid overload.)*

- Monitor for signs and symptoms of metabolic acidosis:

- Rapid, shallow respirations
- Headaches
- Nausea and vomiting
- Low plasma pH
- Behavioral changes, drowsiness, lethargy

(Acidosis results from the kidney's inability to excrete hydrogen ions, phosphates, sulfates, and ketone bodies. Bicarbonate loss results from decreased renal resorption. Hyperkalemia, hyperphosphatemia, and decreased bicarbonate levels aggravate metabolic acidosis. Excessive ketone bodies cause headaches, nausea, vomiting, and abdominal pain. Respiratory rate and depth increase in an attempt to increase CO_2 excretion and thus reduce acidosis. Acidosis affects the CNS and can increase neuromuscular irritability because of the cellular exchange of hydrogen and potassium [Porth 2007].)

- For a client with metabolic acidosis, ensure adequate caloric intake while limiting fat and protein intake. Consult with a dietitian for an appropriate diet. *(Restricting fats and protein helps prevent accumulation of acidic end products.)*
- Assess for signs and symptoms of hypocalcemia, hypokalemia, and alkalosis as acidosis is corrected. *(Rapid correction of acidosis may cause rapid excretion of calcium and potassium and result in rebound alkalosis.)*
- Consult with the primary provider to initiate bicarbonate/acetate dialysis if the preceding measures do not correct metabolic acidosis:
  - Bicarbonate dialysis for severe acidosis: dialysate – $NaHCO_3$ = 100 mEq/L
  - Bicarbonate dialysis for moderate acidosis: dialysate – $NaHCO_3$ = 60 mEq/L

(The acetate anion, which the liver converts to bicarbonate, is used in dialysate to combat metabolic acidosis. Bicarbonate dialysis is indicated for clients with liver impairment, lactic acidosis, or severe acid–base imbalance.)

- Monitor for signs and symptoms of hypernatremia with fluid overload:
  - Extreme thirst
  - CNS effects ranging from agitation to convulsion

(Hypernatremia results from excessive sodium intake or increased aldosterone output. Water is pulled from the cells, causing cellular dehydration and producing CNS symptoms. Thirst is a compensatory response aimed at diluting sodium.)

- Maintain prescribed sodium restrictions. *(Hypernatremia must be corrected slowly to minimize CNS deterioration.)*
- Monitor for electrolyte imbalances:
  - Potassium

- Calcium
- Phosphorus
- Sodium
- Magnesium

(Refer to Risk for Complications of Electrolyte Imbalances for specific signs and symptoms and interventions. Renal dysfunction can cause hyperkalemia, hypernatremia, hypocalcemia, hypermagnesemia, or hyperphosphatemia. Diuretic therapy can cause hypokalemia or hyponatremia.)

- Monitor for gastrointestinal (GI) bleeding. *(Refer to Risk for Complications of GI Bleeding for more information and specific interventions. The poor platelet aggregation and capillary fragility associated with high serum levels of nitrogenous wastes may aggravate bleeding. Heparinization required during dialysis in cases of gastric ulcer disease also may precipitate GI bleeding.)*
- Monitor for manifestations of anemia:
  - Dyspnea
  - Fatigue
  - Tachycardia, palpitations
  - Pallor of nail beds and mucous membranes
  - Low hemoglobin and hematocrit levels
  - Easy bruising

  (Chronic renal failure results in decreased red blood cell production and survival time because of elevated uremic toxins.)

- Avoid unnecessary collection of blood specimens. *(Some blood loss occurs with every blood collection.)*
- Instruct client to use a soft toothbrush and to avoid vigorous nose blowing, constipation, and contact sports. *(Trauma prevention reduces the risk of bleeding and infection.)*
- Demonstrate the pressure method to control bleeding should it occur. *(Applying direct, constant pressure on a bleeding site can help prevent excessive blood loss.)*
- Monitor for manifestations of hypoalbuminemia:
  - Serum albumin level <3.5 g/dL; proteinuria (<100–150 mg protein/24 h)
  - Edema formation: pedal, facial, sacral
  - Hypovolemia
  - Increased hematocrit and hemoglobin levels.

  (Refer to Risk for Complications of Negative Nitrogen Balance for more information and interventions. When albumin leaks into the urine because of changes in the glomerular electrostatic barrier or because of peritoneal dialysis, the liver responds by increasing production of plasma proteins. When the loss is great, the liver cannot compensate, and hypoalbuminemia results.)

- Monitor for hypervolemia. Evaluate daily:

- Weight
- Fluid intake and output records
- Circumference of the edematous parts
- Laboratory data: hematocrit, serum sodium, and plasma protein in specific serum albumin

(As glomerular filtration rate decreases and the functioning nephron mass continues to diminish, the kidneys lose the ability to concentrate urine and to excrete sodium and water, resulting in hypervolemia.)

- Monitor for signs and symptoms of congestive heart failure and decreased cardiac output:
  - Gradual increase in heart rate
  - Increasing dyspnea
  - Diminished breath sounds, rales
  - Decreased systolic blood pressure
  - Presence of or increase in S_3 and/or S_4 heart sounds
  - Gallop rhythm
  - Peripheral edema
  - Distended neck veins

(Congestive heart failure can result from increased cardiac output, hypervolemia, dysrhythmias, and hypertension, reducing the ability of the left ventricle to eject blood, with subsequent decreased cardiac output and increased pulmonary vascular congestion.)

- Encourage adherence to strict fluid restrictions: 800–1000 mL/24 h, or 24-h urine output plus 500 mL. *(Fluid restrictions are based on urine output. In an anuric client, restriction usually is 800 mL/day, which accounts for insensible losses from metabolism, the GI tract, perspiration, and respiration.)*
- Collaborate with physician, advanced practice nurse, or dietitian to plan an appropriate diet. Encourage adherence to a low-sodium diet (2–4 g/day). *(Sodium restrictions should be adjusted based on urine sodium excretion.)*
- If hemodialysis or peritoneal dialysis is initiated, follow institutional protocols.

NEUROLOGIC/SENSORY SYSTEMS

▶ Risk for Complications of Neurologic/Sensory Dysfunction

DEFINITION

Describes a person experiencing or at high risk to experience various neurologic or sensory dysfunctions.

AUTHOR'S NOTE

The nurse can use this generic collaborative problem to describe a person at risk for several types of neurologic or sensory problems (e.g., a client recovering from cranial surgery or who has sustained multiple trauma). For such a person, using *Risk for Complications of Neurologic/Sensory Dysfunction* directs nurses to monitor neurologic and sensory function based on focus assessment findings. Should a complication occur, the nurse would add the applicable specific collaborative problem (e.g., *Risk for Complications of Increased Intracranial Pressure*) to the client's problem list to describe nursing management of the complication.

▶ Risk for Complications of Increased Intracranial Pressure

DEFINITION

Describes a person experiencing or at high risk to experience increased pressure (>15 mm Hg) exerted by cerebrospinal fluid within the brain's ventricles or the subarachnoid space.

HIGH-RISK POPULATIONS

- Intracerebral mass (lesions, hematomas, tumors, abscesses)
- Blood clots
- Blockage of venous outflow
- Head injuries
- Reye's syndrome
- Meningitis
- Premature birth
- Cranial surgery

Nursing Goals

The nurse will manage and minimize episodes of increased intracranial pressure (ICP).

Indicators

Alert, oriented, calm or no change in usual cognitive status
No seizures
Appropriate speech
Pupils equal; reactive to light and accommodation
Intact extraocular movements
Pulse 60–100 beats/min
Respirations 16–20 breaths/min
BP >90/60, <140/90 mm Hg
Stable pulse pressure (difference between diastolic and systolic readings)
No nausea/vomiting
Mild to no headache
ICP monitoring to maintain the range indicated.

General Interventions and Rationales

- Monitor for signs and symptoms of increased ICP.
- Assess the following (Glasgow Coma Scale [GCS]) (Hickey, 2006)
  - Best eye opening response: spontaneously, to auditory stimuli, to painful stimuli, or no response
  - Best motor response: obeys verbal commands, localizes pain, flexion–withdrawal, flexion–decorticate, extension–decerebrate, or no response
  - Best verbal response: oriented to person, place, and time; confused conversation; inappropriate speech; incomprehensible sounds; or no response

  (Deficiencies of cerebral blood supply resulting from hemorrhage, hematoma, cerebral edema, thrombus, or emboli compromise cerebral tissue. These responses evaluate the client's ability to integrate commands with conscious and involuntary movement. The nurse can assess cortical function by evaluating eye opening and motor response. No response may indicate damage to the midbrain.)
- Assess for changes in vital signs:
  - Pulse changes: slowing rate to 60 beats/min or lower or increasing rate to 100 beats/min or higher *(Bradycardia is a late sign of brain stem ischemia. Tachycardia may indicate hypothalamic ischemia and sympathetic discharge.)*

- Respiratory irregularities: slowing rate with lengthening apneic periods *(Respiratory patterns vary depending on the site of impairment. Cheyne-Stokes breathing [a gradual increase followed by a gradual decrease, then a period of apnea] points to damage in both cerebral hemispheres, midbrain, and upper pons. Central neurogenic hyperventilation occurs with midbrain and upper pontine lesions. Ataxic breathing [irregular with random sequence of deep and shallow breaths] indicates pontine dysfunction. Hypoventilation and apnea occur with medullary lesions.)*
- Rising blood pressure and/or widening pulse pressure
- Bradycardia, increased systolic blood pressure, and increased pulse pressure. *(These are late signs [known as Cushings Response] [Hickey, 2006] of brain stem ischemia leading to cerebral herniation.)*
- Assess pupillary responses. *(Changes indicate pressure on oculomotor or optic nerves.)*
  - Inspect the pupils with a bright pinpoint light to evaluate size, configuration, and reaction to light. Compare both eyes for similarities and differences. *(The oculomotor nerve [cranial nerve III] in the brain stem regulates pupil reactions.)*
  - Evaluate gaze to determine whether it is conjugate (paired, working together) or if eye movements are abnormal. *(Conjugate eye movements are regulated from parts of the cortex and brain stem.)*
  - Evaluate the ability of the eyes to adduct and abduct. *(Cranial nerve VI, or the abducens nerve, regulates abduction and adduction of the eyes. Cranial nerve IV, or the trochlear nerve, also regulates eye movement.)*
- Note any other signs and symptoms:
  - Vomiting *(Vomiting results from pressure on the medulla, which stimulates the brain's vomiting center.)*
  - Headache: constant, increasing in intensity, or aggravated by movement
  - Straining *(Compression of neural tissue increases ICP and causes pain.)*
  - Subtle changes (e.g., lethargy, restlessness, forced breathing, purposeless movements, changes in mentation; *These signs may be the earliest indicators of cranial pressure changes.*)
- Elevate the head of the bed 30 to 45 degrees unless contraindicated. *(Slight head elevation can aid venous drainage to reduce cerebrovascular congestion, thereby decreasing ICP. Positioning is very dependent upon the type of surgery done and the approach used and should always be clarified before repositioning.)*
- Avoid the following situations or maneuvers, which can increase ICP (Porth, 2007):

- Carotid massage *(This slows the heart rate and reduces systemic circulation, which is followed by a sudden increase in circulation.)*
- Neck flexion or extreme rotation; if intubated, do not use securing device with circumferential wrapping (Bhardwaj, Mirski, & Ulatowski, 2004) *(This inhibits jugular venous drainage, which increases cerebrovascular congestion and ICP.)*
- Digital anal stimulation, breath-holding, straining *(These can initiate the Valsalva maneuver, which impairs venous return by constricting the jugular veins, thus increasing ICP.)*
- Extreme flexion of the hips and knees *(Flexion increases intrathoracic pressure, which inhibits jugular venous drainage, increasing cerebrovascular congestion and, thus, ICP.)*
- Rapid position changes
- Seizures (Bhardwaj et al., 2004)

- Consult with the physician or nurse practitioner for stool softeners, if needed. *(Stool softeners prevent constipation and straining during defecation, which can trigger the Valsalva maneuver.)*
- Maintain a quiet, calm, softly lit environment. Schedule several lengthy periods of uninterrupted rest daily. Cluster necessary procedures and activities to minimize interruptions. *(These measures promote rest and decrease stimulation, both of which can help decrease ICP.)*
- Avoid sequential performance of activities that increase ICP (e.g., coughing, suctioning, repositioning, bathing). *(Research has validated that such sequential activities can cause a cumulative increase in ICP [Porth, 2007].)*
- Monitor temperature. As indicated, initiate external hypothermia or hyperthermia measures per orders and institutional protocol. *(Impaired hypothalamic function can interfere with temperature regulation, necessitating intervention. Hypothermia may reduce ICP, whereas hyperthermia may increase it. Prevent shivering, which can increase ICP [Bhardwaj et al., 2004].)*
- Limit suctioning time to 10 s at a time; hyperoxygenate client both before and after suctioning. *(These measures help prevent hypercapnia, which can increase cerebral vasodilation and raise ICP, and prevent hypoxia, which may increase cerebral ischemia.)*
- Consult with physician or advanced practice nurse about administering prophylactic lidocaine before suctioning. *(This measure may help prevent acute intracranial hypertension [Morton et al., 2005].)*
- Maintain optimal ventilation through proper positioning and suctioning as needed. *(These measures help prevent hypoxemia and hypercapnia; suctioning when not needed causes agitation and increases ICP [Bhardwaj et al., 2004].)*

- Carefully monitor hydration status; evaluate fluid intake and output, serum osmolality, and urine specific gravity and osmolality. (*Dehydration from diuretic therapy can cause hypotension and decreased cardiac output.*)
- If using an ICP monitoring device, refer to the procedure manual for guidelines (e.g., ventriculostomy, subarachnoid bolt, epidural monitor).

▶ Risk for Complications of Seizures

DEFINITION

Describes a person experiencing or at high risk to experience paroxysmal episodes of involuntary muscular contraction (tonus) and relaxation (clonus).

HIGH-RISK POPULATIONS

- Perinatal injuries
- Family history of seizure disorder
- Cerebral cortex lesions
- Head injury
- Infectious disorder (e.g., meningitis)
- Cerebral circulatory disturbance (e.g., cerebral palsy, stroke)
- Brain tumor
- Alcohol overdose or withdrawal
- Drug overdose or withdrawal (e.g., theophylline)
- Electrolyte imbalances (e.g., hypocalcemia, pyridoxine deficiency)
- Hypoglycemia
- High fever
- Eclampsia
- Metabolic abnormalities (renal, hepatic, electrolyte)
- Poisoning (mercury, lead, carbon monoxide)

Nursing Goals

The nurse will manage and minimize seizure episode

Indicators
No seizures

General Interventions and Rationales

- Determine whether the client senses an aura before onset of seizure activity. If so, reinforce safety measures to take during

an aura (e.g., lie down, pull car over to roadside and shut off ignition).
- If seizure activity occurs, observe and document the following (Hickey, 2006):
  - Where seizure began
  - Type of movements, parts of body involved
  - Changes in pupil size or position
  - Urinary or bowel incontinence
  - Duration
  - Unconsciousness (duration)
  - Behavior after seizure
  - Weakness, paralysis after seizure
  - Sleep after seizure (postictal period)

  (Progression of seizure activity may assist in identifying its anatomic focus.)
- Provide privacy during and after seizure activity. *(To protect the client from embarrassment)*
- During seizure activity, take measures to ensure adequate ventilation (e.g., loosen clothing). *Do not* try to force an airway or tongue blade through clenched teeth. *(Strong clonic/tonic movements can cause airway occlusion. Forced airway insertion can cause injury.)*
- During seizure activity, gently guide movements to prevent injury. Do not attempt to restrict movements. *(Physical restraint could result in musculoskeletal injury.)*
- If the client is sitting when seizure activity occurs, ease him or her to the floor and place something soft under his or her head. *(These measures help prevent injury.)*
- After seizure activity subsides, position client on the side. *(This position helps prevent aspiration of secretions.)*
- Allow person to sleep after seizure activity; reorient on awakening. *(The person may experience amnesia; reorientation can help him or her regain a sense of control and can help reduce anxiety.)*
- If person continues to have generalized convulsions, notify physician or advanced practice nurse and initiate protocol:
  - Establish airway.
  - Suction PRN.
  - Administer oxygen through nasal catheter.
  - Initiate an IV line.

  (Status epilepticus is a medical emergency with a 10% mortality rate. Impaired respiration can cause systemic and cerebral hypoxia. IV administration of a rapid-acting anticonvulsant [e.g., diazepam] is indicated [Hickey, 2006].)
- Keep the bed in a low position with the siderails up, and pad the siderails with blankets. *(These precautions help prevent injury from fall or trauma.)*

- If the client's condition is chronic, evaluate the need for teaching self-management techniques. Use the nursing diagnosis *Risk for Ineffective Self-Health Management related to insufficient knowledge of condition, medication regimen, safety measures, and community resources* (see Section 2).

GASTROINTESTINAL/HEPATIC/ BILIARY SYSTEM

Gastrointestinal/Hepatic/Biliary System
Risk for Complications of Gastrointestinal/Hepatic/Biliary Dysfunction
Risk for Complications of Paralytic Ileus
Risk for Complications of GI Bleeding
Risk for Complications of Hepatic Dysfunction
Risk for Complications of Hyperbilirubinemia

▶ Risk for Complications of Gastrointestinal/Hepatic/Biliary Dysfunction

DEFINITION

Describes a person experiencing or at high risk to experience compromised function in the gastrointestinal (GI), hepatic, or biliary systems. (*Note:* These three systems are grouped together for classification purposes. In a clinical situation, the nurse would use either *Risk for Complications of Gastrointestinal Dysfunctional, Risk for Complications of Hepatic Dysfunction, Risk for Complications of Bleeding* or *Risk for Complications of Biliary Dysfunction* to specify the applicable system.)

AUTHOR'S NOTE

The nurse can use these generic collaborative problems to describe a person at risk for various problems affecting the GI, hepatic, or biliary systems. Doing so focuses nursing

(continued)

■■■ **AUTHOR'S NOTE** *(Continued)*
interventions on monitoring GI, hepatic, or biliary status to detect and diagnose abnormal functioning. Should a complication develop, the nurse would add the applicable specific collaborative problem (e.g., *Risk for Complications of GI Bleeding, Risk for Complications of Hepatic Dysfunction*) to the problem list, specifying appropriate nursing management.

▶ Risk for Complications of Paralytic Ileus

DEFINITION

Describes a person experiencing or at high risk to experience neurogenic or functional bowel obstruction.

HIGH-RISK POPULATIONS

- Thrombosis or embolus to mesenteric vessels
- Any major surgery with use of general anesthesia and subsequent limitation of mobility, as well as minor surgery of the abdomen
- Postoperative status (bowel, retroperitoneal, or spinal cord surgery)
- Electrolyte imbalances (e.g., hypokalemia)
- Hypokalemia
- Postshock status
- Hypovolemia
- Post-trauma (e.g., spinal cord injury)
- Strangulated hernias
- Congenital bowel deformities
- Uremia
- Spinal cord lesion

Nursing Goals

The nurse will manage and minimize complications of paralytic ileus.

Indicators
Bowel sounds present
No nausea and vomiting
No abdominal distention

General Interventions and Rationales

- In a postoperative client, monitor bowel function, looking for:
  - Bowel sounds in all quadrants returning within 24 to 48 h of surgery
  - Flatus and defecation resuming by the second or third post-operative day

  (Surgery and anesthesia decrease innervation of the bowel, reducing peristalsis and possibly leading to transient paralytic ileus [Porth, 2007].)
- Do not allow client any fluids until bowel sounds are present. When indicated, begin with small amounts of clear liquids only. Monitor client's response to resumption of fluid and food intake, and note the nature and amount of any emesis or stools. *(The client will not tolerate fluids until bowel sounds resume.)*
- Monitor for signs of paralytic ileus—primarily pain, typically localized, sharp, and intermittent; hiccups; nausea/vomiting; constipation; distended abdomen; rebound tenderness. *(Intraoperative manipulation of abdominal organs and the depressive effects of narcotics and anesthetics on peristalsis can cause paralytic ileus, typically developing between the third and fifth postoperative day.)*
- If paralytic ileus is related to hypovolemia, refer to *Risk for Complications of Hypovolemia* for more information and specific interventions.

▶ Risk for Complications of GI Bleeding

DEFINITION

Describes a person experiencing or at high risk to experience GI bleeding.

HIGH-RISK POPULATIONS

- Prolonged mechanical ventilation
- Disorders of GI, hepatic, and biliary systems
- Transfusion of 5 U (or more) of blood
- Recent stress (e.g., trauma, sepsis), prolonged mechanical ventilation
- Esophageal varices
- Peptic ulcer
- Colon cancer
- Platelet deficiency
- Coagulopathy
- Shock, hypotension

- Major surgery (>3 h)
- Head injury
- Severe vascular disease
- Burns (>35% of body)
- Daily use of aspirin or nonsteroidal anti-inflammatory drugs (NSAIDs)

Infants/Children (Hockenberry & Wilson, 2009)

- Neonate to 6 months (hemorrhagic disease, anal fissure, stress ulcers, enterocolitis, vascular malformations, intussusception, lymphonodular hyperplasia)
- 6 months to 5 years (same as above, epistaxis, esophagitis, varices, gastritis, Meckel's diverticulum, Henoch-Schönlein purpura, polyps)
- 5 to 18 years (same as above, Mallory-Weiss tear, peptic ulcer, chronic ulcerative colitis, Crohn's disease, hemorrhoids)

Nursing Goals

The nurse will manage and minimize complications of GI bleeding

Indicators

Negative stool occult blood
Calm, oriented
Refer to *Risk for Complications of Hypovolemia* for indicators

General Interventions and Rationales

- Initiate prophylaxis protocol for persons on mechanical ventilation. *(These individuals are high risk for GI bleeding.)*
- Monitor for signs and symptoms of GI bleeding:
  - Nausea
  - Hematemesis
  - Blood in stool
  - Decreased hematocrit or hemoglobin
  - Hypotension, tachycardia
  - Diarrhea or constipation
  - Anorexia

  (Clinical manifestations depend on the amount and duration of GI bleeding. Early detection enables prompt intervention to minimize complications.)
- Monitor vital signs often, particularly blood pressure and pulse. *(Careful monitoring can detect early changes in blood volume.)*
- Consult with physician/advanced practice nurse for the specific prescription for titration ranges of pH and antacid administration.

- If NG intubation is prescribed, use a large-bore (18-gauge) tube and follow protocols for insertion and client care. *(An NG tube can remove irritating gastric secretions, blood, and clots and can reduce abdominal distention.)*
- Follow the protocol for gastric lavage, if ordered. *(Lavage provides local vasoconstriction and may help control GI bleeding.)*
- Monitor hemoglobin, hematocrit, red blood cell count, platelets, prothrombin time, partial thromboplastin time, type blood and cross match, and blood urea nitrogen (BUN) values. *(These values reflect the effectiveness of therapy.)*
- If hypovolemia occurs, refer to *RC of Hypovolemia* for more information and specific interventions.

▶ Risk for Complications of Hepatic Dysfunction

DEFINITION

Describes a person experiencing or at high risk to experience progressive liver dysfunction.

> ■■■■ **AUTHOR'S NOTE**
> In 2006 NANDA accepted the nursing diagnosis *Risk for Impaired Liver Function*. This author maintains that this is a collaborative problem. Nurses can choose to use either terminology. Students should consult with their faculty for direction.

HIGH-RISK POPULATIONS

Infections

- Hepatitis A, B, C, D, E, non-A, non-B, non-C
- Herpes simplex virus (types 1 and 2)
- Epstein-Barr virus
- Varicella zoster
- Dengue fever virus
- Rift Valley fever virus

Drugs/Toxins

- Industrial substances (chlorinated hydrocarbons, phosphorus)
- *Amanita phalloides* (mushrooms)
- Aflatoxin (herb)

- Medications (isoniazid, rifampin, halothane, methyldopa, tetracycline, valproic acid, monoamine oxidase inhibitors, phenytoin, nicotinic acid, tricyclic antidepressants, isoflurane, ketoconazole, cotrimethoprim, sulfasalazine, pyrimethamine, octreotide, antivirals)
- Acetaminophen toxicity
- Cocaine
- Alcohol

Hypoperfusion (Shock Liver)
- Venous obstructions
- Budd-Chiari syndrome
- Veno-occlusive disease
- Ischemia

Metabolic Disorders
- Hyperbilirubinemia
- Wilson's disease
- Tyrosinemia
- Heat stroke
- Galactosemia
- Nutritional deficiencies

Surgery
(Traumatized liver)
- Jejunoileal bypass
- Partial hepatectomy
- Liver transplant failure

Other
- Reye's syndrome
- Acute fatty liver of pregnancy
- Massive malignant infiltration
- Autoimmune hepatitis
- Rh incompatibility
- Ingestion of raw contaminated fish
- Thalassemia

Nursing Goals

The nurse will manage and minimize the complications of hepatic dysfunction.

Indicators
Prothrombin time (PT) 11–12.5 sec
Partial prothrombin time (PTT) 60–70 sec

Aspartate aminotransferase (AST) male 7–21 u/L, female 6–18
u/L
Alanine aminotransferase (ALT) 5–35 u/L
Alkaline phosphatase 30–150 u/L
Serum electrolytes within normal range

General Interventions and Rationales

- Monitor for signs and symptoms of hepatic dysfunction:
  - Anorexia, indigestion *(GI effects result from circulating toxins.)*
  - Jaundice *(Yellowed skin and sclera result from excessive bilirubin production.)*
  - Petechiae, ecchymoses *(These skin changes reflect impaired synthesis of clotting factors.)*
  - Clay-colored stools *(This can result from decreased bile in stools.)*
  - Elevated liver function tests (e.g., serum bilirubin, serum transaminase) *(Elevated values indicate extensive liver damage.)*
  - Prolonged prothrombin time *(This reflects reduced production of clotting factors.)*
- With hepatic dysfunction, monitor for hemorrhage. *(The liver has a central role in hemostasis. Decreased platelet count results from impaired production of new platelets from the bone marrow. Decreased clearance of old platelets by the reticuloendothelial system also results. In addition, synthesis of coagulation factors [II, V, VII, IX, and X] is impaired, resulting in bleeding. The most frequent site is the upper GI tract. Other sites include the nasopharynx, lungs, retroperitoneum, kidneys, and intracranial and skin puncture sites [Porth, 2002].)*
- Teach client to report any unusual bleeding (e.g., in the mouth after brushing teeth). *(Mucous membranes are prone to injury because of their high surface vascularity.)*
- Monitor for portal systemic encephalopathy by assessing:
  - General appearance and behavior
  - Orientation
  - Speech patterns
  - Laboratory values: blood pH and ammonia level
  (Profound liver failure results in accumulation of ammonia and other toxic metabolites in the blood. The blood–brain barrier permeability increases, and both toxins and plasma proteins leak from capillaries to the extracellular space, causing cerebral edema.)
- Monitor for signs and symptoms of (refer to the index under each electrolyte for specific signs and symptoms):
  - Hypoglycemia *(Hypoglycemia is caused by loss of glycogen stores in the liver from damaged cells and decreased serum concentrations of glucose, insulin, and growth hormones.)*
  - Hypokalemia *(Potassium losses occur from vomiting, NG suctioning, diuretics, or excessive renal losses.)*

- Hypophosphatemia *(The loss of potassium ions causes the proportional loss of magnesium ions. Increased phosphate loss, transcellular shifts, and decreased phosphate intake contribute to hypophosphatemia.)*
- Monitor for acid–base disturbances. Hepatocellular necrosis can result in accumulation of organic anions, resulting in metabolic acidosis. *(People with ascites often have metabolic alkalosis from increased bicarbonate levels resulting from increased sodium/hydrogen exchange in the distal tubule.)*
- Assess for side effects of medications. Avoid administering narcotics, sedatives, and tranquilizers and exposing the client to ammonia products. *(Liver dysfunction results in decreased metabolism of certain medications [e.g., opiates, sedatives, tranquilizers], increasing the risk of toxicity from high drug blood levels. Ammonia products should be avoided because of the client's already high serum ammonia level.)*
- Monitor for signs and symptoms of renal failure. (Refer to *Risk for Complications of Renal Failure* for more information.) *(Obstructed hepatic blood flow results in decreased blood to the kidneys, impairing glomerular filtration and leading to fluid retention and decreased urinary output.)*
- Monitor for hypertension. *(Fluid retention and overload can cause hypertension.)*
- Teach client and family to report signs and symptoms of complications, such as:
  - Increased abdominal girth *(It may indicate worsening portal hypertension.)*
  - Rapid weight loss or gain *(Weight loss points to negative nitrogen balance; weight gain points to fluid retention.)*
  - Bleeding *(Unusual bleeding indicates decreased prothrombin time and clotting factors.)*
  - Tremors *(They can result from impaired neurotransmission because of failure of the liver to detoxify enzymes that act as false neurotransmitters.)*
  - Confusion *(This can result from cerebral hypoxia caused by high serum ammonia levels resulting from the liver's impaired ability to convert ammonia to urea.)*

▶ Risk for Complications of Hyperbilirubinemia

DEFINITION

Describes a neonate with or at high risk for development of excessive serum bilirubin levels (>0.15 mg/dL).

HIGH-RISK POPULATIONS

Newborn

- Birthweight <1500 g
- Preterm delivery
- Male sex
- Hypothermia
- Asphyxia
- Hypoalbuminemia
- Sepsis
- Meningitis
- Polycythemia (Hct > 65%)
- Drugs that affect albumin binding
- Congenital hypothyroidism
- Bruising
- Poor feeding
- Inborn errors of metabolism

Maternal

- Oxytocin
- Forceps or vacuum delivery
- Blood incompatibilities
- Diabetes
- East Asian heritage
- Gestational hypertension
- Family history of jaundice, liver disease, anemia, or splenectomy

Nursing Goals

The nurse will manage and minimize complications of hyperbilirubinemia

Indicators
Bilirubin level < 0.15 mg/dL

General Interventions and Rationales

- Prevent cold stress. *(Metabolism of brown adipose tissue releases nonesterified free fatty acids, which compete with bilirubin for albumin-binding sites.)*
- Ensure adequate hydration and intake. *(Optimal fluid and feedings facilitate bilirubin excretion.)*
- Differentiate physiologic jaundice from pathologic jaundice. Physiologic jaundice requires no treatment, whereas pathologic jaundice does.

- Physiologic jaundice:
  - Benign
  - Onset 3 to 6 days (breast-feeding jaundice)
  - Onset 5 to 15 days (breast milk jaundice)
- Pathologic jaundice:
  - Rapidly rises
  - Onset first 24 h of life
- Screen for high-risk infants.
- Evaluate for presence of jaundice.
  - Face (early sign of bilirubin level >5 mg/dL)
  - Trunk/sternum (seen with levels >10 mg/dL)
  - Lower body (seen with levels >15 mg/dL)
- Assess for ecchymoses, abrasions, or petechiae. *(Extravasated hemoglobin in the tissue will add to normal hemoglobin breakdown and increase bilirubin production.)*
- Monitor for bilirubin-induced neurologic dysfunction. *(Bilirubin deposits in the basal ganglia and at nerve terminals cause encephalopathy in 25% of preterm infants and 2% of healthy term infants.)*
  - Behavior change: lethargy, somnolence progressing to convulsions and coma
  - Muscle tone abnormalities
  - Shrill, high-pitched cry
  - Poor sucking
- Initiate phototherapy according to protocol, if indicated. *(Phototherapy breaks down bilirubin into water-soluble products that can be excreted.)*
- If phototherapy is performed, ensure optimal hydration. Weigh infant daily to assess fluid status. *(Phototherapy increases fluid loss through diaphoresis.)*
- Protect infant's eyes during phototherapy treatment. Use Plexiglas shields; ensure that lids are closed before applying shields. Provide periods out of light with eye shields removed. *(These precautions help ensure safe treatment.)*
- Monitor for eye discharge, excessive pressure on lids, and corneal irritation. *(These complications may result from use of eye shields.)*
- Turn infant frequently during phototherapy. *(Any areas not exposed to light will remain jaundiced.)*
- Monitor temperature, checking it at least every 4 h. *(A nude infant is vulnerable to hypothermia; use of radiant warmers increases the risk of hyperthermia.)*
- Prepare parents for home phototherapy. *(Term infants older than 48 h with bilirubin levels >14 mg/dL but <18 mg/mL are candidates.)*

- Explain procedure.
  - Teach warning signs of neurotoxicity.
  - Provide written instructions.
  - Arrange for daily home health nurse visits.

MUSCULAR/SKELETAL SYSTEM

Muscular/Skeletal System
Risk for Complications of Muscular/Skeletal Dysfunction
Risk for Complications of Joint Dislocation

▶ Risk for Complications of Muscular/Skeletal Dysfunction

DEFINITION

Describes a person experiencing or at high risk to experience various musculoskeletal problems.

■■■ AUTHOR'S NOTE

The nurse can use this generic collaborative problem to describe people at risk for several types of musculoskeletal problems (e.g., all clients who have sustained multiple trauma). This collaborative problem focuses nursing management on assessing musculoskeletal status to detect and to diagnose abnormalities.

Because musculoskeletal problems typically affect daily functioning, the nurse must assess the client's functional patterns for evidence of impairment. Findings may have significant implications—for instance, a casted leg that prevents a woman from assuming her favorite sleeping position and impairs her ability to perform housework. After identifying any such problems, the nurse should use nursing diagnoses to address specific responses of actual or potential altered functioning.

▶ Risk for Complications of Joint Dislocation

DEFINITION

Describes a person experiencing or at high risk to experience displacement of a bone from its position in a joint.

HIGH-RISK POPULATIONS

- Total hip replacement
- Total knee replacement
- Fractured hip, knee, shoulder

For Infants/Children

- Birth trauma (e.g., breech, firstborn)
- Sports
- Cerebral palsy (hip)

Nursing Goals

The nurse will manage and minimize complications of joint dislocation.

Indicators

Hip in abduction or neutral position
Aligned affected extremity

General Interventions and Rationales

- Maintain correct positioning.
  - Hip: Maintain the hip in abduction, neutral rotation, or slight external rotation.
  - Hip: Avoid hip flexion over 60 degrees.
  - Knee: Slightly elevated from hip; avoid using bed knee gatch or placing pillows under the knee (to prevent flexion contractures). Place pillows under the calf.
  (Specific positions are used to prevent prosthesis dislocation.)
- Assess for signs of joint (hip, knee) dislocation:
  - *Hip*
    - Acute groin pain in operative hip
    - Shortening of leg with external rotation
  - *Hip, Knee, Shoulder*
    - "Popping" sound heard by client
    - Bulge at surgical site
    - Inability to move
    - Pain with mobility

(Until the surrounding muscles and joint capsule heal, joint dislocation may occur if positioning exceeds the limits of the prosthesis, as in flexing or hyperextending the knee or abducting the hip >45 degrees.)

- The client may be turned toward either side unless contraindicated. Always maintain an abduction pillow when turning; limit the use of Fowler's position. *(If proper positioning is maintained, including the abduction pillow, clients may safely be turned toward the operative and nonoperative side. This promotes circulation and decreases the potential for pressure ulcer formation as a result of immobility. A prolonged Fowler's position can dislocate the prosthesis.)*
- Monitor for shoulder joint dislocation/subluxation. *(Total shoulder arthroplasty has a higher risk of joint dislocation/subluxation because the shoulder is capable of movement in three planes [flexion/extension, abduction/adduction, internal/external rotation].)*

REPRODUCTIVE SYSTEM

Reproductive System
Risk for Complications of Pregnancy, Postpartum or Fetal
    Functioning
Risk for Complications of Prenatal Bleeding
Risk for Complications of Nonreassuring Fetal Status
Risk for Complications of Postpartum Bleeding

▶ Risk for Complications of Pregnancy, Postpartum or Fetal Functioning

DEFINITION

Describes a person experiencing or at high risk to experience a problem in reproductive system functioning.

■■■ AUTHOR'S NOTE
This generic collaborative problem provides a category under which to classify more specific collaborative problems affecting the reproductive system. Unlike the other generic
(continued)

■■■ **AUTHOR'S NOTE** *(Continued)*
collaborative problems (e.g., *Risk for Complications of Respiratory Dysfunction, Risk for Complications of Cardiac Dysfunction*),
it is of little clinical use by itself. So, instead of adding this
generic collaborative problem to a client's problem list,
the nurse should use the appropriate specific collaborative
problem, such as *Risk for Complications of Nonreassuring Fetal
Status* or *Risk for Complications of Postpartum Bleeding*.

▶ Risk for Complications of Prenatal Bleeding

DEFINITION

Describes a woman experiencing or at high risk to experience
bleeding during pregnancy.

HIGH-RISK POPULATIONS

- Incompetent cervix
- Spontaneous therapeutic abortion
- Ectopic pregnancy
- Gestational trophoblastic disease (hydatidiform mole)
- Cervical carcinoma
- Cervicitis
- Genital tract trauma
- Disseminated intravascular coagulation

For Placenta Previa (Late Pregnancy) (Simpson & Creehan, 2007)

- Previous placenta previa
- Previous cesarean section
- Induced or spontaneous abortions involving suction curettage
- Multiparity
- Uterine abnormalities
- Advanced maternal age (>35 years)
- Cigarette smoking
- Multiple gestation
- Fetal hydrops
- Large placenta
- Uterine anomalies
- Fibroid tumors
- Endometritis
- African-American or Asian ethnicity

For Abruptio Placentae (Late Pregnancy) (Simpson & Creehan, 2007)

- Hypertension
- Very short umbilical cord
- Trauma
- Precipitous labor
- Uterine abnormalities
- Poor nutrition, especially folic acid deficiency
- Partial abruption of current pregnancy
- History of abruption
- Preterm premature rupture of membranes <34 weeks' gestation
- Prior cesarean delivery
- High parity
- Oxytocin induction resulting in uterine tachysystole
- Cocaine/amphetamine use
- Cigarette smoking
- Rapid decompression of the uterus such as in the birth of the first of multiple fetuses or with polyhydramnios
- Uterine fibroids at the placental implantation site
- Use of intrauterine pressure catheters during labor

Nursing Goals

The nurse will manage and minimize complications of prenatal bleeding.

Indicators

Refer to Risk for Complications of Bleeding.

General Interventions and Rationales

- Teach the client to report unusual bleeding immediately.
- If bleeding occurs, notify physician or midwife and monitor:
  - Amount, character, color
  - Cramps, contractions, pain, or tenderness
  - Vital signs, hematocrit, urine output
- Monitor fetal heart tones (refer to *Risk for Complications of Non-reassuring Fetal Status* for specific guidelines).
- Do not perform vaginal or rectal examinations until placenta previa has been ruled out. *(These procedures can tear the placenta, causing life-threatening hemorrhage.)*
- Maintain client in a lateral recumbent position. *(This position displaces the uterus, which reduces compression on the vena cava. This improves maternal cardiac output and increases perfusion to the fetus.)*

- Administer oxygen by face mask at a rate of 10 L/min, as indicated. *(Supplemental oxygen therapy increases maternal circulating oxygen to the fetus.)*
- If signs of shock occur, refer to *Risk for Complications of Hypovolemic Shock* for more information on nursing management.
- Refer to the nursing diagnosis *Grieving* for interventions to provide support.

▶ Risk for Complications of Nonreassuring Fetal Status

DEFINITION

Describes a fetus experiencing or at high risk to experience a disruption of the physiologic exchange of nutrients, oxygen, and metabolites (Simpson & Creehan, 2007; Feinstein, Torgerson & Atterbury, 2003; Gilbert, 2007).

HIGH-RISK POPULATIONS

Fetal Factors

- Prematurity
- Intrauterine growth retardation
- Atresia of umbilical cord
- Cord compression
- Placental insufficiency
- Infection
- Multiple gestation
- Congenital anomalies
- Dysmaturity
- Acute hemolytic crisis
- Rh disease

Maternal Factors

- Chronic hypertension, pregnancy-associated hypertension
- Diabetes mellitus
- Third-trimester bleeding
- Maternal hypoxia (e.g., respiratory insufficiency)
- Maternal infection
- Hypotension
- Seizures
- Uterine tachysystole
- Prolonged uterine contractions
- Abruptio placentae

- Cardiovascular disease
- Substance abuse
- Malnutrition

Nursing Goals

The nurse will manage and minimize episodes of nonreassuring fetal status.

Indicators
Refer to assessment criteria under Interventions.

General Interventions and Rationales

- Determine baseline fetal heart tones and evaluate as reassuring if:
  - Rate of 110–160 bpm, regular rhythm
  - Presence of moderate variability (normal fetal rate has a fine irregularity of 6–25 bpm)
  - Presence of accelerations
  - Absence of decrease from baseline
  - Early decelerations (transient slowing of fetal heart rate with compression of the contraction causing parasympathetic stimulation)
- Monitor for nonreassuring fetal heart rate or rhythm, including:
  - Absent baseline variability (undetectable from baseline)
  - Minimal baseline variability (<5 bpm)
  - Tachycardia (>160 bpm)
  - Bradycardia (<110 bpm)
  - Late decelerations (visually apparent gradual decrease of FHR below baseline; the onset, nadir and recovery of the deceleration occur after the onset, peak and recovery of the contraction)
  - Variable decelerations, caused by compression of the umbilical cord
  - Sinusoidal pattern (smooth, repetitive undulation of baseline)

  (Fetal hypoxia, maternal drugs, maternal anemia, or dysrhythmias can cause changes in fetal heart rate [Feinstein, Torgerson & Atterbury, 2003].)
- If tachycardia occurs, assess:
  - Maternal temperature *(Fetal tachycardia occurs when maternal core temperature rises. It may increase before the mother's temperature can be measured orally or rectally.)*
  - Maternal intake, output, and urine specific gravity *(Maternal dehydration can cause fetal tachycardia.)*

- Maternal anxiety level *(Severe anxiety can increase fetal heart rate.)*
- Maternal medication use *(Certain medications used by the mother can cause increased fetal heart rate [e.g., atropine, terbutaline, ritodrine hydrochloride, scopolamine].)*
- Increase maternal hydration *(Maternal dehydration can cause fetal tachycardia.)*
- Notify the physician or advanced practice nurse of the situation and your assessment findings.
- Position the mother on her left side. *(This position decreases occlusion of the inferior vena cava by displacing the uterus, promoting venous return to the heart.)*
- If decreased variability occurs, evaluate possible causes, which can include:
  - Sleeping fetus
  - Effects of narcotics or sedatives
  - Fetal hypoxia
  - Maternal position
- If nonreassuring fetal heart patterns continue, notify the physician or advanced practice nurse and take the following steps (Feinstein, Torgerson & Atterbury, 2003):
  - Change maternal position from side to side.
  - Administer oxygen by face mask at a flow rate of 10 L/min, according to protocol. *(This increases oxygen delivery to the fetus.)*
  - Discontinue oxytocin infusion.
- Initiate continuous electronic fetal monitoring.
- Coach mother on breathing techniques to reduce anxiety and decrease hyperventilation.
- If the mother's condition worsens or if fetal pH is 7.2 or below, anticipate a cesarean section and assist as indicated.
- If mild variable decelerations occur, change the mother's position from supine to lateral or from one side to the other. *(Position shifts may relieve cord compression.)*
- If severe variable decelerations occur, take the following steps:
  - Notify the physician or advanced practice nurse.
  - Discontinue oxytocin infusion.
  - Perform a vaginal examination to assess for cord prolapse.
  - Shift the mother's position to left side lying and evaluate fetal heart rate; if not improved, turn the mother on her right side.
  - If these position changes do not improve fetal heart rate, or if cord is prolapsed, help the mother assume a knee–chest position. *(This reduces pressure on the cord and increases perfusion to the fetus.)*

- Administer oxygen by face mask at a rate of 10 L/min, according to protocol. (*This increases oxygen delivery to the fetus.*)
- Assess for improvement in fetal heart rate within 1 min.
- Anticipate an emergency vaginal delivery or cesarean section if the mother's condition worsens, if cord prolapse occurs, and/or if fetal pH is 7.2 or lower.

▶ Risk for Complications of Postpartum Bleeding

DEFINITION

Describes a woman who is experiencing or is at high risk to experience acute blood loss greater than 500 mL after vaginal birth or greater than 1000 mL after cesarean birth within the first 24 h postpartum (primary hemorrhage) or occurring after 24 h and before the 6th week postpartum (secondary hemorrhage).

HIGH-RISK POPULATIONS (SIMPSON & CREEHAN, 2007)

- Problematic third stage of labor
- Overdistended uterus (e.g., due to hydramnios, large fetus, multiple gestation)
- Prolonged labor
- Precipitous labor/birth
- Oxytocin induction/augmentation
- Multiparity
- Maternal exhaustion
- Instrumented delivery
- History of uterine atony
- Uterine fibroids
- History of postpartum hemorrhage
- Excessive analgesic or anesthesia use
- Preeclampsia
- Retained placental fragments
- Trauma to genital tract
- Maternal systemic disease (leukemia, thrombocytopenia, blood dyscrasia)
- Chorioamnionitis
- Asian or Hispanic ethnicity

Nursing Goals

The nurse will manage and minimize postpartum bleeding.

Indicators
Refer to Risk for Complications of Bleeding
Firm uterus

General Interventions and Rationales

- Assess the uterine fundus every 5 min for the first hour postpartum and PRN thereafter for the first 24 h; evaluate:
  - Height (normally should be at the level of the umbilicus immediately after delivery; midway between the umbilicus and symphysis 1 to 2 hours after delivery; then 1 cm above the uterus at 12 hours after delivery.)
  - Size (when contracted, should be about the size of a large grapefruit)
  - Consistency (should feel firm)
  (A boggy or relaxed uterus will not control bleeding by compression of the uterine muscle fibers.)
- If the uterus is relaxed or relaxing, massage it with firm but gentle circular strokes until it contracts. *(Massage stimulates the uterine muscle to contract.)*
- Avoid routine massage or overmassaging the uterus. *(Unnecessary massage can cause pain and muscle fatigue, with subsequent uterine relaxation.)*
- Monitor blood pressure and pulse every 15 min for 1 h, then every 30 min for the next hour, and then once every hour until the mother's condition stabilizes. *(Careful vital sign monitoring provides accurate evaluation of hemodynamic status.)*
- Monitor perineal blood loss. Keep a record of the number of pads used and the amount of saturation. *(Continuous seepage of blood with a firm uterus can indicate cervical or vaginal lacerations. Bleeding after the first 24 hours can indicate retained placental fragments or subinvolution.)*
- Obtain hemoglobin and hematocrit levels. Report a decrease to the physician or midwife. *(A decrease in the hemoglobin value of 1.0–1.5 g/dL and a four-point drop in hematocrit indicate a blood loss of 450–500 mL.)*
- Monitor bladder size and urine output with the same frequency as for vital signs. *(A distended bladder can displace the uterus and increase uterine atony.)*
- If bleeding becomes excessive, if the uterus fails to contract, or if vital sign changes occur, notify the physician or advanced practice nurse.
- If the woman exhibits signs of shock, refer to *RC of Hypovolemic Shock* for nursing interventions.

Diagnostic Clusters

Diagnostic
Clusters

MEDICAL CONDITIONS

▪▪▪▪▪▪▪ Cardiovascular/Hematologic/ Peripheral Vascular Disorders

Cardiac Conditions

Angina Pectoris

Collaborative Problems
Refer to Heart Failure

Nursing Diagnoses*

Anxiety related to chest pain secondary to effects of hypoxia
Fear related to present status and unknown future
Disturbed Sleep Pattern related to treatments and environment
Risk for Constipation related to bed rest, change in lifestyle, and medications
Activity Intolerance related to deconditioning secondary to fear of recurrent angina
Risk for Disturbed Self-Concept related to perceived and/or actual role changes
Risk for Impaired Home Maintenance related to angina or fear of angina
Risk for Interrupted Family Processes related to impaired ability of person to assume role responsibilities
Risk for Ineffective Sexuality Patterns related to fear of angina and altered self-concept
Grieving related to actual or perceived losses secondary to cardiac condition
Risk for Ineffective Self-Health Management related to insufficient knowledge of condition, home activities, diet, and medications

*List includes nursing diagnoses that may be associated with the medical diagnosis.

Heart Failure

Collaborative Problems

†△ RC of Deep vein thrombosis
▲ RC of Hypoxia
△ RC of Cardiogenic shock
✻ RC of Hepatic failure
✻ RC of Multiple organ failure
✻ RC of Hepatic insufficiency

Nursing Diagnoses✻

▲ Activity Intolerance related to insufficient oxygen for activities of daily living
△ Imbalanced Nutrition: Less Than Body Requirements related to nausea; anorexia secondary to venous congestion of gastrointestinal tract and fatigue
△ Ineffective Peripheral Tissue Perfusion related to venous congestion secondary to right-sided heart failure
▲ Anxiety related to breathlessness
✻ Fear related to progressive nature of condition
✻ Risk for Impaired Home Maintenance related to inability to perform activities of daily living secondary to breathlessness and fatigue
✻ (Specify) Self-Care Deficit related to dyspnea and fatigue
△ Disturbed Sleep Pattern related to nocturnal dyspnea and inability to assume usual sleep position
▲ Risk for Excessive Fluid Volume: Edema related to decreased renal blood flow secondary to right-sided heart failure
△ Powerlessness related to progressive nature of condition
△ Risk for Ineffective Self-Health Management related to insufficient knowledge of low-salt diet, drug therapy (diuretic, digitalis), activity program, and signs and symptoms of complications

---

▲ This diagnosis was reported to be monitored for or managed frequently (75% to 100%).
△ This diagnosis was reported to be monitored for or managed often (50% to 74%).
✻ This diagnosis was not included in the validation study.
† RC of (Risk for Complications of) is collaborative problems, not nursing diagnoses.
These symbols repeat throughout the chapter; however, the footnote will only appear once.

Endocarditis, Pericarditis (Rheumatic, Infectious)

See also *Corticosteroid Therapy*. If child, see *Rheumatic Fever*.

Collaborative Problems

RC of Congestive heart failure
RC of Valvular stenosis
RC of Cerebrovascular accident
RC of Emboli (pulmonary, cerebral, renal, splenic, heart)
RC of Cardiac tamponade

Nursing Diagnoses

Activity Intolerance related to insufficient oxygen secondary to decreased cardiac output
Risk for Ineffective Respiratory Function related to decreased respiratory depth secondary to pain
Pain related to friction rub and inflammation process
Risk for Ineffective Self-Health Management related to insufficient knowledge of etiology, prevention, antibiotic prophylaxis, and signs and symptoms of complications

Acute Coronary Syndrome (Myocardial Infarction, Uncomplicated)

Collaborative Problems

▲ RC of Dysrhythmias
▲ RC of Cardiogenic shock
▲ RC of Thromboembolism
RC of Recurrent myocardial infarction

Nursing Diagnoses

▲ Anxiety related to acute pain secondary to cardiac tissue ischemia
✳ Fear related to pain, present status, and unknown future
✳ Disturbed Sleep Pattern related to treatments and environment
Risk for Constipation related to decreased peristalsis secondary to medication effects, decreased activity, and change in diet
▲ Activity Intolerance related to insufficient oxygen for activities of daily living secondary to cardiac tissue ischemia
✳ Risk for Disturbed Self-Concept related to perceived or actual role changes

Risk for Impaired Home Maintenance related to angina or fear of angina

▲ Anxiety/Fear (individual, family) related to unfamiliar situation, unpredictable nature of condition, negative effect on lifestyle, possible sexual dysfunction

✳ Risk for Interrupted Family Processes related to impaired ability of ill person to assume role responsibilities

✳ Risk for Ineffective Sexuality Patterns related to fear of angina and altered self-concept

△ Grieving related to actual or perceived losses secondary to cardiac condition

△ Risk for Ineffective Self-Health Management related to insufficient knowledge of hospital routines, treatments, conditions, medications, diet, activity progression, signs and symptoms of complications, reduction of risks, follow-up care, community resources

Hematologic Conditions

Anemia

Collaborative Problems

RC of Bleeding
RC of Cardiac failure
RC of Iron overload (repeated transfusion)

Nursing Diagnoses

Activity Intolerance related to impaired oxygen transport secondary to diminished red blood cell count

Risk for Infection related to decreased resistance secondary to tissue hypoxia and/or abnormal white blood cells (neutropenia, leukopenia)

Risk for Injury: Bleeding tendencies related to thrombocytopenia and splenomegaly

Risk for Impaired Oral Mucous Membrane related to gastrointestinal mucosal atrophy

Risk for Ineffective Self-Health Management related to insufficient knowledge of condition, nutritional requirements, and drug therapy

Aplastic Anemia

Collaborative Problems

RC of Fatal aplasia

RC of Pancytopenia
RC of Bleeding
RC of Hypoxia
RC of Sepsis

Nursing Diagnoses

Activity Intolerance related to insufficient oxygen secondary to
diminished red blood cell count
Risk for Infection related to increased susceptibility secondary to
leukopenia
Risk for Impaired Oral Mucous Membrane related to tissue
hypoxia and vulnerability
Risk for Ineffective Self-Health Management related to
insufficient knowledge of causes, prevention, and signs and
symptoms of complications

Pernicious Anemia

See also *Anemia*.

Nursing Diagnoses

Impaired Oral Mucous Membrane related to sore red tongue
secondary to papillary atrophy and inflammatory changes
Diarrhea/Constipation related to gastrointestinal mucosal
atrophy
Risk for Imbalanced Nutrition: Less Than Body Requirements
related to anorexia secondary to sore mouth
Risk for Ineffective Self-Health Management related to
insufficient knowledge of chronicity of disease and vitamin B
treatment

Disseminated Intravascular Coagulation (DIC)

See also *Underlying Disorders (e.g., Obstetric, Infections, Burns),
Anticoagulant Therapy*.

Collaborative Problems

RC of Bleeding
RC of Renal failure
RC of Microthrombi (renal, cardiac, pulmonary, cerebral,
gastrointestinal)

Nursing Diagnoses

Fear related to treatments, environment, and unpredictable
outcome

Interrupted Family Processes related to critical nature of the situation and uncertain prognosis

Anxiety related to insufficient knowledge of causes and treatment

Polycythemia Vera (This diagnosis was not included in the validation study)

Collaborative Problems

RC of Thrombus formation
RC of Bleeding
RC of Hypertension
RC of Congestive heart failure
RC of Peptic ulcer
RC of Gout

Nursing Diagnoses

Imbalanced Nutrition: Less Than Body Requirements related to anorexia, nausea, and vasocongestion

Activity Intolerance related to insufficient oxygen secondary to pulmonary congestion and tissue hypoxia

Risk for Infection related to hypoxia secondary to vasocongestion

Risk for Ineffective Self-Health Management related to insufficient knowledge of fluid requirements, exercise program, and signs and symptoms of complications

Peripheral Vascular Conditions

Deep Vein Thrombosis

See also *Anticoagulant Therapy*, if indicated.

Collaborative Problems

▲ RC of Pulmonary embolism
▲ RC of Chronic leg edema
△ RC of Chronic stasis ulcers

Nursing Diagnoses

Risk for Constipation related to decreased peristalsis secondary to immobility

△ Risk for Ineffective Respiratory Function related to immobility

△ Risk for Impaired Skin Integrity related to chronic ankle edema

▲ Acute Pain related to impaired circulation for ambulation

△ Risk for Ineffective Self-Health Management related to insufficient knowledge of prevention of recurrence of deep vein thrombosis and signs and symptoms of complications

Hypertension

Collaborative Problems

RC of Retinal hemorrhage
RC of Cerebrovascular accident
RC of Cerebral hemorrhage
RC of Renal failure

Nursing Diagnoses

Risk for Noncompliance related to negative side effects of prescribed therapy versus the belief that no treatment is needed without the presence of symptoms

Risk for Ineffective Sexuality Patterns related to decreased libido or erectile dysfunction secondary to medication side effects

Risk for Ineffective Self-Health Management related to insufficient knowledge of condition, diet restrictions, medications, risk factors, and follow-up care

Varicose Veins (This diagnosis was not included in the validation study.)

Collaborative Problems

RC of Vascular rupture
RC of Bleeding
RC of Thrombosis

Nursing Diagnoses

Chronic Pain related to engorgement of veins
Risk for Ineffective Self-Health Management related to insufficient knowledge of condition, treatment options, and risk factors

Peripheral Arterial Disease (Atherosclerosis, Arteriosclerosis)

Collaborative Problems

RC of Stroke (cerebrovascular accident)
RC of Ischemic ulcers

RC of Claudication
RC of Acute arterial thrombosis
RC of Hypertension

Nursing Diagnoses

Risk for Impaired Tissue Integrity related to compromised
circulation
Chronic Pain related to muscle ischemia during prolonged
activity
Risk for Injury related to decreased sensation secondary to
chronic atherosclerosis
Risk for Infection related to compromised circulation
Risk for Injury related to effects of orthostatic hypotension
Activity Intolerance related to claudication
Risk for Ineffective Self-Health Management related to
insufficient knowledge of condition, management of
claudication, risk factors, foot care, and treatment plan

Raynaud's Disease

Collaborative Problems

RC of Acute arterial occlusion
RC of Ischemic ulcers
RC of Gangrene

Nursing Diagnoses

Acute Pain related to ischemia secondary to acute vasospasm
Risk for Impaired Tissue Integrity: Ischemic ulcers related to
vasospasm
Fear related to potential loss of work secondary to work-related
aggravating factors
Risk for Ineffective Self-Health Management related to
insufficient knowledge of condition, risk factors, and self-care

Venous Stasis Ulcers (Postphlebitis Syndrome)

Collaborative Problem

▲ RC of Cellulitis
✣ RC of Thrombosis

Nursing Diagnoses

✣ Ineffective Peripheral Tissue Perfusion related to dependent
position of legs

✳ Risk for Infection related to compromised circulation

▲ Chronic Pain related to ulcers and débridement treatments

△ Risk for Disturbed Body Image related to chronic open wounds and response of others to appearance

△ Risk for Ineffective Self-Health Management related to lack of knowledge of condition, prevention of complications, risk factors, and treatment

▰▰▰▰▰ Respiratory Disorders

Adult Respiratory Distress Syndrome

See also *Mechanical Ventilation* (under *Diagnostic and Therapeutic Procedures*).

Collaborative Problems

RC of Electrolyte imbalances
RC of Hypoxemia

Nursing Diagnoses

Anxiety related to implications of condition and critical care setting

Powerlessness related to condition and treatments (ventilator, monitoring)

Chronic Obstructive Pulmonary Disease (Emphysema, Bronchitis)

Collaborative Problems

▲ RC of Hypoxemia

△ RC of Right-sided heart failure

Nursing Diagnoses

▲ Ineffective Airway Clearance related to excessive and tenacious secretions

△ Risk for Imbalanced Nutrition: Less Than Body Requirements related to anorexia secondary to dyspnea, halitosis, and fatigue

▲ Activity Intolerance related to insufficient oxygen for activities and fatigue

Impaired Verbal Communication related to dyspnea

▲ Anxiety related to breathlessness and fear of suffocation

△ Powerlessness related to feeling of loss of control and lifestyle restrictions

△ Disturbed Sleep Pattern related to cough, inability to assume recumbent position, and environmental stimuli

△ Risk for Ineffective Self-Health Management related to insufficient knowledge of condition, treatments, prevention of infection, breathing exercises, risk factors, signs and symptoms of complications

Pleural Effusion

See also underlying disorders (*Heart Disease, Cirrhosis, Malignancy*).

Collaborative Problems

RC of Respiratory failure
RC of Pneumothorax (post-thoracentesis)
RC of Hypoxemia
RC of Hemothorax

Nursing Diagnoses

Activity Intolerance related to insufficient oxygen for activities of daily living

Risk for Imbalanced Nutrition: Less Than Body Requirements related to anorexia secondary to pressure on abdominal structures

Impaired Comfort related to accumulation of fluid in pleural space

(Specify) Self-Care Deficits related to fatigue and dyspnea

Pneumonia

Collaborative Problems

▲ RC of Respiratory insufficiency
△ RC of Septic shock
△ RC of Paralytic ileus

Nursing Diagnoses

Risk for Hyperthermia related to infectious process

▲ Activity Intolerance related to insufficient oxygen for activities of daily living

△ Risk for Impaired Oral Mucous Membrane related to mouth breathing, frequent expectoration, and decreased fluid intake secondary to malaise

✳ Risk for Deficient Fluid Volume related to increased insensible fluid loss secondary to fever and hyperventilation

△ Risk for Imbalanced Nutrition: Less Than Body Requirements related to anorexia, dyspnea, and abdominal distention secondary to air swallowing

▲ Ineffective Airway Clearance related to pain, increased tracheobronchial secretions, and fatigue

✳ Risk for Infection Transmission related to communicable nature of the disease

✳ Impaired Comfort related to hyperthermia and malaise

✳ Risk for Impaired Skin Integrity related to prescribed bed rest

△ Risk for Ineffective Self-Health Management related to lack of knowledge of condition, infection transmission, prevention of recurrence, diet, signs and symptoms of recurrence, and follow-up care

Pulmonary Embolism

See also *Anticoagulant Therapy*.

Collaborative Problem

RC of Hypoxemia

Nursing Diagnoses

Risk for Impaired Skin Integrity related to immobility and prescribed bed rest

Risk for Ineffective Self-Health Management related to insufficient knowledge of anticoagulant therapy and signs and symptoms of complications

▪▪▪▪▪ Metabolic/Endocrine Disorders

Addison's Disease
Collaborative Problems

RC of Addisonian crisis (shock)

RC of Electrolyte imbalances (sodium, potassium)

RC of Hypoglycemia

Nursing Diagnoses

Risk for Imbalanced Nutrition: Less Than Body Requirements related to anorexia and nausea

Risk for Deficient Fluid Volume related to excessive loss of
sodium and water secondary to polyuria

Diarrhea related to increased excretion of sodium and water

Risk for Disturbed Self-Concept related to appearance changes
secondary to increased skin pigmentation and decreased
axillary and pubic hair (female)

Risk for Injury related to postural hypotension secondary to
fluid/electrolyte imbalances

Risk for Ineffective Self-Health Management related to
insufficient knowledge of disease, signs and symptoms
of complications, risks for crisis (infection, diarrhea,
decreased sodium intake, diaphoresis), overexertion, dietary
management, identification (card, medallion), emergency kit,
and pharmacologic management

Aldosteronism, Primary

Collaborative Problems

RC of Hypokalemia
RC of Alkalosis
RC of Hypertension
RC of Hypernatremia

Nursing Diagnoses

Impaired Comfort related to excessive urine excretion and
polydipsia

Risk for Deficient Fluid Volume related to excessive urinary
excretion

Risk for Ineffective Self-Health Management related to
insufficient knowledge of condition, surgical treatment, and
effects of corticosteroid therapy

Cirrhosis (Laënnec's Disease)

See also *Substance Abuse*, if indicated.

Collaborative Problems

▲ RC of Bleeding
△ RC of Hypokalemia
△ RC of Portal systemic encephalopathy
✳ RC of Negative nitrogen balance
▲ RC of Medication toxicity (opiates, short-acting barbiturates,
major tranquilizers)
△ RC of Renal insufficiency

✳ RC of Anemia
✳ RC of Esophageal varices

Nursing Diagnoses

▲ Pain related to liver enlargement and ascites
△ Diarrhea related to excessive secretion of fats in stool secondary to liver dysfunction
✳ Risk for Injury related to decreased prothrombin production and synthesis of substances used in blood coagulation
▲ Imbalanced Nutrition: Less Than Body Requirements related to anorexia, impaired protein, fat, glucose metabolism, and impaired storage of vitamins (A, C, K, D, E)
✳ Risk for Ineffective Respiratory Function related to pressure on diaphragm secondary to ascites
✳ Risk for Disturbed Self-Concept related to appearance changes (jaundice, ascites)
△ Risk for Infection related to leukopenia secondary to enlarged, overactive spleen and hypoproteinemia
△ Impaired Comfort: Pruritus related to accumulation of bilirubin pigment and bile salts on skin
▲ Risk for Impaired Tissue Integrity related to edema and ascites secondary to portal hypertension
△ Risk for Ineffective Self-Health Management related to insufficient knowledge of pharmacologic contraindications, nutritional requirements, signs and symptoms of complications, and risks of alcohol ingestion

Cushing's Syndrome

Collaborative Problems

RC of Hypertension
RC of Congestive heart failure
RC of Psychosis
RC of Electrolyte imbalance (sodium, potassium)

Nursing Diagnoses

Disturbed Self-Concept related to physical changes secondary to disease process (moon face, thinning of hair, truncal obesity, virilism)
Risk for Infection related to excessive protein catabolism and depressed leukocytic phagocytosis secondary to hyperglycemia
Risk for Injury: Fractures related to osteoporosis
Risk for Impaired Skin Integrity related to loss of tissue, edema, and dryness

Ineffective Sexuality Patterns related to loss of libido and
cessation of menses (female) secondary to excessive
adrenocorticotropic hormone production

Risk for Ineffective Self-Health Management related to
insufficient knowledge of disease and diet therapy (high
protein, low cholesterol, low sodium)

Diabetes Mellitus

Collaborative Problems

Acute Complications:

▲ RC of Ketoacidosis (DKA)
△ RC of Hyperosmolar hyperglycemic nonketotic coma
(HHNC)
▲ RC of Hypoglycemia
▲ RC of Infections

Chronic Complications:

Macrovascular
▲ RC of Cardiac artery disease
▲ RC of Peripheral vascular disease
Microvascular
△ RC of Retinopathy
▲ RC of Neuropathy
△ RC of Nephropathy

Nursing Diagnoses

△ Risk for Injury related to decreased tactile sensation, diminished visual acuity, and hypoglycemia
△ Fear (client, family) related to diagnosis of diabetes, potential complications of diabetes, insulin injection, negative effect on lifestyle
△ Risk for Ineffective Coping (client, family) related to chronic disease, complex self-care regimen, and uncertain future
▲ Imbalanced Nutrition: More Than Body Requirements related to intake in excess of activity expenditures, lack of knowledge, and ineffective coping
Risk for Ineffective Sexuality Patterns (male) related to erectile problems secondary to peripheral neuropathy or psychological conflicts
△ Risk for Ineffective Sexuality Patterns (female) related to frequent genitourinary problems and physical and psychological stressors of diabetes

△ Powerlessness related to the future development of complications of diabetes (blindness, amputations, kidney failure, painful neuropathy)

✳ Risk for Loneliness related to visual impairment/blindness

△ Risk for Noncompliance related to the complexity and chronicity of the prescribed regimen

△ Risk for Ineffective Self-Health Management related to insufficient knowledge of condition, self-monitoring of blood glucose, medications, American Diabetes Association exchange diet, treatment of hypoglycemia, weight control, sick-day care, exercise program, foot care, signs and symptoms of complications, and community resources

Hepatitis (Viral)

Collaborative Problems

✳ RC of Hepatic failure

✳ RC of Coma

✳ RC of Subacute hepatic necrosis

✳ RC of Fulminant hepatitis

✳ RC of Portal systemic encephalopathy

△ RC of Hypokalemia

△ RC of Bleeding

△ RC of Drug toxicity

△ RC of Renal failure

△ RC of Progressive liver degeneration

Nursing Diagnoses

✳ Fatigue related to reduced metabolism by liver

▲ Risk for Infection Transmission related to contagious nature of virus type A and type B

▲ Imbalanced Nutrition: Less Than Body Requirements related to anorexia, epigastric distress, and nausea

✳ Risk for Deficient Fluid Volume related to lack of desire to drink

△ Impaired Comfort related to accumulation of bilirubin pigment and bile salts

✳ Risk for Injury related to reduced prothrombin synthesis and reduced vitamin K absorption

△ Pain related to swelling of inflamed liver

✳ Deficient Diversional Activity related to the monotony of confinement and isolation precautions

△ Risk for Ineffective Self-Health Management related to insufficient knowledge of condition, rest requirements, precautions to prevent transmission, nutritional requirements, and contra-indications

Hyperthyroidism (Thyrotoxicosis, Graves' Disease)

Collaborative Problems

RC of Thyroid storm
RC of Cardiac dysrhythmias

Nursing Diagnoses

Imbalanced Nutrition: Less Than Body Requirements related to intake less than metabolic needs secondary to excessive metabolic rate

Activity Intolerance related to fatigue and exhaustion secondary to excessive metabolic rate

Diarrhea related to increased peristalsis secondary to excessive metabolic rate

Impaired Comfort related to heat intolerance and profuse diaphoresis

Risk for Impaired Corneal Tissue Integrity related to inability to close eyelids secondary to exophthalmos

Risk for Injury related to tremors

Risk for Hyperthermia related to lack of metabolic compensatory mechanism secondary to hyperthyroidism

Risk for Ineffective Self-Health Management related to insufficient knowledge of condition, treatment regimen, pharmacologic therapy, eye care, dietary management, and signs and symptoms of complications

Hypothyroidism (Myxedema)

Collaborative Problems

RC of Atherosclerotic heart disease
RC of Normochromic, normocytic anemia
RC of Acute organic psychosis
RC of Myxedemic coma
RC of Metabolic
RC of Hematologic

Nursing Diagnoses

Imbalanced Nutrition: More Than Body Requirements related to intake greater than metabolic needs secondary to slowed metabolic rate

Activity Intolerance related to insufficient oxygen secondary to slowed metabolic rate

Constipation related to decreased peristaltic action secondary to decreased metabolic rate and decreased physical activity

Impaired Skin Integrity related to edema and dryness secondary to decreased metabolic rate and infiltration of fluid into interstitial tissues

Impaired Comfort related to cold intolerance secondary to decreased metabolic rate

Risk for Impaired Social Interaction related to listlessness and depression

Risk for Ineffective Self-Health Management related to insufficient knowledge of condition, treatment regimen, dietary management, signs and symptoms of complications, pharmacologic therapy, and contraindications

Obesity

Nursing Diagnoses

Ineffective Coping related to increased food consumption secondary to response to external stressors

Chronic Low Self-Esteem related to feelings of self-degradation and the response of others to the condition

Risk-Prone Health Behavior related to multiple factors resulting in imbalance between caloric intake and energy expenditure

Pancreatitis

Collaborative Problems

△ RC of Hypovolemia/shock

✳ RC of Hemotologic

✳ RC of Acute Respiratory Distress Syndrome

△ RC of Hypercalcemia

▲ RC of Hyperglycemia

✳ RC of Sepsis

✳ RC of Acute renal failure

Nursing Diagnoses

▲ Acute Pain related to nasogastric suction, distention of pancreatic capsule, and local peritonitis

Risk for Deficient Fluid Volume related to decreased intake secondary to nausea and vomiting

▲ Imbalanced Nutrition: Less Than Body Requirements related to vomiting, anorexia, and impaired digestion secondary to decreased pancreatic enzymes

△ Diarrhea related to excessive excretion of fats in stools secondary to insufficient pancreatic enzymes

△ Ineffective Denial related to inability to accept the consequences of one's alcohol abuse or dependency

△ Risk for Ineffective Self-Health Management related to insufficient knowledge of disease process, treatments, contraindications, dietary management, and follow-up care

▪▪▪▪▪ Gastrointestinal Disorders

Esophageal Disorders (Esophagitis, Hiatal Hernia)

Collaborative Problems

RC of Bleeding
RC of Gastric ulcers

Nursing Diagnoses

Risk for Imbalanced Nutrition: Less Than Body Requirements related to anorexia, heartburn, and dysphagia

Impaired Comfort: Heartburn related to regurgitation and eructation

Risk for Ineffective Self-Health Management related to insufficient knowledge of condition, dietary management, hazards of alcohol and tobacco, positioning after meals, pharmacologic therapy, and weight reduction (if indicated)

Gastroenterocolitis/Enterocolitis

Collaborative Problem

RC of Fluid/electrolyte imbalances

Nursing Diagnoses

Risk for Deficient Fluid Volume related to vomiting and diarrhea

Acute Pain related to abdominal cramping, diarrhea, and vomiting secondary to vascular dilatation and hyperperistalsis

Risk for Ineffective Self-Health Management related to insufficient knowledge of condition, dietary restrictions, and signs and symptoms of complications

Hemorrhoids/Anal Fissure (Nonsurgical)

Collaborative Problems

RC of Bleeding
RC of Bowel strangulation
RC of Thrombosis

Nursing Diagnoses

Acute Pain related to pressure on defecation
Risk for Constipation related to fear of pain on defecation
Risk for Ineffective Self-Health Management related to
   insufficient knowledge of condition, bowel routine, diet
   instructions, exercise program, and perianal care

Inflammatory Bowel Disease (Crohn's Disease, Ulcerative Colitis)

Collaborative Problems

▲ RC of Gastrointestinal bleeding
▲ RC of Fluid/electrolyte imbalances
▲ RC of Anemia
▲ RC of Intestinal obstruction
△ RC of Renal calculi
△ RC of Fistula/fissure/abscess

Nursing Diagnoses

▲ Chronic Pain related to intestinal inflammatory process
▲ Diarrhea related to intestinal inflammatory process
✳ Constipation related to inadequate dietary intake of fiber
✳ Risk for Impaired Skin Integrity (Perianal) related to diarrhea
   and chemical irritants
△ Risk for Ineffective Coping related to chronicity of condition
   and lack of definitive treatment
▲ Imbalanced Nutrition: Less Than Body Requirements related to dietary restrictions, nausea, diarrhea, and abdominal
   cramping associated with eating or painful ulcers of the oral
   mucous membrane
△ Risk for Ineffective Self-Health Management related to insufficient knowledge of condition, diagnostic tests, prognosis,
   treatment, and signs and symptoms of complications

Peptic Ulcer Disease

Collaborative Problems

▲ RC of Bleeding
▲ RC of Perforation
△ RC of Pyloric obstruction

Nursing Diagnoses

▲ Acute/Chronic Pain related to lesions secondary to increased gastric secretions
▲ Constipation/Diarrhea related to effects of medications on bowel function
△ Risk for Ineffective Self-Health Management related to insufficient knowledge of disease process, contraindications, signs and symptoms of complications, and treatment regimen

■■■■■ Renal/Urinary Tract Disorders

Acute Kidney Failure

Collaborative Problems

▲ RC of Fluid overload
▲ RC of Metabolic acidosis
▲ RC of Electrolyte imbalances
✱ RC of Hypertension
✱ RC of Pulmonary edema
✱ RC of Dysrthmias
✱ RC of Gastrointestinal Bleeding

Nursing Diagnoses

△ Imbalanced Nutrition: Less Than Body Requirements related to anorexia, nausea, vomiting, loss of taste, loss of smell, stomatitis, and unpalatable diet
▲ Risk for Infection related to invasive procedures
✱ Anxiety related to present status and unknown prognosis
✱ Risk for Ineffective Self-Health Management related to insufficient knowledge of condition, dietary restriction, daily recording, pharmacologic therapy, signs and symptoms of complications, follow-up visits, and community resources

Chronic Kidney Disease

See also *Peritoneal Dialysis* and *Hemodialysis*, if indicated.

Collaborative Problems

▲ RC of Fluid/electrolyte imbalances
△ RC of Gastrointestinal bleeding
✳ RC of Hyperparathyroidism
✳ RC of Pathologic fractures
✳ RC of Malnutrition
▲ RC of Anemia
▲ RC of Fluid overload
△ RC of Hypoalbuminemia
△ RC of Polyneuropathy
△ RC of Congestive heart failure
✳ RC of Pulmonary edema
△ RC of Metabolic acidosis
△ RC of Pleural effusion
  RC of Pericarditis, cardiac tamponade

Nursing Diagnoses

△ Imbalanced Nutrition: Less Than Body Requirements related to anorexia, nausea/vomiting, loss of taste/smell, stomatitis, and unpalatable diet
  Ineffective Sexuality Patterns related to decreased libido, impotence, amenorrhea, sterility, fatigue
✳ Disturbed Self-Concept related to effects of limitation on achievement of developmental tasks
✳ Risk for Caregiver Role Strain related to long-term care needs secondary to disability and treatment requirements
✳ Impaired Comfort related to (examples) fatigue, headaches, fluid retention, anemia
✳ Fatigue related to insufficient oxygenation secondary to anemia
△ Impaired Comfort: Pruritus related to calcium phosphate or urate crystals on skin
▲ Risk for Infection related to invasive procedures
△ Powerlessness related to progressively disabling nature of illness
▲ Risk for Ineffective Self-Health Management related to insufficient knowledge of condition, dietary restriction, daily recording, pharmacologic therapy, signs and symptoms of complications, follow-up visits, and community resources

Neurogenic Bladder

Collaborative Problems

RC of Renal calculi
RC of Autonomic dysreflexia

Nursing Diagnoses

Risk for Impaired Skin Integrity related to constant irritation from urine

Risk for Infection related to retention of urine or introduction of urinary catheter

Risk for Loneliness related to embarrassment from wetting self in front of others and fear of odor from urine

Overflow Incontinence related to chronically overfilled bladder with loss of sensation of bladder distention *or*

Reflex Incontinence related to absence of sensation to void and loss of ability to inhibit bladder contraction *or*

Urge Incontinence related to disruption of the inhibitory efferent impulses secondary to brain or spinal cord dysfunction

Risk for Dysreflexia related to reflex stimulation of sympathetic nervous system secondary to loss of autonomic control

Risk for Ineffective Self-Health Management related to insufficient knowledge of etiology of incontinence, management, bladder retraining programs, signs and symptoms of complications, and community resources

Urinary Tract Infections (Cystitis, Pyelonephritis, Glomerulonephritis)

See also *Acute Kidney Failure*.

Nursing Diagnoses

Chronic Pain related to inflammation and tissue trauma

Impaired Comfort related to inflammation and infection

Risk for Imbalanced Nutrition: Less Than Body Requirements related to anorexia secondary to malaise

Risk for Ineffective Coping related to the chronicity of the condition

Risk for Ineffective Self-Health Management related to insufficient knowledge of prevention of recurrence (adequate fluid intake, frequent voiding, hygiene measures [post-toileting], and voiding after sexual activity), signs and symptoms of recurrence, and pharmacologic therapy

Urolithiasis (Renal Calculi)

Collaborative Problems

△ RC of Pyelonephritis

▲ RC of Renal insufficiency

Nursing Diagnoses

▲ Acute Pain related to inflammation secondary to irritation of calculi and smooth muscle spasms

✽ Diarrhea related to renointestinal reflexes

△ Risk for Ineffective Self-Health Management related to insufficient knowledge of prevention of recurrence, dietary restrictions, and fluid requirements

▪▪▪▪▪ Neurologic Disorders

Brain Tumor

Because this disorder can cause alterations varying from minimal to profound, the following possible nursing diagnoses reflect individuals with varying degrees of involvement.

See also *Surgery (General, Cranial)*; *Cancer.*

Collaborative Problems

RC of Increased intracranial pressure
RC of Paralysis
RC of Hyperthermia
RC of Motor losses
RC of Sensory losses
RC of Cognitive losses

Nursing Diagnoses

Risk for Injury related to gait disorders, vertigo, or visual disturbances, secondary to compression/displacement of brain tissue
Anxiety related to implications of condition and uncertain future
(Specify) Self-Care Deficit related to inability to perform/difficulty in performing activities of daily living secondary to sensory–motor impairments

Imbalanced Nutrition: Less Than Body Requirements related to dysphagia and fatigue

Grieving related to actual/perceived loss of function and uncertain future

Impaired Physical Mobility related to sensory–motor impairment

Acute Pain related to compression/displacement of brain tissue and increased intracranial pressure

Interrupted Family Processes related to the nature of the condition, role disturbances, and uncertain future

Disturbed Self-Concept related to interruption in achieving/failure to achieve developmental tasks (childhood, adolescence, young adulthood, middle age)

Risk for Deficient Fluid Volume related to vomiting secondary to increased intracranial pressure

Risk for Injury related to impaired/uncontrolled sensory–motor function

Cerebrovascular Accident

Because this disorder can cause alterations varying from minimal to profound, the following possible nursing diagnoses reflect individuals with varying degrees of involvement.

Collaborative Problems

▲ RC of Increased intracranial pressure
▲ RC of Pneumonia
▲ RC of Atelectasis

Nursing Diagnoses

❋ Disturbed Sensory Perception: (specify) related to hypoxia and compression or displacement of brain tissue
▲ Impaired Physical Mobility related to decreased motor function of (specify) secondary to damage to upper motor neurons
▲ Impaired Communication related to dysarthria or aphasia
▲ Risk for Injury related to visual field, motor, or perception deficits
❋ Activity Intolerance related to deconditioning secondary to fatigue and weakness
❋ Disuse Syndrome
△ Continuous Incontinence related to loss of bladder tone, loss of sphincter control, or inability to perceive bladder cues
▲ (Specify) Self-Care Deficit related to impaired physical mobility or confusion

▲ Impaired Swallowing related to muscle paralysis or paresis secondary to damage to upper motor neurons

△ Grieving (Family, Individual) related to loss of function and inability to meet role responsibilities

△ Risk for Impaired Social Interaction related to difficulty communicating and embarrassment regarding disabilities

△ Risk for Deficient Fluid Volume related to dysphagia, difficulty in obtaining fluids secondary to weakness or motor deficits

△ Risk for Impaired Home Maintenance related to altered ability to maintain self at home secondary to sensory/motor/cognitive deficits and lack of knowledge by caregivers of home care, reality orientation, bowel/bladder program, skin care, signs and symptoms of complications, and community resources

▲ Functional Incontinence related to inability or difficulty in reaching toilet secondary to decreased mobility or motivation

△ Unilateral Neglect related to (specify site) secondary to right hemispheric brain damage

✳ Risk for Caregiver Role Strain related to complex care requirements secondary to (specify sensory or motor deficits)

△ Risk for Disturbed Self-Concept related to effects of prolonged debilitating condition on achieving developmental tasks and lifestyle

✳ Risk for Ineffective Self-Health Management related to insufficient knowledge of condition, pharmacologic therapy, self-care activities of daily living, home care, speech therapy, exercise program, community resources, self-help groups, and signs and symptoms of complications

✳ Wandering related to impaired cerebral function secondary to cerebrovascular accident

Nervous System Disorders (Degenerative, Demyelinating, Inflammatory, Myasthenia Gravis, Multiple Sclerosis, Muscular Dystrophy, Parkinson's Disease, Guillain-Barré Syndrome, Amyotrophic Lateral Sclerosis)

Because the responses associated with these disorders can range from minimal to profound, the following possible diagnoses reflect individuals with varying degrees of involvement.

Collaborative Problems

RC of Renal failure
RC of Pneumonia
RC of Atelectasis
RC of Acute Respiratory Dysfunction
RC of Autonomic Nervous System Dysfunction
RC of Peripheral Nervous System Dysfunction
RC of Decreased Cardiac Output

Nursing Diagnoses

Risk for Disturbed Self-Concept related to the effects of prolonged debilitating condition on lifestyle and on achieving developmental tasks

Risk for Injury related to visual disturbances, unsteady gait, sensory losses, weakness, or uncontrolled movements

Impaired Verbal Communication related to dysarthria secondary to ataxia of muscles of speech

Risk for Imbalanced Nutrition: Less Than Body Requirements related to dysphagia/chewing difficulties secondary to cranial nerve impairment

Activity Intolerance related to fatigue and difficulty in performing activities of daily living

Disuse Syndrome

Impaired Physical Mobility related to effects of muscle rigidity, tremors, and slowness of movement on activities of daily living

Impaired Swallowing related to cerebellar lesions

Fatigue related to extremity weakness, spasticity, fear of injury, and stressors

Overflow Incontinence related to sensory/motor deficits

Chronic Sorrow (Client, Family) related to nature of disease and uncertain prognosis

Ineffective Sexuality Patterns (female) related to loss of libido, fatigue, and decreased perineal sensation

Interrupted Family Processes related to nature of disorder, role disturbances, and uncertain future

Risk for Deficient Diversional Activity related to inability to perform usual job-related/recreational activities

Risk for Loneliness related to mobility difficulties and associated embarrassment

Impaired Home Maintenance related to inability to care for/difficulty in caring for self/home secondary to disability or unavailable or inadequate caregiver

Parental Role Conflict related to disruptions secondary to disability

Caregiver Role Strain related to continuous, multiple care needs

(Specify) Self-Care Deficits related to (examples) headaches, muscular spasms, joint pain, fatigue, paresis/paralysis

Powerlessness related to the unpredictable nature of the condition (e.g., remissions/exacerbations)

(Specify) Incontinence: related to poor sphincter control and spastic bladder

Ineffective Airway Clearance related to impaired ability to cough

Risk for Ineffective Self-Health Management related to insufficient knowledge of condition, treatments, prevention of infection, stress management, aggravating factors, signs and symptoms of complications, and community resources

Presenile Dementia (Alzheimer's Disease, Huntington's Disease)

See also *Nervous System Disorders*.

Nursing Diagnoses

Risk for Injury related to lack of awareness of environmental hazards

Chronic Confusion related to inability to evaluate reality secondary to cerebral neuron degeneration

Impaired Physical Mobility related to gait instability

Risk for Interrupted Family Processes related to effects of condition on relationships, role responsibilities, and finances

Impaired Home Maintenance related to inability to care for/ difficulty in caring for self/home or inadequate or unavailable caregiver

Unilateral Neglect related to (specify site) secondary to neurologic pathology

(Specify) Self-Care Deficit related to (specify)

Decisional Conflict related to placement of person in a care facility

Caregiver Role Strain related to multiple care needs and insufficient resources

Wandering related to impaired cerebral function secondary to Alzheimer's dementia

Seizure Disorders (Epilepsy)

If the client is a child, see also *Developmental Problems/Needs*.
RC of Staus Epilepticus

Nursing Diagnoses

❋ Risk for Injury related to uncontrolled tonic-clonic movements during seizure episode

▲ Risk for Ineffective Airway Clearance related to relaxation of tongue and gag reflexes secondary to disruption in muscle innervation

Risk for Loneliness related to fear of embarrassment secondary to having a seizure in public

❋ Risk for Delayed Growth and Development related to interruption in achieving/failure to achieve developmental tasks (adolescence, young adulthood, middle age)

❋ Risk for Impaired Oral Mucous Membrane related to effects of drug therapy on oral tissue

❋ Fear related to unpredictable nature of seizures and embarrassment

△ Risk for Ineffective Self-Health Management related to insufficient knowledge of condition, medication, activity, care during seizures, environmental hazards, and community resources

Spinal Cord Injury†

Collaborative Problems

△ RC of Electrolyte imbalances

❋ RC of Spinal shock

❋ RC of Neurogenic shock

❋ RC of Respiratory complications

△ RC of Paralytic ileus

△ RC of Gastrointestinal bleeding

▲ RC of Thrombophlebitis

△ RC of Fracture/dislocation

△ RC of Cardiovascular Insufficiency

▲ RC of Hypoxemia

▲ RC of Urinary retention

❋ RC of Pyelonephriris

△ RC of Renal insufficiency

Nursing Diagnoses

▲ Self-Care Deficit related to sensory/motor deficits secondary to level of spinal cord injury

❋ Impaired Verbal Communication related to impaired ability to speak secondary to tracheostomy

✳ Fear related to possible abandonment by others, changes in role responsibilities, effects of injury on lifestyle, multiple tests and procedures, or separation from support systems

△ Interrupted Family Processes related to adjustment requirements, role disturbances, and uncertain future

✳ Risk for Aspiration related to inability to cough secondary to level of injury

△ Risk for Impaired Home Maintenance related to insufficient knowledge of the effects of altered skin, bowel, bladder, respiratory, thermoregulation, and sexual function and their management, signs and symptoms of complications, follow-up care, and community resources

▲ Anxiety related to perceived effects of injury on lifestyle and unknown future

▲ Chronic Sorrow related to loss of body function and its effects on lifestyle

✳ Risk for Loneliness (individual/family) related to disability or requirements for the caregiver(s)

✳ Risk for Caregiver Role Strain related to continuous, multiple care needs, inadequate resources, and coping mechanisms

△ Risk for Disturbed Self-Concept related to effects of disability on achieving developmental tasks and lifestyle

✳ Risk for Deficient Fluid Volume related to difficulty obtaining liquids

✳ Risk for Imbalanced Nutrition: More Than Body Requirements related to imbalance of intake versus activity expenditures

✳ Risk for Imbalanced Nutrition: Less Than Body Requirements related to anorexia and increased metabolic requirements

✳ Risk for Deficient Diversional Activity related to effects of limitations on ability to participate in recreational activities
  • Reflex Urinary Incontinence or Overflow Urinary Incontinence
  • Related to bladder atony secondary to sensory–motor deficits

✳ Disuse Syndrome

✳ Risk for Injury related to impaired ability to control movements and sensory–motor deficits

✳ Risk for Infection related to urinary stasis, repeated catheterizations, and invasive procedures (skeletal tongs, tracheostomy, venous lines, surgical sites)

△ Risk for Ineffective Sexuality Patterns related to physiologic, sensory, and psychological effects of disability on sexuality or function

△ Bowel Incontinence (Reflex) related to lack of voluntary sphincter control secondary to spinal cord injury at the 11th thoracic vertebra (T_{11})

△ Bowel Incontinence (Areflexia) related to lack of voluntary sphincter control secondary to spinal cord injury involving sacral reflex arc (S_2–S_4)

△ Risk for Dysreflexia related to reflex stimulation of sympathetic nervous system secondary to loss of autonomic control

✳ Risk for Ineffective Self-Health Management related to insufficient knowledge of condition, treatment regimen, rehabilitation, and assistance devices

Unconscious Individual

See also *Mechanical Ventilation*, if indicated.

Collaborative Problems

✳ RC of Respiratory insufficiency
▲ RC of Pneumonia
▲ RC of Atelectasis
▲ RC of Fluid/electrolyte imbalances
✳ RC of Negative nitrogen balance
✳ RC of Bladder distention
✳ RC of Seizures
✳ RC of Stress ulcers
✳ RC of Increased intracranial pressure
△ RC of Sepsis
▲ RC of Thrombophlebitis
✳ RC of Renal calculi
△ RC of Urinary tract infection

Nursing Diagnoses

✳ Risk for Infection related to immobility and invasive devices (tracheostomy, Foley catheter, venous lines)
✳ Risk for Impaired Corneal Tissue Integrity related to corneal drying secondary to open eyes and lower tear production
✳ Family Anxiety/Fear related to present state of individual and uncertain prognosis
✳ Risk for Impaired Oral Mucous Membrane related to inability to perform own mouth care and pooling of secretions
▲ Continuous Incontinence related to unconscious state
△ Disuse Syndrome
△ Powerlessness (family) related to feelings of loss of control and restrictions on lifestyle

Risk for Ineffective Airway Clearance related to stasis of secretions secondary to inadequate cough and decreased mobility

▪▪▪▪▪▪ Sensory Disorders

Ophthalmic Disorders (Cataracts, Detached Retina, Glaucoma, Inflammations)

See also *Cataract Extractions*; *Scleral Buckle/Vitrectomy*.

Collaborative Problem

RC of Increased intraocular pressure

Nursing Diagnoses

Risk for Injury related to visual limitations

Acute Pain related to (examples) inflammation (lid, lacrimal structures, conjunctiva, uveal tract, retina, cornea, sclera), infection, increased intraocular pressure, ocular tumors

Risk for Noncompliance related to negative side effects of prescribed therapy versus the belief that no treatment is needed without the presence of symptoms

Risk for Loneliness related to fear of injury or embarrassment outside home environment

Risk for Impaired Home Maintenance related to impaired ability to perform activities of daily living secondary to impaired vision

(Specify) Self-Care Deficit related to impaired vision

Anxiety related to actual or possible vision loss and perceived impact of chronic illness on lifestyle

Risk for Disturbed Self-Concept related to effects of visual limitations

Risk for Ineffective Self-Health Management related to insufficient knowledge of condition, eye care, medications, safety measures, activity restrictions, and follow-up care

Otic Disorders (Infections, Mastoiditis, Trauma)

Nursing Diagnoses

Risk for Injury related to disturbances of balance and impaired ability to detect environmental hazards

Impaired Verbal Communication related to difficulty understanding others secondary to impaired hearing

Risk for Impaired Social Interaction related to difficulty in participating in conversations

Risk for Loneliness related to the lack of contact with others secondary to fear and embarrassment of hearing losses

Acute Pain related to inflammation, infection, tinnitus, or vertigo

Fear related to actual or possible loss of hearing

Risk for Ineffective Self-Health Management related to insufficient knowledge of condition, medications, prevention of recurrence, hazards (swimming, air travel, showers), signs and symptoms of complications, and hearing aids

■■■■ Integumentary Disorders

Dermatologic Disorders (Dermatitis, Psoriasis, Eczema)

Nursing Diagnoses

Impaired Skin Integrity related to lesions and inflammatory response

Impaired Comfort related to dermal eruptions and pruritus

Risk for Impaired Social Interaction related to fear of embarrassment and negative reactions of others

Risk for Disturbed Self-Concept related to appearance and response of others

Risk for Ineffective Self-Health Management related to insufficient knowledge of condition, topical agents, and contraindications

Pressure Ulcers†

Collaborative Problem

△ RC of Sepsis

Nursing Diagnoses

▲ Risk for Infection related to exposure of ulcer base to fecal/urinary drainage

▲ Impaired Tissue Integrity related to mechanical destruction of tissue secondary to pressure, shear, and friction

❋ Impaired Home Maintenance related to complexity of care or unavailable caregiver

▲ Imbalanced Nutrition: Less Than Body Requirements related to anorexia secondary to (specify)

▲ Impaired Physical Mobility related to imposed restrictions, deconditioned status, loss of motor control, or altered mental status

✳ Excess Fluid Volume: Edema related to (specify)

✳ Continuous Incontinence related to (specify)

△ Risk for Ineffective Self-Health Management related to insufficient knowledge of etiology, prevention, treatment, and home care

Skin Infections (Impetigo, Herpes Zoster, Fungal Infections)

Herpes Zoster

Collaborative Problems

RC of Postherpetic neuralgia
RC of Keratitis
RC of Uveitis
RC of Corneal ulceration
RC of Blindness

Nursing Diagnoses

Impaired Skin Integrity related to lesions and pruritus
Impaired Comfort related to dermal eruptions and pruritus
Risk for Infection Transmission related to contagious nature of the organism
Risk for Ineffective Self-Health Management related to insufficient knowledge of condition (causes, course), prevention, treatment, and skin care

Thermal Injuries (Burns, Severe Hypothermia)

Acute Period
Collaborative Problems

▲ RC of Hypovolemia/shock
✳ RC of Fluid overload
✳ RC of Anemia
△ RC of Negative nitrogen balance
▲ RC of Electrolyte imbalance
△ RC of Metabolic acidosis
▲ RC of Respiratory Insufficiency
▲ RC of Sepsis
✳ RC of Emboli

▲ RC of Graft rejection/infection
✳ RC of Hypothermia
△ RC of Curling's ulcer
△ RC of Paralytic ileus
✳ RC of Stress diabetes
✳ RC of Pneumonia
△ RC of Renal insufficiency
✳ RC of Compartment syndrome

Nursing Diagnoses

▲ Risk for Infection related to loss of protective layer secondary to thermal injury
▲ Imbalanced Nutrition: Less Than Body Requirements related to increased caloric requirement secondary to thermal injury and inability to ingest sufficient quantities to meet increased requirements
✳ Impaired Physical Mobility related to acute pain secondary to thermal injury and treatments
△ (Specify) Self-Care Deficit related to impaired range-of-motion ability secondary to pain
✳ Fear related to painful procedures and possibility of death
✳ Risk for Loneliness related to infection control measures and separation from family and support systems
△ Disuse Syndrome
✳ Disturbed Sleep Pattern related to position restrictions, pain, and treatment interruptions
✳ Risk for Disturbed Sensory Perception related to (examples) excessive environmental stimuli, stress, imposed immobility, sleep deprivation, protective isolation
▲ Grieving (family, individual) related to actual or perceived impact of injury on life, appearance, relationships, lifestyle
▲ Anxiety related to sudden injury, treatments, uncertainty of outcome, and pain
✳ Anxiety related to pain secondary to thermal injury treatments and immobility
▲ Acute Pain related to thermal injury treatments and immobility

Postacute Period
If individual is a child, see also *Developmental Problems/Needs*.

Collaborative Problems

RC of Same as in acute period

Nursing Diagnoses

△ Deficient Diversional Activity related to monotony of confinement

❊ Risk for Loneliness related to embarrassment and response of others to injury

❊ Powerlessness related to inability to control situation

△ Risk for Disturbed Self-Concept related to effects of thermal injury on achieving developmental tasks (child, adolescent, adult)

❊ Fear related to uncertain future and effects of injury on lifestyle, relationships, occupation

❊ Impaired Home Maintenance related to long-term requirements of treatments

△ Risk for Ineffective Self-Health Management related to insufficient knowledge of exercise program, wound care, nutritional requirements, pain management, signs and symptoms of complications, and burn prevention and follow-up care

▨▨▨▨▨▨ Musculoskeletal/ Connective Tissue Disorders

Fractured Jaw

Collaborative Problems

RC of Dislocation

Nursing Diagnoses

Risk for Aspiration related to inadequate cough secondary to pain and fixative devices

Impaired Oral Mucous Membrane related to difficulty in performing oral hygiene secondary to fixation devices

Impaired Verbal Communication related to fixation devices

Acute Pain related to tissue trauma and fixation device

Risk for Imbalanced Nutrition: Less Than Body Requirements related to inability to ingest solid food secondary to fixation devices

Risk for Ineffective Self-Health Management related to insufficient knowledge of mouth care, nutritional requirements, signs and symptoms of infection, and procedure for emergency wire cutting (e.g., vomiting)

Fractures

See also *Casts*.

Collaborative Problems

▲ RC of Neurovascular compromise
▲ RC of Fat embolism
▲ RC of Bleeding/hematoma formation
✳ RC of Osteomyelitis
✳ RC of Compartment syndrome
✳ RC of Contracture
▲ RC of Thromboemboli

Nursing Diagnoses

✳ Acute Pain related to tissue trauma and immobility
▲ Impaired Physical Mobility related to tissue trauma secondary to fracture
✳ Disuse Syndrome
✳ Risk for Infection related to invasive fixation devices
▲ (Specify) Self-Care Deficit related to limitation of movement secondary to fracture
✳ Deficient Diversional Activity related to boredom of confinement secondary to immobilization devices
✳ Risk for Impaired Home Maintenance related to (examples) fixation device, impaired physical mobility, unavailable support system
✳ Interrupted Family Processes related to difficulty of ill person in assuming role responsibilities secondary to limited motion
△ Risk for Ineffective Self-Health Management related to insufficient knowledge of condition, signs and symptoms of complications, activity restrictions

Low Back Pain

Collaborative Problems

RC of Herniated nucleus pulposus

Nursing Diagnoses

Pain related to (examples) acute lumbosacral strain, weak muscles, osteoarthritis of spine, unstable lumbosacral ligaments, spinal stenosis, intervertebral disk problem
Impaired Physical Mobility related to decreased mobility and flexibility secondary to muscle spasm

Risk for Ineffective Coping related to effects of chronic pain on lifestyle

Risk for Interrupted Family Processes related to impaired ability to meet role responsibilities (financial, home, social)

Risk for Ineffective Self-Health Management related to insufficient knowledge of condition, exercise program, noninvasive pain relief methods (relaxation, imagery), proper posture and body mechanics, and risk factors (smoking, inactivity, overweight)

Osteoporosis

Collaborative Problems

RC of Fractures
RC of Kyphosis
RC of Paralytic ileus

Nursing Diagnoses

Acute/Chronic Pain related to muscle spasm and fractures

Ineffective Self-Health Management related to insufficient daily physical activity

Imbalanced Nutrition: Less Than Body Requirements related to inadequate dietary intake of calcium, protein, and vitamin D

Impaired Physical Mobility related to limited range of motion secondary to skeletal changes

Fear related to unpredictable nature of condition

Risk for Ineffective Self-Health Management related to insufficient knowledge of condition, risk factors, nutritional therapy, and prevention

Inflammatory Joint Disease

Collaborative Problems

RC of Septic arthritis
RC of Sjögren's syndrome
RC of Neuropathy
RC of Anemia, leukopenia
RC of Avascular necrosis
RC of Cardiopulmonary effects
RC of Diabetes mellitus
RC of Septic shock

Nursing Diagnoses

Chronic Pain related to local and systemic inflammatory lesions

(Specify) Self-Care Deficit related to loss of motion, muscle weakness, pain, stiffness, or fatigue

Powerlessness related to physical and psychological changes imposed by the disease

Ineffective Coping related to the stress imposed by unpredictable exacerbations

(Specify) Self-Care Deficit related to limitations secondary to disease process

Fatigue related to effects of chronic inflammatory process

Risk for Impaired Oral Mucous Membrane related to effects of medications or Sjögren's syndrome

Impaired Home Maintenance related to impaired ability to perform household responsibilities secondary to limited mobility and pain

Disturbed Sleep Pattern related to pain or secondary to fibrositis

Impaired Physical Mobility related to pain and limited joint motion

Ineffective Sexuality Patterns related to pain, fatigue, difficulty in assuming positions, and lack of adequate lubrication (female) secondary to disease process

Risk for Loneliness related to ambulation difficulties and fatigue

Interrupted Family Processes related to difficulty/inability of ill person to assume role responsibilities secondary to fatigue and limited motion

Risk for Ineffective Self-Health Management related to insufficient knowledge of condition, pharmacologic therapy, home care, stress management, and quackery

▪▪▪▪▪ Infectious/Immunodeficient Disorders

Lupus Erythematosus (Systemic)

See also *Rheumatic Diseases*; *Corticosteroid Therapy*.

Collaborative Problems

RC of Sepsis

RC of Polymyositis, Serositis, Pericarditis, Pleuritis

RC of Vasculitis

RC of Hematologic abnormalities

RC of Raynaud's disease

RC of Neuropsychiatric disorders

Nursing Diagnoses

Powerlessness related to unpredictable course of disease

Ineffective Coping related to unpredictable course and altered appearance

Risk for Loneliness related to embarrassment and the response of others to appearance

Risk for Disturbed Self-Concept related to inability to achieve developmental tasks secondary to disabling condition and changes in appearance

Risk for Injury related to increased dermal vulnerability secondary to disease process

Fatigue related to decreased mobility and effects of chronic inflammation

Risk for Ineffective Self-Health Management related to insufficient knowledge of condition, rest versus activity requirements, pharmacologic therapy, signs and symptoms of complications, risk factors, and community resources

Meningitis/Encephalitis

Collaborative Problems

RC of Fluid/electrolyte imbalances

RC of Cerebral edema

RC of Adrenal damage

RC of Circulatory collapse

RC of Bleeding

RC of Seizures

RC of Sepsis

RC of Alkalosis

RC of Increased intracranial pressure

Nursing Diagnoses

Risk for Infection Transmission related to contagious nature of organism

Acute Pain related to headache, fever, neck pain secondary to meningeal irritation

Activity Intolerance related to fatigue and malaise secondary to infection

Risk for Impaired Skin Integrity related to immobility, dehydration, and diaphoresis

Risk for Impaired Oral Mucous Membrane related to dehydration and impaired ability to perform mouth care

Risk for Imbalanced Nutrition: Less Than Body Requirements related to anorexia, fatigue, nausea, and vomiting

Risk for Ineffective Respiratory Function related to immobility and pain

Risk for Injury related to restlessness and disorientation secondary to meningeal irritation

Interrupted Family Processes related to critical nature of situation and uncertain prognosis

Anxiety related to treatments, environment, and risk of death

Risk for Ineffective Self-Health Management related to insufficient knowledge of condition, treatments, pharmacologic therapy, rest/activity balance, signs and symptoms of complications, follow-up care, and prevention of recurrence

Sexually Transmitted Infections/Diseases

Nursing Diagnoses

Risk for Infection Transmission related to lack of knowledge of the contagious nature of the disease and reports of high-risk behaviors

Anxiety related to nature of the condition and its implications for lifestyle with genital herpes/warts diagnosis

Grieving related to loss of trust in partner secondary to infidelity

Acute Pain related to inflammatory process

Risk for Loneliness related to fear of transmitting disease to others, e.g., genital herpes, HIV

Risk for Ineffective Self-Health Management related to insufficient knowledge of condition, modes of transmission, consequences of repeated infections, and prevention of recurrences

Acquired Immunodeficiency Syndrome (AIDS) (Adult)

See also *End-Stage Cancer*.

Collaborative Problems

▲ RC of Opportunistic infections
▲ RC of Myelosuppression
▲ RC of Sepsis
✳ RC of Neuropathy
✳ RC of Peripheral Nephropathy

Nursing Diagnoses

✳ Chronic Pain related to headache, fever secondary to inflammation of cerebral tissue

▲ Fatigue related to effects of disease, stress, chronic infections, and nutritional deficiency

❋ Risk for Impaired Skin Integrity related to perineal and anal tissue excoriation secondary to diarrhea and chronic genital candidal or herpes lesions

❋ Imbalanced Nutrition: Less Than Body Requirements related to chronic diarrhea, gastrointestinal malabsorption, fatigue, anorexia, or oral/esophageal lesions

▲ Risk for Infection Transmission related to contagious nature of blood and body secretions

△ Risk for Loneliness related to fear of rejection or actual rejection of others secondary to fear

❋ Hopelessness related to nature of the condition and poor prognosis

△ Powerlessness related to unpredictable nature of condition

▲ Interrupted Family Processes related to the nature of the AIDS condition, role disturbance, and uncertain future

△ Anxiety related to perceived effects of illness on lifestyle and unknown future

△ Chronic Sorrow related to loss of body function and its effects on lifestyle

▲ Risk for Infection related to increased susceptibility secondary to compromised immune system

▲ Risk for Impaired Oral Mucous Membrane related to compromised immune system

❋ Risk for Caregiver Role Strain related to multiple needs of ill person and chronicity

△ Risk for Ineffective Self-Health Management related to insufficient knowledge of condition, medications, home care, infection control, and community resources

▦▦▦ Neoplastic Disorders

Cancer

Cancer: Initial Diagnosis
See also specific types.

Nursing Diagnoses

▲ Anxiety related to unfamiliar hospital environment, uncertainty about outcomes, feelings of helplessness and hopelessness, and insufficient knowledge about cancer and treatment

▲ Grieving related to potential loss of body function and the perceived losses associated with cancer on lifestyle

- ❋ Powerlessness related to uncertainty about prognosis and outcome of cancer treatment
- ▲ Interrupted Family Processes related to fears associated with recent cancer diagnosis, disruptions associated with treatments, financial problems, and uncertain future
- △ Decisional Conflict related to treatment modality choices
- △ Risk for Disturbed Self-Concept related to changes in lifestyle, role responsibilities, and appearance
- △ Risk for Loneliness related to fear of rejection or actual rejection secondary to fear
- △ Risk for Spiritual Distress related to conflicts centering on the meaning of life, cancer, spiritual beliefs, and death
- ❋ Risk for Ineffective Self-Health Management related to insufficient knowledge of cancer, cancer treatment options, diagnostic tests, effects of treatment, treatment plan, and support services

Cancer: General (Applies to Malignancies in Varied Sites and Stages)

Nursing Diagnoses

Impaired Oral Mucous Membranes related to (examples) disease process, therapy, radiation, chemotherapy, inadequate oral hygiene, and altered nutritional/hydration status

Risk for Ineffective Sexuality Patterns related to (examples) fear, grieving, changes in body image, anatomic changes, pain, fatigue (treatments, disease), or change in role responsibilities

Acute/Chronic Pain related to disease process and treatments

Diarrhea related to (examples) disease process, chemotherapy, radiation, and medications

Constipation related to (examples) disease process, chemotherapy, radiation therapy, immobility, dietary intake, and medications

Disturbed Self-Concept related to (examples) anatomic changes, role disturbances, uncertain future, disruption of lifestyle

(Specify) Self-Care Deficit related to fatigue, pain, or depression

Risk for Infection related to altered immune system

Imbalanced Nutrition: Less Than Body Requirements related to anorexia, fatigue, nausea, and vomiting secondary to disease process and treatments

Risk for Injury related to disorientation, weakness, sensory/perceptual deterioration, or skeletal/muscle deterioration

Disuse Syndrome

Risk for Deficient Fluid Volume related to (examples) altered ability/desire to obtain fluids, weakness, vomiting, diarrhea, depression, and fatigue

Risk for Impaired Home Maintenance related to (examples) lack of knowledge, lack of resources (support system, equipment, finances), motor deficits, sensory deficits, cognitive deficits, and emotional deficits

Risk for Impaired Social Interaction related to fear of rejection or actual rejection of others after diagnosis

Powerlessness related to inability to control situation

Interrupted Family Processes related to (examples) stress of diagnosis/treatments, role disturbances, and uncertain future

Grieving (Family, Individual) related to actual, perceived, or anticipated losses associated with diagnosis

Risk for Ineffective Self-Health Management related to insufficient knowledge of disease, misconceptions, treatments, home care, and support agencies

Cancer: End-Stage

See also specific types.

Collaborative Problems

RC of Hypercalcemia
RC of Intracerebral metastasis
RC of Malignant effusions
RC of Opioid toxicity
RC of Pathologic fractures
RC of Spinal cord compression
RC of Superior vena cava syndrome
RC of Negative nitrogen imbalance
RC of Myelosuppression
RC of Bowel Obstruction
RC of Hepatoxicity
RC of Increased Intracranial pressure
RC of Cardiotoxicity

Nursing Diagnoses

See also *Cancer (General)*.

Imbalanced Nutrition: Less Than Body Requirements related to decreased oral intake, increased metabolic demands of tumor, and altered lipid metabolism

Impaired Comfort related to pruritus secondary to dry skin and biliary obstruction

Ineffective Airway Clearance related to inability to cough up secretions secondary to weakness, increased viscosity, and pain

Impaired Physical Mobility related to pain, sedation, weakness, fatigue, and edema

(Specify) Self-Care Deficit related to fatigue, weakness, sedation, pain, or decreased sensory/perceptual capacity

Activity Intolerance related to hypoxia, fatigue, malnutrition, and decreased mobility

Grieving related to terminal illness, impending death, functional losses, and withdrawal of, or from, others

Hopelessness related to overwhelming functional losses or impending death

Disturbed Self-Concept related to dependence on others to meet basic needs and decrease in functional ability

Powerlessness related to change from curative status to palliative status

Caregiver Role Strain related to multiple care needs and concern about ability to manage home care

Risk for Spiritual Distress related to fear of death, overwhelming grief, belief system conflicts, and unresolved conflicts

Death Anxiety related to effects of disease process

Risk for Impaired Home Maintenance related to insufficient knowledge of home care, pain management, signs and symptoms of complications, and community resources available

Colorectal Cancer

See also *Cancer (General)*.

Nursing Diagnoses

Risk for Ineffective Sexuality Patterns (Male) related to inability to have or sustain an erection secondary to surgical procedure on perineal structures

Risk for Ineffective Self-Health Management related to insufficient knowledge of ostomy care, supplies, dietary management, signs and symptoms of complications, and community services

■■■■■■ Surgical Procedures

General Surgery

Preoperative Period
Nursing Diagnoses

Fear related to surgical experience, loss of control, and unpredictable outcome

Anxiety related to preoperative procedures (surgical permit, diagnostic studies, Foley catheter, diet and fluid restrictions, medications, skin preparation, waiting area for family) and postoperative procedures (disposition [recovery room, intensive care unit], medications for pain, coughing/turning/leg exercises, tube/drain placement, nothing by mouth [NPO]/diet restrictions, bed rest)

Postoperative Period
Collaborative Problems

† RC of Urinary retention
  RC of Bleeding
  RC of Hypovolemia/shock
  RC of Pneumonia
  RC of Peritonitis
  RC of Thrombophlebitis
  RC of Paralytic ileus
  RC of Evisceration/dehiscence

Nursing Diagnoses

Risk for Infection related to site for bacterial invasion
Risk for Ineffective Respiratory Function related to postanesthesia state, postoperative immobility, and pain
Acute Pain related to incision, flatus, and immobility
Risk for Constipation related to decreased peristalsis secondary to the effects of anesthesia, immobility, and pain medication
Risk for Imbalanced Nutrition: Less Than Body Requirements related to increased protein/vitamin requirements for wound healing and decreased intake secondary to pain, nausea, vomiting, and diet restrictions
Risk for Ineffective Self-Health Management related to insufficient knowledge of home care, incisional care, signs and symptoms of complications, activity restriction, and follow-up care

Amputation (Lower Extremity)

Preoperative Period
See also *Surgery (General)*.

Nursing Diagnoses

▲ Anxiety related to insufficient knowledge of postoperative routines, postoperative sensations, and crutch-walking techniques

Postoperative Period
Collaborative Problems

- ▲ RC of Edema of stump
- ▲ RC of Bleeding
- ▲ RC of Hematoma site
- ❊ RC of Delayed wound healing

Nursing Diagnoses

- ❊ Disuse Syndrome
- ▲ Grieving related to loss of limb and its effects on lifestyle
- ▲ Acute/Chronic Pain related to phantom limb sensations secondary to peripheral nerve stimulation or abnormal impulses to central nervous system
- ▲ Risk for Injury related to altered gait and hazards of assistive devices
- △ Risk for Impaired Home Maintenance related to architectural barriers
- △ Risk for Disturbed Body Image related to perceived negative effects of amputation and response of others to appearance
- ▲ Risk for Injury related to contracture formation secondary to impaired movement and pain
- △ Risk for Ineffective Self-Health Management related to insufficient knowledge of activities of daily living adaptations, stump care, prosthesis care, gait training, and follow-up care

Aneurysm Resection (Abdominal Aortic)

See also *Surgery (General)*.

Preoperative Period
Collaborative Problems

- ▲ RC of Rupture of aneurysm

Postoperative Period
Collaborative Problems

- ▲ RC of Distal vessel thrombosis or emboli
- ▲ RC of Kidney failure
- △ RC of Mesenteric ischemia/thrombosis
- △ RC of Spinal cord ischemia

Nursing Diagnoses

- ▲ Risk for Infection related to location of surgical incision
- ❊ Risk for Ineffective Sexuality Patterns (male) related to possible loss of ejaculate and erections secondary to surgery

△ Risk for Ineffective Self-Health Management related to insufficient knowledge of home care, activity restrictions, signs and symptoms of complications, and follow-up care

Anorectal Surgery

See also *Surgery (General)*.

Preoperative Period
See *Hemorrhoids/Anal Fissure*.

Postoperative Period
Collaborative Problems

RC of Bleeding
RC of Urinary retention

Nursing Diagnoses

Risk for Constipation related to fear of pain
Risk for Infection related to surgical incision and fecal contamination
Risk for Ineffective Self-Health Management related to insufficient knowledge of wound care, prevention of recurrence, nutritional requirements (diet, fluid), exercise program, and signs and symptoms of complications

Arterial Bypass Graft of Lower Extremity (Aortic, Iliac, Femoral, Popliteal)

See also *Surgery (General)*; *Anticoagulant Therapy*.

Postoperative Period
Collaborative Problems

▲ RC of Thrombosis of graft
△ RC of Compartment syndrome
  RC of Lymphocele
▲ RC of Disruption of anastomosis

Nursing Diagnoses

▲ Risk for Infection related to location of surgical incision
▲ Acute Pain related to increased tissue perfusion to previous ischemic tissue
△ Risk for Impaired Tissue Integrity related to immobility and vulnerability of heels

△ Risk for Ineffective Self-Health Management related to insufficient knowledge of wound care, signs and symptoms of complications, activity restrictions, and follow-up care

Arthroscopy, Arthrotomy, Meniscectomy, Bunionectomy

See also *Surgery (General)*.

Postoperative Period
Collaborative Problems

RC of Hematoma formation
RC of Neurovascular impairments
RC of Bleeding
RC of Effusion

Nursing Diagnoses

Risk for Ineffective Self-Health Management related to insufficient knowledge of home care, incision care, activity restrictions, signs of complications, and follow-up care

Breast Surgery (Lumpectomy, Mastectomy)

See also *Cancer (General)*; *Surgery (General)*.

Preoperative Period
▲ *Anxiety/Fear related to perceived effects of breast surgery and cancer on (immediate concerns of pain, edema and postdischarge concerns regarding relationships, work and prognosis*

Postoperative Period
Collaborative Problems

▲ RC of Neurovascular compromise

Nursing Diagnoses

▲ Risk for Impaired Physical Mobility (shoulder, arm) related to lymphedema, nerve/muscle damage, and pain
▲ Risk for Injury related to compromised lymph, motor, and sensory function in affected arm
▲ Grieving related to loss of breast and change in appearance
▲ Risk for Ineffective Self-Health Management related to insufficient knowledge of wound care, exercises, breast prosthesis, signs and symptoms of complications, hand/arm precautions, community resources, and follow-up care

Carotid Endarterectomy

See also *Surgery (General)*.

Preoperative Period
Nursing Diagnoses

△ Anxiety related to anticipated surgery and unfamiliarity with preoperative and postoperative routines and postoperative sensations

Postoperative Period
Collaborative Problems

▲ RC of Thrombosis
▲ RC of Hypotension
▲ RC of Hypertension
▲ RC of Bleeding
▲ RC of Cerebral infarction
   RC of Cranial nerve impairment
▲ RC of Facial nerve impairment
▲ RC of Hypoglossal nerve impairment
▲ RC of Glossopharyngeal nerve impairment
△ RC of Vagus nerve impairment
△ RC of Local nerve impairment (peri-incisional numbness of skin)
▲ RC of Respiratory obstruction

Nursing Diagnoses

△ Risk for Injury related to syncope secondary to vascular insufficiency
△ Risk for Ineffective Self-Health Management related to insufficient knowledge of home care, signs and symptoms of complications, risk factors, activity restrictions, and follow-up care

Cataract Extraction

Postoperative Period
Collaborative Problem

▲ RC of Bleeding

Nursing Diagnoses

△ Acute Pain related to surgical procedure
▲ Risk for Infection related to increased susceptibility secondary to surgical interruption of eye surface

▲ Risk for Injury related to visual limitations, presence in unfamiliar environment, limited mobility, and postoperative presence of eye patch

△ Risk for Loneliness related to decreased socialization and altered visual acuity and fear of falling

△ Risk for Impaired Home Maintenance related to inability to perform activities of daily living secondary to activity restrictions and visual limitations

▲ Risk for Ineffective Self-Health Management related to insufficient knowledge of activities permitted and restricted, medications, complications, and follow-up care

Cesarean Section

See *Surgery (General)*; *Postpartum Period*.

Cholecystectomy

See also *Surgery (General)*.

Postoperative Period
Collaborative Problem

RC of Peritonitis

Nursing Diagnoses

Risk for Ineffective Respiratory Function related to high abdominal incision and splinting secondary to pain

Risk for Impaired Oral Mucous Membrane related to NPO state and mouth breathing secondary to nasogastric intubation

Colostomy

See also *Surgery (General)*.

Postoperative Period
Collaborative Problems

▲ RC of Peristomal ulceration/herniation

▲ RC of Stomal necrosis, retraction, prolapse, stenosis, obstruction

Nursing Diagnoses

△ Grieving related to implications of cancer diagnosis

▲ Risk for Disturbed Self-Concept related to effects of ostomy on body image and lifestyle

- △ Risk for Ineffective Sexuality Patterns related to perceived negative impact of ostomy on sexual functioning and attractiveness

  Risk for Sexual Dysfunction related to physiologic impotence secondary to damaged sympathetic nerves (male) or inadequate vaginal lubrication (female)
- △ Risk for Loneliness related to decreased socialization and anxiety about possible odor and leakage from appliance
- ▲ Risk for Ineffective Self-Health Management related to insufficient knowledge of stoma pouching procedure, colostomy irrigation, peristomal skin care, perineal wound care, and incorporation of ostomy care into activities of daily living

Corneal Transplant (Penetrating Keratoplasty)

See also *Surgery (General)*.

Postoperative Period

Collaborative Problems

- ❊ RC of Endophthalmitis
- ▲ RC of Increased intraocular pressure
- ❊ RC of Epithelial defects
- ❊ RC of Graft failure

Nursing Diagnoses

- △ Risk for Infection related to nonintact ocular tissue
- ▲ Acute Pain related to surgical procedure
- ▲ Risk for Ineffective Self-Health Management related to insufficient knowledge of eye care, resumption of activities, medications/medication administration, signs and symptoms of complications, and long-term follow-up care

Coronary Artery Bypass Grafting (CABG)

See also *Surgery (General)*.

Postoperative Period

Collaborative Problems

- ▲ RC of Cardiovascular insufficiency
- ▲ RC of Respiratory insufficiency
- ▲ RC of Renal insufficiency
- ❊ RC of Hyperthermia
- ❊ RC of Postcardiotomy delirium

Nursing Diagnoses

▲ Acute Pain related to surgical incisions, chest tubes, and immobility secondary to lengthy surgery

Impaired Physical Mobility related to surgical incisions, chest tubes, and fatigue

△ Fear related to transfer from intensive environment of the critical care unit and potential for complications

Impaired Verbal Communication related to endotracheal tube (temporary)

△ Interrupted Family Processes related to disruption of family life, fear of outcome (death, disability), and stressful environment (intensive care unit)

△ Risk for Disturbed Self-Concept related to the symbolic meaning of the heart and changes in lifestyle

△ Risk for Ineffective Self-Health Management related to insufficient knowledge of incisional care, pain management (angina, incisions), signs and symptoms of complications, condition, pharmacologic care, risk factors, restrictions, stress management techniques, and follow-up care

Cranial Surgery

See also *Surgery (General)*; *Brain Tumor* for preoperative and postoperative care.

Postoperative Period
Collaborative Problems

▲ RC of Increased intracranial pressure
▲ RC of Cerebral/cerebellar dysfunction
✳ RC of Hypoxemia
▲ RC of Seizures
▲ RC of Brain hemorrhage, hematomas, hygroma
▲ RC of Cranial nerve dysfunctions
✳ RC of Cardiac dysrhythmias
▲ RC of Fluid/electrolyte imbalances
△ RC of Meningitis/encephalitis
▲ RC of Sensory–motor losses
▲ RC of Hypothermia/hyperthermia
△ RC of Antidiuretic hormone secretion disorders
▲ RC of Cerebrospinal fluid leaks
▲ RC of Hygromas
✳ RC of Brain shifts/herniations
✳ RC of Hydrocephalus
✳ RC of Gastrointestinal bleeding

Nursing Diagnoses

▲ Acute Pain related to compression/displacement of brain tissue and increased intracranial pressure

△ Risk for Impaired Corneal Tissue Integrity related to inadequate lubrication secondary to tissue edema

△ Risk for Ineffective Self-Health Management related to insufficient knowledge of wound care, signs and symptoms of complications, restrictions, and follow-up care

Dilatation and Curettage

See also *Surgery (General)—Preoperative and Postoperative.*

Postoperative Period
Collaborative Problems

RC of Bleeding

Nursing Diagnoses

Risk for Ineffective Self-Health Management related to insufficient knowledge of condition, home care, signs and symptoms of complications, and activity restrictions.

Enucleation

Postoperative Period
Collaborative Problems

▲ RC of Bleeding
RC of Abscess

Nursing Diagnoses

△ Risk for Injury related to visual limitations and presence in unfamiliar environment

△ Grieving related to loss of eye and its effects on lifestyle

△ Risk for Disturbed Self-Concept related to effects of change in appearance on lifestyle

△ Risk for Loneliness related to changes in body image and altered vision

△ Risk for Impaired Home Maintenance related to inability to perform activities of daily living secondary to change in visual abilities

△ Risk for Ineffective Self-Health Management related to insufficient knowledge of activities permitted, self-care activities, medications, complications, and plans for follow-up care

Fractured Hip and Femur

See also *Surgery (General)*.

Postoperative Period
Collaborative Problems

- ▲ RC of Hypovolemia/shock
- ▲ RC of Pulmonary embolism
- ▲ RC of Sepsis
- ▲ RC of Fat emboli
- ▲ RC of Compartment syndrome
- △ RC of Peroneal nerve palsy
- ▲ RC of Displacement of hip joint
- ▲ RC of Venous stasis/thrombosis
  RC of Avascular necrosis of femoral head

Nursing Diagnoses

- ▲ (Specify) Self-Care Deficit related to prescribed activity restriction
- ▲ Disuse syndrome
- △ Fear related to anticipated postoperative dependence
- △ Risk for Disturbed Sensory Perceptions related to unfamiliar environment, pain, and immobility
- △ Risk for Ineffective Self-Health Management related to insufficient knowledge of activity restrictions, assistive devices, home care, follow-up care, and supportive services

Hysterectomy (Vaginal, Abdominal)

See also *Surgery (General)*.

Postoperative Period
Collaborative Problems

- ▲ RC of Vaginal bleeding
- ✱ RC of Urinary retention (postcatheter removal)
- ✱ RC of Fistula formation
- ▲ RC of Deep vein thrombosis
- ▲ RC of Trauma (ureter, bladder, rectum)
- ✱ RC of Neurological deficits secondary to epidural therapy

Nursing Diagnoses

- ✱ Risk for Infection related to surgical intervention and presence of urinary catheter
- ▲ Risk for Disturbed Self-Concept related to significance of loss
- ✱ Grieving related to loss of body part and childbearing ability

△ Risk for Ineffective Self-Health Management related to insufficient knowledge of perineal/incisional care, signs of complications, activity restrictions, loss of menses, hormone therapy, and follow-up care

Ileostomy

Postoperative Period
Collaborative Problems

▲ RC of Peristomal ulceration/herniation
▲ RC of Stomal necrosis, retraction, prolapse, stenosis, obstruction
▲ RC of Fluid and electrolyte imbalances
✳ RC of Ileanal Kock pouchitis
✳ RC of Failed nipple valve (Kock Pouch)
✳ RC of Ileal reservoir pouchitis (Kock Pouch)
✳ RC of Cholelithiasis
✳ RC of Urinary calculi

Nursing Diagnoses

▲ Risk for Disturbed Self-Concept related to effects of ostomy on body image
△ Risk for Ineffective Sexuality Patterns related to perceived negative impact of ostomy on sexual functioning and attractiveness
△ Risk for Loneliness related to decreased socialization and anxiety about possible odor and leakage from appliance
△ Risk for Ineffective Self-Health Management related to insufficient knowledge of stoma pouching procedure, peristomal skin care, perineal wound care, and incorporation of ostomy care into activities of daily living
△ Risk for Ineffective Self-Health Management related to insufficient knowledge of care of ileoanal reservoir
Risk for Ineffective Self-Health Management related to insufficient knowledge of intermittent intubation of Kock continent ileostomy

Laminectomy

See also *Surgery (General)*.

Postoperative Period
Collaborative Problems

▲ RC of Neurosensory impairments
✳ RC of Bowel/bladder dysfunction

▲ RC of Paralytic ileus
✳ RC of Cord edema
✳ RC of Skeletal misalignment
△ RC of Cerebrospinal fistula
✳ RC of Hematoma
▲ RC of Urinary retention

Nursing Diagnoses

✳ Risk for Injury related to vertigo secondary to postural hypotension
▲ Acute Pain related to muscle spasms (back, thigh) secondary to surgical trauma
✳ (Specify) Self-Care Deficit related to activity restrictions
▲ Risk for Ineffective Self-Health Management related to insufficient knowledge of home care, brace care, activity restrictions, and exercise program

Radical Neck Dissection (Laryngectomy)

See also *Surgery (General)*; *Cancer (General)*; *Tracheostomy*.

Postoperative Period
Collaborative Problems

✳ RC of Hypoxemia
▲ RC of Flap rejection
▲ RC of Bleeding
▲ RC of Carotid artery rupture
✳ RC of Cranial nerve injury
✳ RC of Infection

Nursing Diagnoses

▲ Risk for Impaired Physical Mobility: Shoulder, head related to removal of muscles, nerves, flap graft reconstruction, and surgical trauma
▲ Risk for Disturbed Self-Concept related to change in appearance
▲ Risk for Ineffective Self-Health Management related to insufficient knowledge of wound care, signs and symptoms of complications, exercises, and follow-up care

Ophthalmic Surgery

See also *Surgery (General)*.

Postoperative Period

Collaborative Problems

△ RC of Wound dehiscence/evisceration
△ RC of Increased intraocular pressure
△ RC of Retinal detachment
❇ RC of Dislocation of lens implant
❇ RC of Choroidal hemorrhage
❇ RC of Endophthalmitis
❇ RC of Hyphema
❇ RC of Hypopyon
△ RC of Blindness

Nursing Diagnoses

△ Risk for Infection related to increased susceptibility secondary to surgical trauma
▲ Risk for Injury related to visual limitations, presence in unfamiliar environment, and presence of postoperative eye patches
▲ Feeding, Bathing Self-Care Deficit related to activity restrictions, visual impairment, or presence of eye patch(es)
▲ Risk for Disturbed Sensory Perceptions related to insufficient input secondary to impaired vision or presence of unilateral/bilateral eye patches
△ Risk for Ineffective Self-Health Management related to insufficient knowledge of activities permitted and restricted, medications, complications, and follow-up care

Otic Surgery (Stapedectomy, Tympanoplasty, Myringotomy, Tympanic Mastoidectomy)

See also *Surgery (General)*.

Postoperative Period

Collaborative Problems

RC of Bleeding
RC of Facial paralysis
RC of Infection
RC of Impaired hearing/deafness

Nursing Diagnoses

Impaired Communication related to decreased hearing
Risk for Loneliness related to embarrassment of not being able to hear in a social setting
Risk for Injury related to vertigo

Risk for Ineffective Self-Health Management related
  to insufficient knowledge of signs and symptoms of
  complications (facial nerve injury, vertigo, tinnitus, gait
  disturbances, and ear discharge), ear care, contraindications,
  and follow-up care

Nephrectomy

See also *Surgery (General).*

Collaborative Problems

▲ RC of Hypovolemia/Shock
▲ RC of Paralytic ileus
▲ RC of Renal insufficiency
△ RC of Pyelonephritis
△ RC of Ureteral stent dislodgement
△ RC of Pneumothorax secondary to thoracic approach

Nursing Diagnoses

△ Impaired Physical Mobility related to distention of renal capsule and incision
▲ Risk for Ineffective Respiratory Function related to pain on
  breathing and coughing secondary to location of incision
▲ Risk for Ineffective Self-Health Management related to insufficient knowledge of hydration requirements, nephrostomy
  care, and signs and symptoms of complications

Renal Transplant

See also *Corticosteroid Therapy*; *Surgery (General).*

Collaborative Problems

▲ RC of Hemodynamic instability
▲ RC of Hypervolemia/hypovolemia
▲ RC of Hypertension/hypotension
▲ RC of Renal insufficiency (donor kidney). Examples:
❋ Ischemic damage before implantation
❋ Hematoma
❋ Rupture of anastomosis
❋ Bleeding at anastomosis
❋ Renal vein thrombosis
❋ Renal artery stenosis
❋ Blockage of ureter (kinks, clots)

✳ Kinking of ureter, renal artery
▲ RC of Rejection of donor tissue
▲ RC of Excessive immunosuppression
▲ RC of Electrolyte imbalances (potassium, phosphate)
▲ RC of Deep vein thrombosis
▲ RC of Sepsis

Nursing Diagnoses

▲ Risk for Infection related to altered immune system secondary to medications
▲ Risk for Impaired Oral Mucous Membrane related to increased susceptibility to infection secondary to immunosuppression
△ Risk for Disturbed Self-Concept related to transplant experience and potential for rejection
▲ Fear related to possibility of rejection and death
▲ Risk for Noncompliance related to complexity of treatment regimen (diet, medications, record-keeping, weight, blood pressure, urine testing) and euphoria (post-transplant)
▲ Risk for Ineffective Self-Health Management related to insufficient knowledge of prevention of infection, activity progression, dietary management, daily recording (intake, output, weights, urine testing, blood pressure, temperature), pharmacologic therapy, daily urine testing (protein), signs and symptoms of rejection/infection, avoidance of pregnancy, follow-up care, and community resources

Thoracic Surgery

See also *Surgery (General)*; *Mechanical Ventilation*.

Postoperative Period
Collaborative Problems

✳ RC of Atelectasis
✳ RC of Pneumonia
▲ RC of Respiratory insufficiency
▲ RC of Pneumothorax, hemothorax
✳ RC of Bleeding
▲ RC of Pulmonary embolism
▲ RC of Subcutaneous emphysema
△ RC of Mediastinal shift
▲ RC of Acute pulmonary edema
△ RC of Thrombophlebitis

Nursing Diagnoses

▲ Acute Pain related to surgical incision, chest tube sites, and immobility secondary to lengthy surgery

▲ Ineffective Airway Clearance related to increased secretions and diminished cough secondary to pain and fatigue

Activity Intolerance related to reduction in exercise capacity secondary to loss of alveolar ventilation

▲ Impaired Physical Mobility related to restricted arm and shoulder movement secondary to pain and muscle dissection and imposed position restrictions

Grieving related to loss of body part and its perceived effects on lifestyle

✲ Risk for Ineffective Self-Health Management related to insufficient knowledge of condition, pain management, shoulder/arm exercises, incisional care, breathing exercises, splinting, prevention of infection, nutritional needs, rest versus activity, respiratory toilet, and follow-up care

Tonsillectomy

See also *Surgery (General)*.

Collaborative Problems

RC of Airway obstruction
RC of Aspiration
RC of Bleeding

Nursing Diagnoses

Risk for Deficient Fluid Volume related to decreased fluid intake secondary to pain on swallowing

Risk for Imbalanced Nutrition: Less Than Body Requirements related to decreased intake secondary to pain on swallowing

Risk for Ineffective Self-Health Management related to insufficient knowledge of rest requirements, nutritional needs, signs and symptoms of complications, pain management, positioning, and activity restrictions

Total Joint Replacement (Hip, Knee, or Shoulder Replacement)

See also *Surgery (General)*.

Postoperative Period
Collaborative Problems

▲ RC of Fat emboli
❊ RC of Bleeding/hematoma formation
▲ RC of Dislocation/subluxation of joint
❊ RC of Stress fractures
▲ RC of Neurovascular compromise
❊ RC of Synovial herniation
▲ RC of Thromboemboli
▲ RC of Sepsis

Nursing Diagnoses

▲ Risk for Impaired Skin Integrity related to immobility and incision
❊ Activity Intolerance related to fatigue, pain, and impaired gait
❊ Impaired Home Maintenance related to postoperative flexion restrictions
▲ Risk for Constipation related to activity restriction
▲ Risk for Injury related to altered gait and assistive devices
△ Risk for Ineffective Self-Health Management related to insufficient knowledge of activity restrictions, use of supportive devices, rehabilitative program, follow-up care, apparel restrictions, signs of complications, supportive services, and prevention of infection

Transurethral Resection (Prostate [Benign Hypertrophy or Cancer], Bladder Tumor)

See also *Surgery (General)*.

Postoperative Period
Collaborative Problems

RC of Oliguria/anuria
RC of Bleeding
RC of Perforated bladder (intraoperative)
RC of Hyponatremia
RC of Sepsis
RC of Occlusion of drainage devices
RC of Prostatectomy
RC of Clot formation

Nursing Diagnoses

Acute Pain related to bladder spasms, clot retention, or back and leg pain

Risk for Ineffective Self-Health Management related to
insufficient knowledge of fluid requirements, activity
restrictions, catheter care, urinary control, follow-up, and
signs and symptoms of complications

Urostomy

See also *Surgery (General)*.

Postoperative Period
Collaborative Problems

△ RC of Internal urine leakage
▲ RC of Urinary tract infection
▲ RC of Peristomal ulceration/herniation
▲ RC of Stomal necrosis, retraction, prolapse, stenosis, obstruc-
tion

Nursing Diagnoses

△ Risk for Disturbed Self-Concept related to effects of ostomy
on body image
Risk for Ineffective Sexuality Patterns related to perceived
negative impact of ostomy on sexual functioning and attractiveness
✳ Risk for Ineffective Sexuality Patterns related to erectile dysfunction (male) or inadequate vaginal lubrication (female)
△ Risk for Loneliness related to anxiety about possible odor and
leakage from appliance
▲ Risk for Ineffective Self-Health Management related to insufficient knowledge of stoma pouching procedure, colostomy
irrigation, peristomal skin care, perineal wound care, incorporation of ostomy care into activities of daily living
△ Risk for Ineffective Self-Health Management related to insufficient knowledge of intermittent self-catheterization of Kock
continent urostomy

Radical Vulvectomy

See also *Surgery (General)*; *Anticoagulant Therapy*.

Postoperative Period
Collaborative Problems

▲ RC of Hypovolemia/shock
▲ RC of Urinary retention
▲ RC of Sepsis
△ RC of Pulmonary embolism
▲ RC of Thrombophlebitis

Nursing Diagnoses

▲ Acute Pain related to effects of surgery and immobility
▲ Grieving related to loss of body function and its effects on lifestyle
△ Risk for Ineffective Sexuality Patterns related to negative impact of surgery on sexual functioning and attractiveness
△ Risk for Ineffective Self-Health Management related to insufficient knowledge of home care, wound care, self-catheterization, and follow-up care

OBSTETRIC/GYNECOLOGIC CONDITIONS

■■■■■ Prenatal Period (General)

Nursing Diagnoses

Nausea related to elevated estrogen levels, decreased blood sugar, or decreased gastric motility and pressure on cardiac sphincter from enlarged uterus

Constipation related to decreased gastric motility and pressure of uterus on lower colon

Activity Intolerance related to fatigue and dyspnea secondary to pressure of enlarging uterus on diaphragm and increased blood volume

Risk for Impaired Oral Mucous Membranes related to hyperemic gums secondary to estrogen and progesterone levels

Risk for Injury related to syncope//hypotension secondary to peripheral venous pooling secondary to peripheral venous pooling

Risk for Ineffective Self-Health Management related to insufficient knowledge of (examples) effects of pregnancy on body systems (cardiovascular, integumentary, gastrointestinal, urinary, pulmonary, musculoskeletal), psychosocial domain, sexuality/sexual function, family unit (spouse, children), fetal growth and development, nutritional requirements, hazards of smoking, excessive alcohol intake, drug abuse, excessive caffeine intake, excessive weight gain, signs and symptoms of complications (vaginal bleeding, cramping, gestational diabetes, excessive edema, preeclampsia), preparation for childbirth (classes, printed references)

Abortion, Induced

Preprocedure Period
Nursing Diagnoses

Anxiety related to significance of decision, procedure, and post procedure care

Post procedure Period
Collaborative Problems

RC of Bleeding
RC of Infection

Nursing Diagnoses

Risk for Ineffective Coping related to unresolved emotional responses (guilt) to societal, moral, religious, and familial opposition

Risk for Interrupted Family Processes related to effects of procedure on relationships (disagreement about decisions, previous conflicts [personal, marital], or adolescent identity problems)

Risk for Ineffective Self-Care Management related to insufficient knowledge of self-care (hygiene, breast care), nutritional needs, expected bleeding, cramping, signs and symptoms of complications, resumption of sexual activity, contraception, sex education as indicated, comfort measures, expected emotional responses, follow-up appointment, and community resources

Extrauterine Pregnancy (Ectopic Pregnancy)

Collaborative Problems

RC of Bleeding
RC of Shock
RC of Sepsis
RC of Acute pain

Nursing Diagnoses

Grieving related to loss of fetus
Fear related to possibility of not being able to have successful pregnancies

Hyperemesis Gravidarum

Collaborative Problems

RC of Negative nitrogen balance

Nursing Diagnoses

Risk for Imbalanced Nutrition: Less Than Body Requirements
related to loss of nutrients and fluid secondary to vomiting
Risk for Deficient Fluid Volume related to prolonged vomiting
Self-Health Management related to insufficient knowledge
of condition, signs and symptoms to monitor for, home
management strategies and when to access medical care.

Gestational Hypertension

See also *Prenatal Period*; *Postpartum Period* See also *RC of
Nonassuring Fetal Status*.

Collaborative Problems

RC of Malignant hypertension
RC of Seizures
RC of Proteinuria
RC of Visual disturbances
RC of Coma
RC of Renal failure
RC of Cerebral edema
RC of Fetal compromise

Nursing Diagnoses

Fear related to the effects of condition on self, pregnancy, and
infant
Risk for Injury related to vertigo, visual disturbances, or seizures
Risk for Ineffective Self-Health Management related to
insufficient knowledge of dietary restrictions, signs and
symptoms of complications, conservation of energy,
pharmacologic therapy, comfort measures for headaches and
backaches and when to access medical care

Pregnant Adolescent

See also *General Prenatal*, *Intrapartum Period*, and *Postpartum
Period*.

Prenatal
Collaborative Problems

RC of Gestational hypertension

Nursing Diagnoses

Interrupted Family Processes related to stressors associated with adolescent pregnancy and future implications for family

Risk for Imbalanced Nutrition: Less Than Body Requirements related to maternal growth needs and lower nutritional stores secondary to adolescence

Disturbed Self-Concept related to pregnancy-associated body changes and conflict with adolescent and parenting roles

Risk for Loneliness related to negative response of peer group to pregnancy

Risk for Infection related to insufficient knowledge of prevention of urinary tract infection and increased vulnerability secondary to effects of pregnancy on renal and ureteral anatomy

Postpartum
Nursing Diagnoses

Risk for Impaired Parenting related to conflicting developmental tasks of adolescence and parenthood

Decisional Conflict related to caregiver of infant, adoption options, or living arrangements

Uterine Bleeding During Pregnancy (Placenta Previa, Abruptio Placentae, Uterine Rupture, Nonmalignant Lesions, Hydatidiform Mole)

See also *Postpartum Period.*

Collaborative Problems

RC of Hypovolemia/shock
RC of Disseminated intravascular coagulation
RC of Renal failure
RC of Nonassuring fetal status
RC of Sepsis

Nursing Diagnoses

Fear related to effects of bleeding on pregnancy and infant
Impaired Physical Mobility related to increased bleeding in response to activity

Grieving related to anticipated possible loss of pregnancy and
    loss of expected child
Fear related to possibility of subsequent future complications of
    pregnancy

■■■■■■ Intrapartum Period (General)

Collaborative Problems

RC of Hemorrhage (placenta previa, abruptio placentae)
RC of Nonassuring fetal status
RC of Hypertension
RC of Uterine rupture

Nursing Diagnoses

Acute Pain related to uterine contractions during labor
Fear related to unpredictability of uterine contractions and
    possibility of having an impaired baby
Anxiety related to insufficient knowledge of relaxation/breathing
    exercises, positioning and procedures (preparations [bowel,
    skin], frequent assessments, anesthesia [regional, inhalation])

■■■■■■ Postpartum Period

General Postpartum Period
Collaborative Problems

RC of Hemorrhage
RC of Uterine atony
RC of Retained placental fragments
RC of Lacerations
RC of Hematomas
RC of Urinary retention

Nursing Diagnoses

Risk for Infection related to bacterial invasion secondary to
    trauma during labor, delivery, and episiotomy
Risk for Ineffective Breastfeeding related to inexperience or pain
    secondary to engorged breasts
Acute Pain related to trauma to perineum during labor and
    delivery, hemorrhoids, engorged breasts, and involution of
    uterus

Risk for Constipation related to decreased intestinal peristalsis (post delivery) and decreased activity

Risk for Impaired Parenting related to (examples) inexperience, feelings of incompetence, powerlessness, unwanted child, disappointment with child, or lack of role models

Stress Incontinence related to tissue trauma during delivery

Risk for Situational Low Self-Esteem related to changes that persist after delivery (skin, weight, lifestyle)

Risk for Ineffective Self-Health Management related to insufficient knowledge of postpartum routines, hygiene (breast, perineum), exercises, sexual counseling (contraception), nutritional requirements (infant, maternal), infant care, stresses of parenthood, adaptation of father, sibling, parent–infant bonding, postpartum emotional responses, sleep/rest requirements, household management, community resources, management of discomforts (breast, perineum), and signs and symptoms of complications

▬▬■■■ Miscarriage, Spontaneous

Nursing Diagnoses

Fear related to possibility of subsequent miscarriages

Grieving related to loss of pregnancy

▬▬■■■ Mastitis (Lactational)

Collaborative Problems

RC of Abscess

Nursing Diagnoses

Acute Pain related to inflammation of breast tissue

Risk for Ineffective Breastfeeding related to interruption secondary to inflammation

Risk for Ineffective Self-Health Management related to insufficient knowledge of need for breast support, breast hygiene, breastfeeding restrictions, and signs and symptoms of abscess formation

■■■■■■ Fetal/Newborn Death

Nursing Diagnoses

Interrupted Family Processes related to emotional trauma of loss
on each family member
Grieving related to loss of infant
Fear related to the possibility of future fetal deaths

■■■■■■ Concomitant Medical Conditions (Cardiac Disease [Prenatal, Postpartum], Diabetes [Prenatal, Postpartum])

Cardiac Disease
See also *Cardiac Disorders*; *Prenatal Period*; *Postpartum Period*.

Collaborative Problems

RC of Congestive heart failure
RC of Gestational hypertension (preeclampsia, eclampsia)
RC of Nonassuring fetal status

Nursing Diagnoses

Fear related to effects of condition on self, pregnancy, and infant
Activity Intolerance related to increased metabolic requirements
(pregnancy) in presence of compromised cardiac function
Impaired Home Maintenance related to impaired ability to
perform role responsibilities during and after pregnancy
Risk for Interrupted Family Processes related to disruption of
activity restrictions and fears of effects on lifestyle
Risk for Ineffective Self-Health Management related to
insufficient knowledge of dietary requirements, prevention
of infection, conservation of energy, signs and symptoms of
complications, and community resources

■■■■■■ Diabetes (Prenatal)

See also *Prenatal Period*; *Diabetes Mellitus*; *Postpartum Period*.

Collaborative Problems

RC of Hypoglycemia/hyperglycemia
RC of Hydramnios
RC of Acidosis
RC of Gestational hypertension

Nursing Diagnoses

Risk for Impaired Skin Integrity related to excessive skin stretching secondary to hydramnios

Risk for Infection related to susceptibility to monilial infection

Acute Pain related to cerebral edema or hyperirritability

Risk for Ineffective Self-Health Management related to insufficient knowledge of effects of pregnancy on diabetes, effects of diabetes on pregnancy, nutritional requirements, insulin requirements, signs and symptoms of complications, and need for frequent blood/urine samples

Diabetes (Postpartum)

See also *Postpartum Period (General)*.

Collaborative Problems

RC of Hypoglycemia

RC of Hyperglycemia

RC of Hemorrhage (secondary to uterine atony from excessive amniotic fluid)

RC of Gestational hypertension

Nursing Diagnoses

Anxiety related to separation from infant secondary to the special care needs of infant

Risk for Infection of perineal area related to depleted host defenses and depressed leukocytic phagocytosis secondary to hyperglycemia

Risk for Ineffective Self-Health Management related to insufficient knowledge of risks of future pregnancies, birth control methods, types contraindicated, and special care requirements for infant

▪▪▪▪▪▪ Endometriosis

Collaborative Problems

RC of Hypermenorrhea

RC of Polymenorrhea

Nursing Diagnoses

Chronic Pain related to response of displaced endometrial tissue (abdominal, peritoneal) to cyclic ovarian hormonal stimulation

Ineffective Sexuality Patterns related to painful intercourse or infertility

Anxiety related to unpredictable nature of disease

Risk for Ineffective Self-Health Management related to insufficient knowledge of condition, myths, pharmacologic therapy, and potential for pregnancy

▪▪▪▪▪▪ Pelvic Inflammatory Disease

Collaborative Problems

RC of Septicemia

RC of Abscess formation

RC of Pneumonia

RC of Pulmonary embolism

Nursing Diagnoses

Acute Pain related to malaise, increased temperature secondary to infectious process

Risk for Deficient Fluid Volume related to inadequate intake, fatigue, pain, and fluid losses secondary to elevated temperature

Chronic Pain related to inflammatory process

Risk for Ineffective Coping: Depression related to chronicity of condition and lack of definitive diagnosis/treatment

Risk for Ineffective Self-Health Management related to insufficient knowledge of condition, nutritional requirements, signs and symptoms of complications, prevention of sexually transmitted diseases, and sleep/rest requirements

▪▪▪▪▪▪ Neonatal Conditions

Neonate, Normal

Collaborative Problems

RC of Hypothermia

RC of Hypoglycemia

RC of Hyperbilirubinemia

RC of Bradycardia

Nursing Diagnoses

Risk for Infection related to vulnerability of infant, lack of normal flora, environmental hazards, and open wound (umbilical cord, circumcision)

Risk for Ineffective Airway Clearance related to oropharynx
secretions

Risk for Impaired Skin Integrity related to susceptibility to
nosocomial infection and lack of normal skin flora

Ineffective Thermoregulation related to newborn extrauterine
transition

Risk for Ineffective Infant's Health Management related to
insufficient knowledge of (specify) (see *Postpartum Period*)

Neonate, Premature

See also *Family of High-Risk Neonate*.

Collaborative Problems

RC of Cold stress
RC of Apnea
RC of Bradycardia
RC of Hypoglycemia
RC of Acidosis
RC of Hypocalcemia
RC of Sepsis
RC of Seizures
RC of Pneumonia
RC of Hyperbilirubinemia

Nursing Diagnoses

Risk for Constipation related to decreased intestinal motility and
immobility

Risk for Aspiration related to immobility and increased
secretions

Risk for Infection related to vulnerability of infant, lack of
normal flora, environmental hazards, and open wounds
(umbilical cord, circumcision)

Risk for Impaired Skin Integrity related to susceptibility to
nosocomial infection (lack of normal skin flora)

Ineffective Thermoregulation related to newborn transition to
extrauterine environment

Ineffective Infant Feeding Pattern related to lethargy secondary
to prematurity

Risk for Sudden Infant Death Syndrome related to increased
vulnerability secondary to prematurity

Neonate, Postmature, Small for Gestational Age (SGA), Large for Gestational Age (LGA)

Collaborative Problems

RC of Asphyxia at birth
RC of Meconium aspiration
RC of Hypoglycemia
RC of Polycythemia (SGA)
RC of Edema (generalized, cerebral)
RC of Central nervous system depression
RC of Renal tubular necrosis
RC of Impaired intestinal absorption
RC of Birth injuries (shoulder) (LGA)

Nursing Diagnoses

Risk for Impaired Skin Integrity related to absence of protective vernix and prolonged exposure to amniotic fluid (LGA)
Ineffective Infant Feeding Pattern related to lethargy

Nursing Diagnoses

Risk for Infection Transmission related to contagious nature of organism
Risk for Injury related to uncontrolled tonic-clonic movements

Neonate with Meningomyelocele

See also *Normal Neonate*; *Family of High-Risk Neonate*.

Collaborative Problems

RC of Hydrocephalus
RC of Neurovascular insufficiency (below lesion)

Nursing Diagnoses

Risk for Trauma related to vulnerability of meningomyelocele
Overflow Incontinence related to effects of spinal cord injury on bladder function
Risk for Impaired Skin Integrity related to inability to move lower extremities

Neonate with Congenital Heart Disease (Preoperative)

See also *Normal Neonate*; *Family of High-Risk Neonate*.

Collaborative Problems

RC of Congestive heart failure
RC of Dysrhythmias
RC of Decreased cardiac output

Nursing Diagnoses

Risk for Ineffective Infant Feeding Pattern related to difficulty
   breathing and fatigue

Neonate of a Diabetic Mother

See also *Neonate, Normal; Family of High-Risk Neonate*.

Collaborative Problems

RC of Hypoglycemia
RC of Hypocalcemia
RC of Polycythemia
RC of Hyperbilirubinemia
RC of Sepsis
RC of Acidosis
RC of Hyaline membrane disease
RC of Respiratory distress syndrome
RC of Venous thrombosis

Nursing Diagnoses

Risk for Deficient Fluid Volume related to increased urinary
   excretion and osmotic diuresis

High-Risk Neonate

See also *Family of High-Risk Neonate*.

Collaborative Problems

RC of Hypoxemia
RC of Shock
RC of Respiratory distress
RC of Seizures
RC of Hypotension
RC of Septicemia

Nursing Diagnoses

Disorganized Infant Behavior related to immature central
   nervous system and excess stimulation

Risk for Infection related to vulnerability of infant, lack of normal flora, environmental hazards, open wounds (umbilical cord, circumcision), and invasive lines

Ineffective Infant Feeding Pattern related to (specify)

Risk for Ineffective Respiratory Function related to increased oropharyngeal secretions

Risk for Impaired Skin Integrity related to susceptibility to nosocomial infection secondary to lack of normal skin flora

Ineffective Thermoregulation related to newborn transition to extrauterine environment

Family of High-Risk Neonate

Nursing Diagnoses

Chronic Sorrow related to realization of present or future loss for family and child

Interrupted Family Processes related to effect of extended hospitalization on family (role responsibilities, finances)

Anxiety related to unpredictable prognosis

Risk for Impaired Parenting related to inadequate bonding secondary to parent–child separation or failure to accept impaired child

Hyperbilirubinemia (Rh Incompatibility, ABO Incompatibility)

See also *Family of High-Risk Neonate*; *Neonate, Normal*.

Collaborative Problems

RC of Anemia

RC of Jaundice

RC of Kernicterus

RC of Hepatosplenomegaly

RC of Hydrops fetalis (cardiac failure, hypoxia, anasarca, and pericardial, pleural, and peritoneal effusions)

RC of Renal failure (phototherapy complications, hyperthermia/hypothermia, dehydration, priapism, "bronze baby" syndrome)

Nursing Diagnoses

Risk for Impaired Corneal Tissue Integrity related to exposure to phototherapy light and continuous wearing of eye pads

Risk for Impaired Skin Integrity related to diarrhea, urinary excretion of bilirubin, and exposure to phototherapy light

Neonate of Narcotic-Addicted Mother

See also *Family of High-Risk Neonate; Neonate, Normal; Substance Abuse by Mother.*

Collaborative Problems

RC of Hyperirritability/seizures
RC of Withdrawal
RC of Hypocalcemia
RC of Hypoglycemia
RC of Sepsis
RC of Dehydration
RC of Electrolyte imbalances

Nursing Diagnoses

Risk for Impaired Skin Integrity related to generalized diaphoresis and marked rigidity
Diarrhea related to increased peristalsis secondary to hyperirritability
Disturbed Sleep Pattern related to hyperirritability
Risk for Injury related to frantic sucking of fists
Risk for Injury related to uncontrolled tremors or tonic-clonic movements
Disturbed Sensory Perceptions related to hypersensitivity to environmental stimuli
Ineffective Infant Feeding Pattern related to lethargy
Risk for Sudden Infant Death Syndrome related to increased vulnerability secondary to maternal drug use

Respiratory Distress Syndrome

See also *High-Risk Neonate; Mechanical Ventilation.*

Collaborative Problems

RC of Hypoxemia
RC of Atelectasis
RC of Acidosis
RC of Sepsis
RC of Hyperthermia

Nursing Diagnoses

Activity Intolerance related to insufficient oxygenation of tissues secondary to impaired respirations

Risk for Infection related to vulnerability of infant, lack of
    normal flora, environmental hazards (personnel, other
    newborns, parents), and open wounds (umbilical cord,
    circumcision)
Risk for Impaired Skin Integrity related to susceptibility to
    nosocomial infection and lack of normal skin flora

Sepsis

See also *Neonate, Normal*; *Family of High-Risk Neonate*; *High-Risk
    Neonate*.

Collaborative Problems

RC of Anemia
RC of Respiratory distress
RC of Hypothermia/hyperthermia
RC of Hypotension
RC of Edema
RC of Seizures
RC of Hepatosplenomegaly
RC of Hemorrhage
RC of Jaundice
RC of Meningitis
RC of Pyarthrosis

Nursing Diagnoses

Risk for Impaired Skin Integrity related to edema and
    immobility
Diarrhea related to intestinal irritation secondary to infecting
    organism
Risk for Injury related to uncontrolled tonic-clonic movements
    and hematopoietic insufficiency

PEDIATRIC/ADOLESCENT DISORDERS

Developmental Problems/Needs Related to Chronic Illness (e.g., Permanent Disability, Multiple Handicaps, Developmental Disability [Mental/Physical], Life-Threatening Illness)

Nursing Diagnoses*

Chronic Sorrow (parental) related to anticipated losses secondary to condition

Interrupted Family Processes related to adjustment requirements for situation: (examples) time, energy (emotional, physical), financial, and physical care

Risk for Impaired Home Maintenance related to inadequate resources, housing, or impaired caregiver(s)

Risk for Parental Role Conflict related to separations secondary to frequent hospitalizations

Risk for Loneliness (child/family) related to decreased socialization due to the disability and the requirements of the caregiver(s)

Risk for Impaired Parenting related to abuse, rejection, overprotection secondary to inadequate resources or coping mechanisms

Decisional Conflict related to illness, health care interventions, and parent–child separation

(Specify) Self-Care Deficit related to illness limitations or hospitalization

Risk for Delayed Growth and Development related to impaired ability to achieve developmental tasks

Caregiver Role Strain related to multiple ongoing care needs secondary to restrictions imposed by disease, disability, or treatments

---

*For additional pediatric medical diagnoses, see the adult diagnoses and Developmental Problems/Needs, for example:

Diabetes mellitus	Neoplastic disorders
Anorexia nervosa	Fractures
(psychiatric disorders)	Congestive heart failure
Spinal cord injury	Pneumonia
Head trauma	

Ineffective Child's Health Management has been used for clinical usefulness since Ineffective Self-Health Management does not apply when the patient is a child

Anxiety/School Phobia

Nursing Diagnoses

Anxiety related to altered self-esteem, change in environment, fear of separation, and negative responses (peers, family)

Ineffective Coping related to inadequate problem-solving skills and denial of problem

Disturbed Self-Esteem related to negative peer responses, perceived mental deficits, and unrealistic expectations in performance

Acquired Immunodeficiency Syndrome (Child)

See also *Acquired Immunodeficiency Syndrome (Adult)*; *Developmental Problems/Needs Related to Chronic Illness.*

Nursing Diagnoses

Risk for Infection Transmission related to exposure to stool and other secretions during diaper changes or failure of child to follow handwashing procedure after toileting

Imbalanced Nutrition: Less Than Body Requirements related to lactose intolerance, need for double the usual recommended daily allowance, anorexia secondary to oral lesions, and malaise

Delayed Growth and Development related to decreased muscle tone secondary to encephalopathy

Interrupted Family Processes related to the impact of the child's condition on role responsibilities, siblings, and finances and negative responses of relatives, friends, and community

Risk for Ineffective Child's Health Management related to insufficient knowledge of modes of transmission, risks of live virus vaccines, avoidance of infections, school attendance, and community resources

Asthma

See also *Developmental Problems/Needs.*

Collaborative Problems

RC of Hypoxemia
RC of Corticosteroid therapy
RC of Respiratory acidosis

Nursing Diagnoses

Ineffective Airway Clearance related to bronchospasm and increased pulmonary secretions

Fear related to breathlessness and recurrences

Risk for Ineffective Child's Health Management related to insufficient knowledge of condition, environmental hazards (smoking, allergens, weather), prevention of infection, breathing/relaxation exercises, signs and symptoms of complications, pharmacologic therapy, fluid requirements, behavioral modification, and daily diary recording of peak flows

Attention Deficit Disorder

Collaborative Problems

RC of Adverse effects of central nervous system stimulants

Nursing Diagnoses

Activity Intolerance related to delayed physical, emotional, or mental capacity and fatigue

Ineffective Coping related to fatigue and delayed development

Delayed Growth and Development related to delayed maturation secondary to genetic, physical, and mental disability

Risk for Injury related to motor deficits and hyperactivity

Disturbed Self-Esteem related to lack of success in school and negative peer interactions

Impaired Social Interaction related to delayed social development and poor peer acceptance

Celiac Disease

See also *Developmental Problems/Needs*.

Collaborative Problems

RC of Severe malnutrition/dehydration

RC of Anemia

RC of Altered blood coagulation

RC of Osteoporosis

RC of Electrolyte imbalances

RC of Metabolic acidosis

RC of Shock

RC of Delayed growth

Nursing Diagnoses

Risk for Imbalanced Nutrition: Less Than Body Requirements related to malabsorption, dietary restrictions, and anorexia

Diarrhea related to decreased absorption in small intestines secondary to damaged villi resulting from toxins from undigested gliadin

Risk for Deficient Fluid Volume related to fluid loss in diarrhea

Risk for Ineffective Child's Health Management related to insufficient knowledge of dietary management, restrictions, and requirements

Cerebral Palsy*

See also *Developmental Problems/Needs.*

Collaborative Problems

RC of Contractures
RC of Seizures
RC of Respiratory infections

Nursing Diagnoses

Risk for Injury related to inability to control movements

Risk for Imbalanced Nutrition: Less Than Body Requirements related to sucking difficulties (infant) and dysphagia

(Specify) Self-Care Deficit related to sensory–motor impairments

Impaired Verbal Communication related to impaired ability to speak words related to facial muscle involvement

Risk for Deficient Fluid Volume related to difficulty obtaining or swallowing liquids

Risk for Deficient Diversional Activity related to effects of limitations on ability to participate in recreational activities

Risk for Ineffective Child's Health Management related to insufficient knowledge of disease, pharmacologic regimen, activity program, education, community services, and orthopedic appliances

---

*Because disabilities associated with cerebral palsy can be varied (hemiparesis, quadriparesis, diplegia, monoplegia, triplegia, paraplegia), the nurse will have to specify clearly the child's limitations in the diagnostic statements.

Child Abuse (Battered Child Syndrome, Child Neglect)

See also *Fractures, Burns; Failure to Thrive*.

Collaborative Problems

RC of Failure to thrive
RC of Malnutrition

Nursing Diagnoses

Disabled Family Coping related to presence of factors that contribute to child abuse: (examples) lack of or unavailability of extended family, economic problems (inflation, unemployment); lack of role model as a child, high-risk children (unwanted, of undesired gender or appearance, physically or mentally handicapped, hyperactive, terminally ill); and high-risk parents (single, adolescent, emotionally disturbed, alcoholic, drug-addicted, or physically ill)

Ineffective Coping (child abuser) related to (examples) history of abuse by own parents and lack of warmth and affection from them, social isolation (few friends or outlets for tensions), marked lack of self-esteem with low tolerance for criticism, emotional immaturity and dependency, distrust of others, inability to admit need for help, high expectations for/of child (perceiving child as a source of emotional gratification), and unrealistic desire for child to give pleasure

Ineffective Coping (nonabusing parent) related to passive and compliant response to abuse

Fear related to possibility of placement in a shelter or foster home

Parental Fear related to responses of others, possible loss of child, and criminal prosecution

Risk for Imbalanced Nutrition: Less Than Body Requirements related to inadequate intake secondary to lack of knowledge or neglect

Impaired Parenting related to insufficient knowledge of parenting skills (discipline, expectations), constructive stress management, signs and symptoms of abuse, high-risk groups, child protection laws, and community services

Cleft Lip and Palate

See also *Developmental Problems/Needs; Surgery (General)*.

Preoperative Period
Nursing Diagnoses

Risk for Imbalanced Nutrition: Less Than Body Requirements related to impaired sucking secondary to cleft lip

Postoperative Period
Collaborative Problems

RC of Respiratory distress
RC of Failure to thrive (organic)

Nursing Diagnoses

Impaired Physical Mobility related to restricted activity secondary to use of restraints

Risk for Ineffective Infant Feeding Patten related to impaired muscle development and impaired sucking.

Risk for Ineffective Infant's Health Management related to insufficient knowledge of condition, feeding and suctioning techniques, surgical site care, risks for otitis media (dental/oral problems), and referral to speech therapist

Communicable Diseases

See also *Developmental Problems/Needs.*

Nursing Diagnoses

Acute Pain related to pruritus, fatigue, malaise, sore throat, and elevated temperature

Risk for Infection Transmission related to contagious agents

Risk for Deficient Fluid Volume related to increased fluid loss secondary to elevated temperature or insufficient oral intake secondary to malaise

Risk for Imbalanced Nutrition: Less Than Body Requirements related to anorexia and sore throat or pain on chewing (mumps)

Risk for Ineffective Airway Clearance related to increased mucus production (whooping cough)

Risk for Ineffective Child's Health Management related to insufficient knowledge of condition, transmission, prevention, immunizations, and skin care

Congenital Heart Disease

See also *Developmental Problems/Needs Related to Chronic Illness.*

Collaborative Problems

RC of Congestive heart failure
RC of Pneumonia
RC of Hypoxemia
RC of Cerebral thrombosis
RC of Digoxin toxicity

Nursing Diagnoses

Activity Intolerance related to insufficient oxygenation secondary
to heart defects

Risk for Imbalanced Nutrition: Less Than Body Requirements
related to inadequate sucking, fatigue, and dyspnea

Risk for Ineffective Child's Health Management related to
insufficient knowledge of condition, prevention of infection,
signs and symptoms of complications, digoxin therapy,
nutrition requirements, and community services

Convulsive Disorders

See also *Developmental Problems/Needs; Mental Disabilities*, if
indicated.

Collaborative Problems

RC of Respiratory arrest

Nursing Diagnoses

Risk for Injury related to uncontrolled movements of seizure
activity

Anxiety related to embarrassment and fear of seizure episodes

Risk for Ineffective Coping related to restrictions, parental
overprotection, and parental indulgence

Risk for Ineffective Child's Health Management related to
insufficient knowledge of condition/cause, pharmacologic
therapy, treatment during seizures, and environmental hazards
(water, driving, heights)

Craniocerebral Trauma

Collaborative Problems

RC of Increased intracranial pressure
RC of Hemorrhage
RC of Tentorial herniation
RC of Cranial nerve dysfunction

Nursing Diagnoses

Acute Pain related to compression/displacement of cerebral tissue

Risk for Injury related to uncontrolled tonic-clonic movements during seizure episode or somnolence

Risk for Ineffective Child's Health Management related to insufficient knowledge of condition, signs and symptoms of complications, post-traumatic syndrome, activity restrictions, and follow-up care

Cystic Fibrosis

See also *Developmental Problems/Needs.*

Collaborative Problems

RC of Bronchopneumonia, atelectasis

RC of Paralytic ileus

Nursing Diagnoses

Ineffective Airway Clearance related to mucopurulent secretions

Risk for Imbalanced Nutrition: Less Than Body Requirements related to need for increased calories and protein secondary to impaired intestinal absorption, loss of fat and fat-soluble vitamins in stools

Constipation/Diarrhea related to excessive or insufficient pancreatic enzyme replacement

Activity Intolerance related to impaired oxygen transport secondary to mucopurulent secretions

Risk for Ineffective Child's Health Management related to insufficient knowledge of condition (genetic transmission), risk of infection, pharmacologic therapy (side effects, ototoxicity, renal toxicity), equipment, nutritional therapy, salt replacement requirements, breathing exercises, postural drainage, exercise program, and community resources (Cystic Fibrosis Foundation)

Down Syndrome

See also *Developmental Problems/Needs*; *Mental Disabilities*, if indicated.

Nursing Diagnoses

Risk for Ineffective Respiratory Function related to decreased respiratory expansion secondary to decreased muscle tone, inadequate mucus drainage, and mouth breathing

Risk for Impaired Skin Integrity related to rough, dry skin
surface and flaccid extremities

Risk for Constipation related to decreased gastric motility

Risk for Imbalanced Nutrition: More Than Body Requirements
related to increased caloric consumption secondary to
boredom in the presence of limited physical activity and
decreased metabolic rate

(Specify) Self-Care Deficit related to physical limitations

Ineffective Infant Feeding Pattern related to neurologic
impairment

Risk for Ineffective Child's Health Management related to
insufficient knowledge of condition, home care, education,
and community services

Dysmenorrhea

Nursing Diagnoses

Acute Pain related to insufficient knowledge of comfort
measures, menstrual physiology, and nutritional management.

Failure to Thrive (Nonorganic)

See also *Developmental Problems/Needs*.

Collaborative Problems

RC of Metabolic dysfunction
RC of Dehydration

Nursing Diagnoses

Imbalanced Nutrition: Less Than Body Requirements related to
inadequate intake secondary to lack of emotional and sensory
stimulation or lack of knowledge of caregiver

Disturbed Sensory Perceptions related to history of insufficient
sensory input from primary caregiver

Insomnia related to anxiety and apprehension secondary to
parental deprivation

Impaired Parenting related to (examples) insufficient knowledge
of parenting skills, impaired caregiver, impaired child, lack
of support system, lack of role model, relationship problems,
unrealistic expectations for child, unmet psychological needs

Impaired Home Maintenance related to difficulty of caregiver
with maintaining a safe home environment

Risk for Ineffective Infant's Health Management related
to insufficient knowledge of growth and development

requirements, feeding guidelines, risk for child abuse, parenting skills, and community agencies

Glomerular Disorders (Glomerulonephritis: Acute, Chronic; Nephrotic Syndrome: Congenital, Secondary, Idiopathic)

See also *Developmental Problems/Needs; Corticosteroid Therapy.*

Collaborative Problems

RC of Anasarca (generalized edema)
RC of Hypertension
RC of Azotemia
RC of Sepsis
RC of Malnutrition
RC of Ascites
RC of Pleural effusion
RC of Hypoalbuminemia

Nursing Diagnoses

Risk for Infection related to increased susceptibility during edematous phase and lowered resistance secondary to corticosteroid therapy

Risk for Impaired Skin Integrity related to (examples) immobility, lowered resistance, edema, or frequent application of collection bags

Imbalanced Nutrition: Less Than Body Requirements related to dietary restrictions, anorexia secondary to fatigue, malaise, and pressure on abdominal structures (edema)

Fatigue related to circulatory toxins, fluid and electrolyte imbalances

Deficient Diversional Activity related to hospitalization and impaired ability to perform usual activities

Risk for Ineffective Child's Health Management related to insufficient knowledge of condition, etiology, course, treatments, signs and symptoms of complications, pharmacologic therapy, nutritional/fluid requirements, prevention of infection, home care, follow-up care, and community services

Hemophilia

See also *Developmental Problems/Needs.*

Collaborative Problems

RC of Hemorrhage

Nursing Diagnoses

Acute/Chronic Pain related to joint swelling and limitations secondary to hemarthrosis

Risk for Impaired Physical Mobility related to joint swelling and limitations secondary to hemarthrosis

Risk for Impaired Oral Mucous Membranes related to trauma from coarse food and insufficient dental hygiene

Risk for Ineffective Child's Health Management related to insufficient knowledge of condition, contraindications (e.g., aspirin), genetic transmission, environmental hazards, and emergency treatment to control bleeding

Hydrocephalus

See also *Developmental Problems/Needs Related to Chronic Illness*.

Collaborative Problems

RC of Increased intracranial pressure
RC of Sepsis (post-shunt procedure)

Nursing Diagnoses

Risk for Impaired Skin Integrity related to impaired ability to move head secondary to size

Risk for Injury related to inability to support large head and strain on neck

Risk for Imbalanced Nutrition: Less Than Body Requirements related to vomiting secondary to cerebral compression and irritability

Risk for Ineffective Child's Health Management related to insufficient knowledge of condition, home care, signs and symptoms of infection, increased intracranial pressure, and emergency treatment of shunt

Infectious Mononucleosis (Adolescent)

Collaborative Problems

RC of Splenetic dysfunction, enlargement
RC of Hepatic dysfunction

Nursing Diagnoses

Activity Intolerance related to fatigue secondary to infectious process

Acute Pain related to sore throat, malaise, and headaches

Risk for Imbalanced Nutrition: Less Than Body Requirements related to sore throat and malaise

Risk for Infection Transmission related to contagious condition

Risk for Ineffective Self-Health Management related to insufficient knowledge of condition, communicable nature, diet therapy, risks of alcohol ingestion (with hepatic dysfunction), signs and symptoms of complications (hepatic, splenic, neurologic, hematologic), and activity restrictions

Legg-Calvé-Perthes Disease

See also *Developmental Problems/Needs*.

Collaborative Problems

RC of Permanently deformed femoral head

Nursing Diagnoses

Acute/Chronic Pain related to joint dysfunction

Risk for Impaired Skin Integrity related to immobilization devices (casts, braces)

(Specify) Self-Care Deficit related to pain and immobilization devices

Risk for Ineffective Self-Health Management related to insufficient knowledge of disease, weight-bearing restrictions, application/maintenance of devices, and pain management at home

Leukemia

See also *Chemotherapy*; *Radiation Therapy*; *Cancer (General)*; *Developmental Problems/Needs*.

Collaborative Problems

RC of Hepatosplenomegaly

RC of Increased intracranial edema

RC of Metastasis (brain, lungs, kidneys, gastrointestinal tract, spleen, liver)

RC of Hypermetabolism

RC of Hemorrhage

RC of Dehydration
RC of Myelosuppression
RC of Lymphadenopathy
RC of Central nervous system involvement
RC of Electrolyte imbalance

Nursing Diagnoses

Risk for Infection related to increased susceptibility secondary to leukemic process and side effects of chemotherapy

Risk for Loneliness related to effects of disease and treatments on appearance and embarrassment

Risk for Injury related to bleeding tendencies secondary to leukemic process and side effects of chemotherapy

Powerlessness related to inability to control situation

Risk for Delayed Growth and Development related to impaired ability to achieve developmental tasks secondary to limitations of disease and treatments

Risk for Ineffective Child's Health Management related to insufficient knowledge of disease process, treatment, signs and symptoms of complications, reduction of risk factors, and community resources

Meningitis (Bacterial)

See also *Developmental Problems/Needs.*

Collaborative Problems

RC of Peripheral circulatory collapse
RC of Disseminated intravascular coagulation
RC of Increased intracranial pressure/hydrocephalus
RC of Visual/auditory nerve palsies
RC of Paresis (hemiparesis, quadriparesis)
RC of Subdural effusions
RC of Respiratory distress
RC of Seizures
RC of Fluid/electrolyte imbalances

Nursing Diagnoses

Risk for Injury related to seizure activity secondary to infectious process

Acute Pain related to nuchal rigidity, muscle aches, immobility, and increased sensitivity to external stimuli secondary to infectious process

Impaired Physical Mobility related to intravenous infusion, nuchal rigidity, and restraining devices

Risk for Impaired Skin Integrity related to immobility

Risk for Ineffective Child 's Health Management related to insufficient knowledge of condition, antibiotic therapy, and diagnostic procedures

Meningomyelocele

See also *Developmental Problems/Needs*.

Collaborative Problems

RC of Hydrocephalus/shunt infections
RC of Increased intracranial pressure
RC of Urinary tract infections

Nursing Diagnoses

Reflex Incontinence related to sensory–motor dysfunction

Risk for Infection related to vulnerability of meningomyelocele sac

Risk for Impaired Skin Integrity related to sensory–motor impairments and orthopedic appliances

(Specify) Self-Care Deficit related to sensory–motor impairments

Impaired Physical Mobility related to lower limb impairments

Parental Grieving related to birth of infant with defects

Risk for Ineffective Child's Health Management related to insufficient knowledge of condition, home care, orthopedic appliances, self-catheterization, activity program, and community services

Mental Disabilities

See also *Developmental Problems/Needs*.

Nursing Diagnoses

(Specify) Self-Care Deficit related to sensory–motor deficits

Impaired Communication related to impaired receptive skills or impaired expressive skills

Risk for Loneliness (family, child) related to fear and embarrassment of child's behavior/appearance

Risk for Ineffective Child's Health Management related to insufficient knowledge of condition, child's potential, home care, and community services

Muscular Dystrophy

See also *Developmental Problems/Needs*.

Collaborative Problems

RC of Seizures
RC of Respiratory infections
RC of Metabolic failure

Nursing Diagnoses

Risk for Injury related to inability to control movements
Risk for Imbalanced Nutrition: Less Than Body Requirements
  related to sucking difficulties (infant) and dysphagia
Ineffective Infant Feeding Pattern related to muscle weakness
  and impaired coordination
(Specify) Self-Care Deficit related to sensory–motor
  impairments
Impaired Verbal Communication related to impaired ability to
  speak secondary to facial muscle involvement
Risk for Impaired Physical Mobility related to muscle weakness
Risk for Imbalanced Nutrition: More Than Body Requirements
  related to increased caloric consumption in presence of
  decreased metabolic needs secondary to limited physical
  activity
Chronic Sorrow (parental) related to progressive, terminal
  nature of disease
Impaired Swallowing related to sensory–motor deficits
Risk for Hopelessness related to progressive nature of disease
Risk for Deficient Diversional Activity related to effects of
  limitations on ability to participate in recreational activities
Risk for Ineffective Child's Health Management related to
  insufficient knowledge of disease, pharmacologic regimen,
  activity program, education, and community services

Obesity

See also *Developmental Problems/Needs*.

Nursing Diagnoses

Ineffective Coping related to increased food consumption in
  response to stressors
Ineffective Self-Health Management related to the need for
  exercise program, nutrition counseling, and behavioral
  modification

Disturbed Self-Concept related to feelings of self-degradation and response of others (peers, family, others) to obesity

Interrupted Family Processes related to responses to and effects of weight loss therapy on parent–child relationship

Risk for Impaired Social Interaction related to inability to initiate and maintain relationships secondary to feelings of embarrassment and negative responses of others

Risk for Ineffective Self-Health Management related to insufficient knowledge of condition, etiology, course, risks, therapies available, destructive versus constructive eating patterns, and self-help groups

Osteomyelitis

See also *Developmental Problems/Needs.*

Collaborative Problems

RC of Infective emboli

RC of Side effects of antibiotic therapy (hematologic, renal, hepatic)

Nursing Diagnoses

Acute Pain related to swelling, hyperthermia, and infectious process of bone

Deficient Diversional Activity related to impaired mobility and long-term hospitalization

Risk for Imbalanced Nutrition: Less Than Body Requirements related to anorexia secondary to infectious process

Risk for Constipation related to immobility

Risk for Impaired Skin Integrity related to mechanical irritation of cast/splint

Risk for Injury: Pathologic fractures related to disease process

Risk for Ineffective Child's Health Management related to insufficient knowledge of condition, wound care, activity restrictions, signs and symptoms of complications, pharmacologic therapy, and follow-up care

Parasitic Disorders

See also *Developmental Problems/Needs.*

Nursing Diagnoses

Risk for Imbalanced Nutrition: Less Than Body Requirements related to anorexia, nausea, vomiting, and deprivation of host nutrients by parasites

Impaired Skin Integrity related to pruritus secondary to
emergence of parasites (pinworms) onto perianal skin, lytic
necrosis, and tissue digestion

Diarrhea related to parasitic irritation to intestinal mucosa

Acute Pain related to parasitic invasion of small intestines

Risk for Infection Transmission related to contagious nature of
parasites

Risk for Ineffective Child's Health Management related to
insufficient knowledge of condition, mode of transmission,
and prevention of reinfection

Pediculosis

Nursing Diagnoses

Risk for Infection related to lesions

Impaired Comfort: Pruritus related to lesions

Risk for Infection Transmission related to insufficient knowledge
of modes of transmission, treatment, and prevention

Risk for Ineffective Child's Health Management related to
insufficient resources, low prioritization of problem, or
repeated infections

Poisoning

See also *Dialysis*, if indicated; *Unconscious Individual*.

Collaborative Problems

RC of Respiratory alkalosis

RC of Metabolic acidosis

RC of Hemorrhage

RC of Fluid/electrolyte imbalances

RC of Burns (acid/alkaline)

RC of Aspiration

RC of Blindness

Nursing Diagnoses

Acute Pain related to heat production secondary to poisoning
(e.g., salicylate)

Fear related to invasive nature of treatments (gastric lavage,
dialysis)

Anxiety (parental) related to uncertainty of situation and feelings
of guilt

Risk for Poisoning related to insufficient knowledge of home treatment of accidental poisoning, and poison prevention (storage, teaching, poisonous plants, locks)

Respiratory Tract Infection (Lower)

See also *Developmental Problems/Needs*; *Adult Pneumonia*.

Collaborative Problems

RC of Hyperthermia
RC of Respiratory insufficiency
RC of Septic shock
RC of Paralytic ileus

Nursing Diagnoses

Acute Pain related to hyperthermia, malaise, and respiratory distress
Risk for Imbalanced Nutrition: Less Than Body Requirements related to anorexia secondary to dyspnea and malaise
Anxiety related to breathlessness and apprehension
Risk for Deficient Fluid Volume related to insufficient intake secondary to dyspnea and malaise
Risk for Ineffective Self-Health Management related to insufficient knowledge of condition, prevention of recurrence, and treatment

Rheumatic Fever

See also *Developmental Problems/Needs*.

Collaborative Problems

RC of Endocarditis

Nursing Diagnoses

Deficient Diversional Activity related to prescribed bed rest
Imbalanced Nutrition: Less Than Body Requirements related to anorexia and malaise
Acute Pain related to arthralgia
Risk for Injury related to choreic movements
Risk for Ineffective Child's Health Management related to insufficient knowledge of condition, signs and symptoms of complications, long-term antibiotic therapy, prevention of recurrence, and risk factors (surgery, e.g., dental)

Rheumatoid Arthritis (Juvenile)

See also *Developmental Problems/Needs*; *Corticosteroid Therapy*.

Collaborative Problems

RC of Pericarditis
RC of Ocular Infections

Nursing Diagnoses

Impaired Physical Mobility related to pain and restricted joint
    movement
Acute Pain related to swollen, inflamed joints and restricted
    movement
Fatigue related to chronic inflammatory process
Risk for Ineffective Child's Health Management related to
    insufficient knowledge of condition, pharmacologic therapy,
    exercise program, rest versus activity, myths, and community
    resources

Reye's Syndrome

See also *Unconscious Individual*, if indicated.

Collaborative Problems

RC of Renal failure
RC of Increased intracranial pressure
RC of Fluid/electrolyte imbalances
RC of Hepatic failure
RC of Shock
RC of Seizures
RC of Coma
RC of Respiratory distress
RC of Diabetes insipidus

Nursing Diagnoses

Parental Anxiety related to diagnosis and uncertain prognosis
Risk for Injury related to uncontrolled tonic-clonic movements
Risk for Infection related to invasive monitoring procedures
Acute Pain related to hyperpyrexia and malaise secondary to
    disease process
Fear related to separation from family, sensory bombardment
    (intensive care, treatments), and unfamiliar experiences

Interrupted Family Processes related to critical nature of syndrome, hospitalization of child, and separation of family members

Grieving related to actual, anticipated, or possible death of child

Risk for Impaired Skin Integrity related to immobility

Risk for Ineffective Child's Health Management related to insufficient knowledge of condition, treatment, and complications

Scoliosis

See also *Developmental Problems/Needs*.

Nursing Diagnoses

Impaired Physical Mobility related to restricted movement secondary to braces

Risk for Impaired Skin Integrity related to mechanical irritation of brace

Risk for Noncompliance related to chronicity and complexity of treatment regimen

Risk for Falls related to restricted range of motion

Risk for Ineffective Child's Health Management related to insufficient knowledge of condition, treatment, exercises, environmental hazards, care of appliances, follow-up care, and community services

Sickle Cell Anemia

See also *Developmental Problems/Needs*.

Collaborative Problems

RC of Sickling crisis of transfusion therapy

RC of Thrombosis and infarction

RC of Cholelithiasis

Nursing Diagnoses

Ineffective Peripheral Tissue Perfusion related to viscous blood and occlusion of microcirculation

Acute Pain related to viscous blood and tissue hypoxia

(Specify) Self-Care Deficit related to pain and immobility of exacerbations

Risk for Ineffective Child's Health Management related to insufficient knowledge of hazards, signs and symptoms of complications, fluid requirements, and hereditary factors

Tonsillitis

See also *Tonsillectomy*, if indicated.

Collaborative Problems

RC of Otitis media
RC of Rheumatic fever (β-hemolytic streptococci)

Nursing Diagnoses

Risk for Deficient Fluid Volume related to inadequate fluid
  intake secondary to pain
Risk for Ineffective Child's Health Management related to
  insufficient knowledge of condition, treatments, nutritional/
  fluid requirements, and signs and symptoms of complications

Wilms' Tumor

See also *Developmental Problems/Needs; Nephrectomy; Cancer
  (General)*.

Collaborative Problems

RC of Metastases to liver, lung, bone, brain
RC of Sepsis
RC of Tumor rupture

Nursing Diagnoses

Anxiety related to (examples) age-related concerns (separation,
  strangers, pain), response of others to visible signs (alopecia),
  and uncertain future
Parental Anxiety related to (examples) unknown prognosis,
  painful procedures, treatments (chemotherapy), and feelings
  of inadequacy
Grieving related to actual, anticipated, or possible death of child
Spiritual Distress related to nature of disease and its possible
  disturbances in belief systems
Risk for Ineffective Child's Health Management related to
  insufficient knowledge of condition, prognosis, treatments
  (side effects), home care, nutritional requirements, follow-up
  care, and community services

Affective Disorders (Depression)

Nursing Diagnoses

Dressing/Grooming Self-Care Deficit related to decreased interest in body, inability to make decisions, and feelings of worthlessness

Ineffective Coping related to internal conflicts (guilt, low self-esteem) or feelings of rejection

Risk for Loneliness related to inability to initiate activities to reduce isolation secondary to low energy levels

Complicated Grieving related to unresolved grief, prolonged denial, and repression

Chronic Low Self-Esteem related to feelings of worthlessness and failure secondary to (specify)

Compromised Family Coping related to marital discord and role conflicts secondary to effects of chronic depression

Powerlessness related to unrealistic negative beliefs about self-worth or abilities

Disturbed Thought Processes related to negative cognitive set (overgeneralizing, polarized thinking, selected abstraction, arbitrary inference)

Ineffective Sexuality Patterns related to decreased sex drive, loss of interest and pleasure

Deficient Diversional Activity related to a loss of interest or pleasure in usual activities and low energy levels

Impaired Home Maintenance related to inability to make decisions or concentrate

Risk for Self-Harm related to feelings of hopelessness and loneliness

Insomnia related to difficulty falling asleep or early morning awakening secondary to emotional stress

Constipation related to sedentary lifestyle, insufficient exercise, or inadequate diet

Risk for Imbalanced Nutrition: More Than Body Requirements related to increased intake versus decreased activity expenditures secondary to boredom and frustration

Risk for Imbalanced Nutrition: Less Than Body Requirements related to anorexia secondary to emotional stress

Risk for Ineffective Self-Health Management related to insufficient knowledge of condition, behavior modification, therapy options (pharmacologic, electroshock), and community resources

Alcoholism

Collaborative Problems

RC of Delirium tremens
RC of Autonomic hyperactivity
RC of Seizures
RC of Alcoholic hallucinosis
RC of Hypertension
RC of Hypoglycemia

Nursing Diagnoses

Imbalanced Nutrition: Less Than Body Requirements related to anorexia

Risk for Deficient Fluid Volume related to abnormal fluid loss secondary to vomiting and diarrhea

Risk for Injury related to disorientation, tremors, or impaired judgment

Risk for Violence related to chemical withdrawal with impulsive behavior, disorientation, tremors, or impaired judgment

Disturbed Sleep Pattern related to irritability, tremors, and nightmares

Anxiety related to loss of control, memory losses, and fear of withdrawal

Ineffective Coping related to inability to manage stressors constructively without drugs/alcohol

Impaired Social Interaction related to alcoholic problematic behavior with emotional immaturity, irritability, high anxiety, impulsive behavior, or aggressive responses

Ineffective Sexuality Patterns related to impotence/loss of libido secondary to altered self-concept and substance abuse

Ineffective Family Coping related to disruption in marital dyad and inconsistent limit setting

Disabled Family Coping related to the destructive effects of alcoholic family member on family functioning and each family member

Risk for Ineffective Self-Health Management related to insufficient knowledge of condition, treatments available, high-risk situations, and community resources

Anorexia Nervosa

Collaborative Problems

RC of Anemia
RC of Hypotension
RC of Dysrhythmias
RC of Amenorrhea

Nursing Diagnoses

Imbalanced Nutrition: Less Than Body Requirements related to exercise in excess of caloric intake, refusal to eat, self-induced vomiting following eating, or laxative abuse

Disturbed Self-Concept related to inaccurate perception of self as obese

Risk for Deficient Fluid Volume related to vomiting and excessive weight loss

Activity Intolerance related to fatigue secondary to malnutrition

Ineffective Coping related to self-induced vomiting, denial of hunger, and insufficient food intake secondary to feelings of loss of control and inaccurate perceptions of body states

Compromised Family Coping related to marital discord and its effect on family members

Constipation related to insufficient food and fluid intake

Impaired Social Interaction related to inability to form relationships with others or fear of trusting relationships with others

Fear related to implications of a maturing body and dissatisfaction with relationships with others

Anxiety and Adjustment Disorders (Phobias, Anxiety States, Traumatic Stress Disorders, Adjustment Reactions)

See also *Substance Abuse Disorders*, if indicated.

Nursing Diagnoses

Impaired Social Interaction related to effects of behavior and actions on forming and maintaining relationships

Anxiety related to irrational thoughts or guilt

Ineffective Coping related to inadequate psychological resources to adapt to a traumatic event

Disturbed Sleep Pattern related to recurrent nightmares

Ineffective Coping related to altered ability to manage stressors constructively secondary to (examples) physical illness, marital discord, business crisis, natural disasters, or developmental crisis

Risk for Ineffective Self-Health Management related to insufficient knowledge of condition, pharmacologic therapy, and legal system regarding violence

Bipolar Disorder (Mania)

Nursing Diagnoses

Defensive Coping related to unrealistic expectations secondary to exaggerated sense of self-importance and abilities

Impaired Social Interaction related to alienation from others secondary to overt hostility, overconfidence, or manipulation of others

Risk for Other Directed Violence related to impaired reality testing, impaired judgment, or compromised ability to control behavior

Disturbed Sleep Pattern related to hyperactivity

Disturbed Thought Processes related to biochemical disturbances

Risk for Deficient Fluid Volume related to altered sodium excretion secondary to lithium therapy

Noncompliance related to feelings of no longer requiring medication

Risk for Ineffective Self-Health Management related to insufficient knowledge of condition, pharmacologic therapy, and follow-up care

Childhood Behavioral Disorders (Attention Deficit Disorders, Learning Disabilities)

Nursing Diagnoses

Impaired Social Interaction related to inattention, impulsivity, or hyperactivity

Chronic Sorrow (parental) related to anticipated losses secondary to condition

Interrupted Family Processes related to adjustment requirements for situation: (examples) time, energy, money, physical care, and prognosis

Risk for Other-Directed Violence related to history of aggressive acts and (specify)

Risk for Impaired Home Maintenance related to inadequate resources, inadequate housing, or impaired caregivers

Risk for Loneliness (child, family) related to disability and
   requirements for caregivers
Risk for Impaired Parenting related to inadequate resources or
   inadequate coping mechanisms
Disturbed Self-Concept related to effects of limitations on
   achievement of developmental tasks

Obsessive–Compulsive Disorder

Nursing Diagnoses

(Specify) Self-Care Deficit related to ritualistic obsessions
   interfering with performance of activities of daily living
Noncompliance related to poor concentration and poor impulse
   control secondary to obsessive thought patterns
Risk for Loneliness related to fear of vulnerability associated
   with need for closeness and embarrassment about ritualistic
   behavior
Anxiety related to the perceived threat of actual or anticipated
   events

Paranoid Disorders

Nursing Diagnoses

Impaired Social Interaction related to feelings of mistrust and
   suspicion of others
Ineffective Denial related to unrealistic expectations secondary
   to inability to accept own feelings and responsibility for
   actions
Risk for Imbalanced Nutrition: Less Than Body Requirements
   related to reluctance to eat secondary to fear of poisoning
Impaired Thought Processes related to unknown etiology, e.g.,
   repressed fears, drug use, abuse
Risk for Loneliness related to fear and mistrust of situations and
   others

Personality Disorders

Examples

Schizoid	Histrionic
Antisocial	Passive–aggressive
Borderline	Paranoid
Narcissistic	Schizotypal
Avoidant	Dependent
Compulsive	

Nursing Diagnoses

Ineffective Coping related to biochemical changes with faulty thinking secondary (specify mental disorder)

Ineffective Coping related to biochemical changes with poor impulse control and low frustration level

Impaired Social Interaction related to unrealistic expectations of relationships and impaired ability to maintain enduring attachments

Ineffective Coping related to resistance (procrastination, stubbornness, intentional inefficiency) in responses to responsibilities (role, social)

Schizophrenic Disorders

Nursing Diagnoses

Risk for Other-Directed Violence related to responding to delusional thoughts or hallucinations

Risk for Self-Mutilation related to responding to delusional thoughts or hallucinations

Impaired Verbal Communication related to incoherent/illogical speech pattern and side effects of medications

Impaired Social Interaction related to biochemical disturbances with preoccupation with egocentric and illogical ideas and extreme suspiciousness

Impaired Home Maintenance related to impaired judgment, inability to self-initiate activity, and loss of skills over long course of illness

Somatoform Disorders (Somatization, Hypochondriasis, Conversion Reactions)

See also *Affective Disorders*, if indicated.

Nursing Diagnoses

Impaired Social Interaction related to effects of multiple somatic complaints and complaining on relationships

Ineffective Coping related to unrealistic fear of having a disease despite reassurance to contrary

Risk for Disabled Family Coping related to chronicity of illness

Noncompliance related to impaired judgments and thought disturbances

Dressing Self-Care Deficit related to loss of skills and lack of interest in body and appearance

Deficient Diversional Activity related to apathy, inability to initiate goal-directed activities, and loss of skills

Disturbed Self-Concept related to feelings of worthlessness and lack of ego boundaries

Risk for Ineffective Self-Health Management related to insufficient knowledge of condition, pharmacologic therapy, tardive dyskinesia, occupational skills, and follow-up care

DIAGNOSTIC AND THERAPEUTIC PROCEDURES

Angioplasty (Percutaneous, Transluminal, Coronary, Peripheral)

Preprocedure Period
Nursing Diagnoses

Anxiety/Fear (individual, family) related to health status, angioplasty procedure, routines, outcome, and possible need for cardiac surgery

Postprocedure Period
Collaborative Problems

▲ RC of Dysrhythmias

▲ RC of Acute coronary occlusion (clot, spasm, collapse)

▲ RC of Myocardial infarction

▲ RC of Arterial dissection or rupture

▲ RC of Hemorrhage/hematoma at angioplasty site

❋ RC of Paresthesia distal to site

❋ RC of Arterial thrombosis

❋ RC of Embolization (peripheral)

Nursing Diagnoses

▲ Impaired Physical Mobility related to prescribed bed rest and restricted movement of involved extremity

▲ Risk for Ineffective Self-Health Management related to insufficient knowledge of care of insertion site, discharge activities, diet, medications, signs and symptoms of complications, exercises, and follow-up care

Anticoagulant Therapy

Collaborative Problem

▲ RC of Hemorrhage

Nursing Diagnoses

△ Risk for Ineffective Self-Health Management related to insufficient knowledge of administration schedule, identification card/band, contraindications, dietary precautions and signs and symptoms of bleeding

Cardiac Catheterization

Postprocedure Period
Collaborative Problems

▲ RC of Systemic (allergic reaction)
▲ RC of Cardiac (dysrhythmias, myocardial infarction, pulmonary edema)
✱ RC of CVA
▲ RC of Circulatory (hematoma formation or hemorrhage at entry site, hypovolemia, thromboembolic phenomenon)

Nursing Diagnoses

✱ Impaired Comfort related to tissue trauma and prescribed postprocedure immobilization
△ Risk for Ineffective Self-Health Management related to insufficient knowledge of site care, signs and symptoms of complications, and follow-up care

Casts

Collaborative Problems

▲ RC of Compartment syndrome
▲ RC of Infection/Sepsis

Nursing Diagnoses

✱ Risk for Injury related to hazards of crutch-walking and impaired mobility secondary to cast
▲ Risk for Impaired Skin Integrity related to pressure of cast on skin surface
▲ (Specify) Self-Care Deficit related to limitation of movement secondary to cast

✳ Risk for Ineffective Respiratory Function related to imposed immobility or restricted respiratory movement secondary to cast (body)
✳ Deficient Diversional Activity related to boredom and inability to perform usual recreational activities
▲ Risk for Ineffective Self-Health Management related to insufficient knowledge of cast care, signs and symptoms of complications, use of assistive devices, and hazards

Chemotherapy

See also *Cancer (General)*.

Collaborative Problems

✳ RC of Necrosis/phlebitis at intravenous site
✳ RC of Thrombocytopenia
✳ RC of Anemia
✳ RC of Leukopenia
△ RC of Peripheral nerve toxicosis
▲ RC of Anaphylactic reaction
△ RC of Central nervous system toxicity
△ RC of Congestive heart failure
▲ RC of Electrolyte imbalance
▲ RC of Extravasation of vesicant drugs
△ RC of Hemorrhagic cystitis
▲ RC of Myelosuppression
▲ RC of Renal insufficiency/calculi

Nursing Diagnoses

✳ Risk for Deficient Fluid Volume related to gastrointestinal fluid losses secondary to vomiting
✳ Risk for Infection related to altered immune system secondary to effects of cytotoxic agents or disease process
✳ Risk for Interrupted Family Processes related to interruptions imposed by treatment and schedule on patterns of living
✳ Risk for Ineffective Sexuality Patterns related to amenorrhea and sterility (temporary/permanent) secondary to effects of chemotherapy on testes/ovaries
✳ Risk for Injury related to bleeding tendencies
▲ Anxiety related to prescribed chemotherapy, insufficient knowledge of chemotherapy, and self-care measures
▲ Fatigue related to effects of anemia, malnutrition, persistent vomiting, and sleep pattern disturbance
△ Risk for Constipation related to autonomic nerve dysfunction secondary to vinca alkaloid administration and inactivity

▲ Diarrhea related to intestinal cell damage, inflammation, and increased intestinal motility

▲ Acute Pain related to gastrointestinal cell damage, stimulation of vomiting center, fear, and anxiety

▲ Risk for Impaired Skin Integrity related to persistent diarrhea, malnutrition, prolonged sedation, and fatigue

▲ Imbalanced Nutrition: Less Than Body Requirements related to anorexia, taste changes, persistent nausea/vomiting, and increased metabolic rate

▲ Impaired Oral Mucous Membrane related to dryness and epithelial cell damage secondary to chemotherapy

△ Disturbed Self-Concept related to change in lifestyle, role, alopecia, and weight loss or gain

Corticosteroid Therapy

Collaborative Problems

△ RC of Peptic ulcer

✳ RC of Pseudotumor cerebri

▲ RC of Steroid-induced diabetes

△ RC of Osteoporosis

△ RC of Hypertension

△ RC of Hypokalemia

Nursing Diagnoses

▲ Risk for Excess Fluid Volume related to sodium and water retention

▲ Risk for Infection related to immunosuppression secondary to corticosteroid therapy

△ Risk for Imbalanced Nutrition: More Than Body Requirements related to increased appetite

△ Risk for Disturbed Body Image related to appearance changes (e.g., abnormal fat distribution, increased production of androgens)

△ Risk for Ineffective Self-Health Management related to insufficient knowledge of administration schedule, adverse reactions, signs and symptoms of complications, hazards of adrenal insufficiency, and potential causes of adrenal insufficiency

Electroconvulsive Therapy (ECT)

Postprocedure Period
Collaborative Problems

RC of Hypertension

RC of Dysrhythmias

Nursing Diagnoses

Risk for Injury related to uncontrolled tonic-clonic movements and disorientation, confusion post-treatment

Acute Pain related to headaches, muscle aches, nausea secondary to seizure activity and tissue trauma

Risk for Aspiration related to post-ECT somnolence

Anxiety related to memory losses and disorientation secondary to effects of ECT on cerebral function

Electronic Fetal Monitoring (Internal)

See also *Intrapartum Period (General)*.

Postinsertion
Collaborative Problems

RC of Fetal scalp laceration
RC of Perforated uterus

Nursing Diagnoses

Impaired Physical Mobility related to restrictions secondary to monitor cords

Enteral Nutrition

Collaborative Problems

▲ RC of Hypoglycemia/hyperglycemia
▲ RC of Hypervolemia
△ RC of Hypertonic dehydration
▲ RC of Electrolyte and trace mineral imbalances
△ RC of Mucosal erosion

Nursing Diagnoses

▲ Risk for Infection related to gastrostomy incision and enzymatic action of gastric juices on skin
▲ Impaired Comfort related to cramping, distention, nausea, vomiting related to type of formula, administration rate, temperature, or route
▲ Diarrhea related to adverse response to formula, rate, or temperature
▲ Risk for Aspiration related to position of tube and of individual

△ Risk for Ineffective Self-Health Management related to insufficient knowledge of nutritional indications/requirements, home care, and signs and symptoms of complications

External Arteriovenous Shunting

Collaborative Problems

▲ RC of Thrombosis
▲ RC of Bleeding

Nursing Diagnoses

▲ Risk for Ineffective Self-Health Management related to insufficient knowledge of catheter care, precautions, emergency measures, prevention of infection, and activity limitations

Hemodialysis

See also *Chronic Kidney Failure*.

Collaborative Problems

✱ RC of Anaphylaxis/Allergies
▲ RC of Fluid imbalances
▲ RC of Electrolyte imbalance (potassium, sodium)
▲ RC of Dialysis Disequilibrium Syndrome
△ RC of Transfusion reaction
▲ RC of Hemorrhage
✱ RC of Disruption of vascular access
△ RC of Dialysate leakage
▲ RC of Clotting
✱ RC of Hemolysis
▲ RC of Hypertension/hypotension
▲ RC of Dialysis disequilibrium syndrome
▲ RC of Air embolism
▲ RC of Sepsis
△ RC of Pyrogen Reaction

Nursing Diagnoses

✱ Risk for Injury to (vascular) access site related to vulnerability
✱ Risk for Infection related to direct access to bloodstream secondary to vascular access
▲ Powerlessness related to need for treatments to live despite effects on lifestyle
▲ Interrupted Family Processes related to the interruptions of role responsibilities caused by the treatment schedule

▲ Risk for Infection Transmission related to frequent contacts with blood and high risk for hepatitis B

✻ Risk for Ineffective Self-Health Management related to insufficient knowledge of rationale of treatment, care of site, precautions, emergency treatments (disconnected, bleeding, clotting), pretreatment instructions, and daily assessments (bruit, blood pressure, weight)

Hemodynamic Monitoring

See also *Medical Conditions* for the specific medical diagnosis.

Collaborative Problems

✻ RC of Sepsis

▲ RC of Hemorrhage

✻ RC of Bleeding back

✻ RC of Vasospasm

✻ RC of Tissue ischemia/hypoxia

▲ RC of Thrombosis/thrombophlebitis

▲ RC of Pulmonary embolism, air embolism

▲ RC of Arterial spasm

Nursing Diagnoses

▲ Risk for Infection related to invasive lines

△ Impaired Physical Mobility related to position restrictions secondary to hemodynamic monitoring

△ Anxiety related to impending procedure, loss of control, and unpredictable outcome

✻ Risk for Ineffective Self-Health Management related to insufficient knowledge of purpose, procedure, and associated care

Hickman Catheter

Collaborative Problems

RC of Air embolism
RC of Bleeding
RC of Thrombosis

Nursing Diagnoses

Risk for Infection related to direct access to bloodstream
Risk for Impaired Home Maintenance related to lack of
  knowledge of catheter management

Long-Term Venous Catheter

Collaborative Problems

△ RC of Pneumothorax
▲ RC of Hemorrhage
△ RC of Embolism/thrombosis
▲ RC of Sepsis

Nursing Diagnoses

▲ Anxiety related to upcoming insertion of catheter and insufficient knowledge of procedure
▲ Risk for Infection related to catheter's direct access to bloodstream
△ Risk for Ineffective Self-Health Management related to insufficient knowledge of home care, signs and symptoms of complications, and community resources

Mechanical Ventilation

See also *Tracheostomy*.

Collaborative Problems

✶ RC of Tracheal necrosis
△ RC of Gastrointestinal bleeding
✶ RC of Tension pneumothorax
△ RC of Oxygen toxicity
▲ RC of Respiratory insufficiency
▲ RC of Atelectasis
✶ RC of Ventilation Acquired Pneumonia (VAP)
△ RC of Decreased cardiac output

Nursing Diagnoses

▲ Impaired Verbal Communication related to effects of intubation on ability to speak
△ Disuse Syndrome
▲ Risk for Infection related to disruption of skin layer secondary to tracheostomy
✶ Interrupted Family Processes related to critical nature of situation and uncertain prognosis
△ Fear related to the nature of the situation, uncertain prognosis of ventilator dependence, or weaning
✶ Risk for Disturbed Sensory Perceptions related to excessive environmental stimuli and decreased input of meaningful stimuli secondary to treatment and critical care unit

▲ Risk for Ineffective Airway Clearance related to increased secretions secondary to tracheostomy, obstruction of inner cannula, or displacement of tracheostomy tube

▲ Powerlessness related to dependency on respirator, inability to talk, and loss of mobility

▲ Risk for Dysfunctional Ventilatory Weaning Response related to unsatisfactory weaning attempts, respiratory muscle fatigue secondary to mechanical ventilation, increased work of breathing, supine position, protein–calorie malnutrition, inactivity, and/or fatigue

✳ Risk for Disturbed Self-Concept related to mechanical ventilation, dependence on achieving developmental tasks, and lifestyle changes

Pacemaker Insertion

Postprocedure Period
Collaborative Problems

▲ RC of Cardiac dysfunction

▲ RC of Pacemaker malfunction

△ RC of Rejection of unit

△ RC of Necrosis near pulse generator site

✳ RC of Hemorrhage (site, rupture of vessel)

Nursing Diagnoses

✳ Acute Pain related to insertion site and prescribed postprocedure immobilization

△ Impaired Physical Mobility related to incisional site pain, activity restrictions, and fear of lead displacements

✳ Risk for Infection related to operative site

△ Risk for Ineffective Self-Health Management related to insufficient knowledge of activity restrictions, precautions, signs and symptoms of complications, electromagnetic interference (microwave ovens, arc welding equipment, gasoline engines, electric motors, antitheft devices, power transmitters), pacemaker function (daily pulse taking, signs of impending battery failure), activity restrictions, and follow-up care

Peritoneal Dialysis

Collaborative Problems

✳ RC of Fluid imbalances

△ RC of Electrolyte imbalances

△ RC of Hemorrhage

- ❋ RC of Sepsis
- ▲ RC of Bowel/bladder perforation
- ▲ RC of Hyperglycemia
- ❋ RC of Peritonitis
- ▲ RC of Inflow/outflow problems
- ▲ RC of Uremia

Nursing Diagnoses

- ▲ Risk for Infection related to access to peritoneal cavity, catheter exit site, and use of high-dextrose concentration in dialysis solution
- ❋ Risk for Injury to catheter site related to vulnerability
- △ Risk for Ineffective Breathing Pattern related to immobility, pressure, and pain
- △ Impaired Comfort related to catheter insertion, instillation of dialysis solution, outflow, suction, and chemical irritation of peritoneum
- △ Imbalanced Nutrition: Less Than Body Requirements related to anorexia
- ❋ Risk for Excessive Fluid Volume related to fluid retention secondary to catheter problems (kinks, blockages) or position
- △ Risk for Interrupted Family Processes related to the effects of interruptions of the treatment schedule on role responsibilities
- △ Powerlessness related to chronic illness and the need for continuous treatment
- ❋ Impaired Home Maintenance related to insufficient knowledge of treatment procedure
- △ Risk for Ineffective Self-Health Management related to insufficient knowledge of rationale for treatment, medications, home dialysis procedure, signs and symptoms of complications, community resources, and follow-up care

Radiation Therapy (External)

Postprocedure Period

Collaborative Problems

- ❋ RC of Cerebral Edema, Increased intracranial pressure (site dependent)
- ▲ RC of Myelosuppression
- ❋ RC of Mucositis, Esophagitis, Pneumonitis
- △ RC of Fluid/Electrolyte imbalances
- △ RC of Inflammation

✳ RC of Pleural effusion (site specific)
✳ RC of Myelitis, parotitis

Nursing Diagnoses

▲ Anxiety related to prescribed radiation therapy and insufficient knowledge of treatments and self-care measures

△ Acute Pain related to stimulation of the vomiting center and damage to the gastrointestinal mucosal cells secondary to radiation

▲ Fatigue related to systemic effects of radiation therapy
Acute Pain related to damage to sebaceous and sweat glands secondary to radiation

△ Risk for Impaired Oral Mucous Membrane related to dry mouth or inadequate oral hygiene

▲ Impaired Skin Integrity related to effects of radiation on epithelial and basal cells and effects of diarrhea on perineal area

▲ Imbalanced Nutrition: Less Than Body Requirements related to decreased oral intake, reduced salivation, mouth discomfort, dysphagia, nausea/vomiting, and increased metabolic rate

△ Disturbed Self-Concept related to alopecia, skin changes, weight loss, sterility, and changes in role, relationships, and lifestyle

△ Grieving related to changes in lifestyle, role, finances, functional capacity, body image, and health losses

△ Interrupted Family Processes related to imposed changes in family roles, relationships, and responsibilities

✳ Diarrhea related to increased peristalsis secondary to irradiation of abdomen/lower back

✳ Risk for Infection related to moist skin reaction

✳ Activity Intolerance related to fatigue secondary to treatments or transportation

✳ Risk for Ineffective Self-Health Management related to insufficient knowledge of skin care and signs of complications

Total Parenteral Nutrition (Hyperalimentation Therapy)

Collaborative Problems

▲ RC of Sepsis
▲ RC of Hyperglycemia
△ RC of Air embolism
✳ RC of Sepsis
✳ RC of Perforation

△ RC of Pneumothorax, hydrothorax, hemothorax

Nursing Diagnoses

▲ Risk for Infection related to catheter's direct access to bloodstream

❊ Risk for Impaired Skin Integrity related to continuous skin surface irritation secondary to catheter and adhesive

❊ Risk for Impaired Oral Mucous Membrane related to inability to ingest food/fluid

△ Risk for Ineffective Self-Health Management related to insufficient knowledge of home care, signs and symptoms of complications, catheter care, and follow-up care (laboratory studies)

Tracheostomy

Postoperative Period

Collaborative Problems

▲ RC of Hypoxemia
▲ RC of Hemorrhage
▲ RC of Tracheal edema

Nursing Diagnoses

▲ Risk for Ineffective Airway Clearance related to increased secretions secondary to tracheostomy, obstruction of inner cannula, or displacement of tracheostomy tube

▲ Risk for Infection related to excessive pooling of secretions and bypassing of upper respiratory defenses

▲ Impaired Verbal Communication related to inability to produce speech secondary to tracheostomy

❊ Risk for Ineffective Sexuality Patterns related to change in appearance, fear of rejection

▲ Risk for Ineffective Self-Health Management related to insufficient knowledge of tracheostomy care, precautions, signs and symptoms of complications, emergency care, and follow-up care

UPDATED DIAGNOSES

 SELF-NEGLECT

DEFINITION (NANDA)

A constellation of culturally framed behaviors involving one or more self-care activities in which there is a failure to maintain a socially accepted standard of health and well-being.

DEFINING CHARACTERISTICS (NANDA)

Inadequate personal hygiene
Inadequate environmental hygiene
Non-adherence to health activities

RELATED FACTORS (NANDA)

Capgras syndrome
Cognitive impairment (e.g., dementia)
Depression
Learning disability
Fear of institutionalization
Frontal lobe dysfunction and executive processing ability
Functional impairment
Lifestyle/Choice
Maintaining control
Malingering
Obsessive-compulsive disorder
Schizotypal personal disorders
Substance abuse
Major life stressor

■■■■ **AUTHOR'S NOTE**
This diagnosis focuses on three problems: self-care problems, home hygiene, and non-compliance. Presently, three nursing diagnoses would more specifically describe the focus as *Self-Care Deficit*, *Impaired Home Maintenance*, and *Ineffective Self-Health Management*. Refer to these diagnoses in the index.

RISK FOR VASCULAR TRAUMA

Risk for Vascular Trauma Related to Infusion of Vesicant
   Medications.

DEFINITION

The state in which an individual is at risk for damage to a vein and
its surrounding tissues related to the presence of a catheter and/
or infused solutions.

RISK FACTORS

Treatment-Related

Catheter type*; catheter width*
Impaired ability to visualize the insertion site
Inadequate catheter fixation*
Infusion rate*; length of insertion time
Nature of solution (e.g., concentration, chemical irritant,
   temperature, pH)

AUTHOR'S NOTE

This new NANDA-I diagnosis represents a risk for all
persons with intravenous catheters. Procedure manuals on
the clinical unit should contain the correct placement, fixation and monitoring of all intravenous sites. Nurses needing
these guidelines should refer to the procedure manual.
There is no need for practicing nurses to have this diagnosis
on the care plan. Students should refer to their fundamentals
of nursing text for specific techniques to start, secure, and
monitor intravenous therapy. Consult with your faculty to
determine if this should be written on your assigned client's
care plan.

---

*May indicate poor clinical practice.

▶ Related to Infusion of Vesicant Medications

NOC
Knowledge Treatment Procedure, Risk Control

Goals
The client will report or be monitored for early signs/symptoms of extravasation.

Indicators:
- Swelling, redness, and lack of blood return
- Stinging, burning, or pain at the injection site

NOC
Intravenous Insertion, Medication Administration: Intravenous, Surveillance, Teaching: Procedure/ Treatment, Venous Access Device (VAD) Maintenance, Chemotherapy Management

Interventions

Prior to Administration of a Prescribed Vesicant Medication, Review the Agency Protocol, Physician Order, and Information About the Medication

If Inexperienced in This Procedure, Consult an Experienced Nurse

Identify Clients at Increased Risk for Extravasation (Elderly, Debilitated, Confused, Unable to Communicate, Diabetics, Fragile Veins, General Vascular Disease).

Avoid Infusing Vesicant Drugs Over Joints, Bony Prominences, Tendons, Neurovascular Bundles, or the Antecubital Fossa, When Venous or Lymphatic Circulation Is Poor, and at Sites that Have Been Previously Irritated

The Drug Is Toxic to Tissues

Prior to Infusion, Check for Blood Return Gently and Check All Needle or Catheter Sites for Leaks, Evidence of Swelling, or Venous Thrombosis

Use the Correct Equipment (IV, Port, Huber-Point Needle)

Assess the Client Every _____ Per Institution's Policy for Swelling; Stinging, Burning, or Pain at the Injection Site; Redness; and Lack of Blood Return

If the Above Signs or Symptoms Occur, Stop Infusion and Contact an Experienced Nurse, Physician, or Nurse Practitioner Immediately

If Extravasation Occurs, Follow Institutional Policy for Discontinuation, Antidote Administration, Diluents, Site Care, Ice Applications, and Elevation of the Extremity

Document the Extravasation Event Including Subjective Complaints and Objective Observations with Times and Actions Taken

REFERENCES/BIBLIOGRAPHY

Acute Pain Management Guideline Panel. (1992). *Acute pain management in infants, children, and adolescents: Operative and medical procedures*. Quick Reference Guide for Clinicians. AHCPR Pub. No. 92-0020. Rockville, MD: Agency for Health Care Policy and Research, Public Health Service, U.S. Department of Health and Human Services.

Algase, D. L. (1999). Wandering: A dementia-compromised behavior. *Journal of Gerontological Nursing, 25*(9), 10–16.

Allender, J. & Spradley, B. (2006). *Community health nursing* (4th ed.). Philadelphia: Lippincott Williams & Wilkins.

American Academy of Pediatrics. (2000). Task force on infant sleep position and Sudden Infant Death Syndrome: Changing concepts of Sudden Infant Death Syndrome; implications for infants sleeping environment and sleep position. *Pediatrics, 105*(3), 650–56.

American Psychiatric Association. (2004). *DSM IV-TR: Diagnostic and statistical manual of mental disorders* (5th ed., text revision). Washington, DC: Author.

American Psychiatric Association. (2000). *Diagnostic and statistical manual of mental disorders* (4th ed., text revision). Washington, DC: Author.

Anetzberger, G. J. (1987). *The etiology of elder abuse by adult offsprings*. Springfield, IL: Charles C. Thomas.

Bamberger, J. D., Unick, J., Klein, P., et al. (2000). Helping the urban poor stay with antiretroviral HIV drug therapy. *American Journal of Public Health, 90*(5), 699–701.

Bandura, A. (1982). Self-efficacy mechanism in human agency. *American Psychology, 37*(3), 122–147.

Barnhouse, A. (1987). *Development of the nursing diagnosis of translocation syndrome with critical care patients*. Unpublished master's thesis. Kent, OH: Kent State University.

Bennett, C. (2003). Urgent urological management of the paraplegic/ quadriplegic patient. *Urologic Nursing, 23*(6), 436–437.

Bennett, R. (2002). Acute gastrointestinal and associated conditions. In R. Barker, J. Burton & P. Zieve (Eds.), *Principles of ambulatory medicine*. Baltimore: Williams & Wilkins.

Bhardwaj, A., Mirski, M. A., & Ulatowski, J. A. (2004). *Handbook of neurocritical care*. Totowa, NJ: Humana Press.

Blackburn, S. (1993). Assessment and management of neuralgic dysfunction. In C. Kenner, A. Brueggemeyer, & L. Gunderson (Eds.), *Comprehensive neonatal nursing*. Philadelphia: W. B. Saunders.

Blackburn, S., & Vandenberg, K. (1993). Assessment and management of neonatal neurobehavioral development. In C. Kenner, A. Brueggemeyer, & L. Gunderson (Eds.), *Comprehensive neonatal nursing*. Philadelphia: W. B. Saunders.

Bodenheimer, T., MacGregor, K., & Sharifi, C. (2005). Helping patients manage their chronic medications. California Healthcare Foundation. Available at http://www.chcf.org/topics/chronicdisease/index.cfm? itemID=111768. Accessed 1/06/2007.

Boyd, M. A. (2005). *Psychiatric nursing: Contemporary practice*. Philadelphia: Lippincott Williams & Wilkins.

Breslin, E. (1992). Dyspnea-limited response in chronic obstructive pulmonary disease: Reduced unsupported arm activities. *Rehabilitation Nursing, 17*(1), 13–20.

Bridges, E. J., & Dukes, M. S. (2005). Cardiovascular aspects of septic shock: Pathophysiology, monitoring, and treatment. *Critical Care Nurse, 25*(2), 14–42.

Burnside, I., & Haight, B. (1994). Reminiscence and life review: Therapeutic interventions for older people. *Nurse Practitioner, 19*(4), 55–60.

Carpenito-Moyet, L. J. (2010). *Nursing diagnosis: Application to clinical practice* (13th ed.). Philadelphia: Lippincott Williams & Wilkins.

Carscadden, J. S. (1993). *On the cutting edge: A guide for working with people who self injure* (pp. 29–34). London, Ontario: London Psychiatric Hospital.

Carson, V. B. (1989). *Spiritual dimensions of nursing practice.* Philadelphia: W. B. Saunders.

Centers for Disease Control and Prevention. (2000). Youth risk behavior surveillance. *MMWR, 49*(5), 1–94.

Centers for Disease Control and Prevention. (2003). Male batterers. Available at www.cdc.gov/ncipc/factsheet/malebat.htm.

Centers for Disease Control and Prevention. (2004). www.cdc.gov/health/tobacco.htm. http://www.bt.cdc.gov/ncidod/dhap/gl_isolation_ptII.htm/

Centers for Disease Control and Prevention. (2008). HIV Transmission Rates in US. Retrieved February 25, 2009 from www.cdc.gov/hiv/topics/surveillance/resources/factsheets/transmission.htm.

Cohen-Mansfield, J., & Werner, P. (1998). Determinants of the effectiveness of one to one social interactions for treating verbally disruptive behaviors. *Journal of Mental Health and Aging, 4*(3), 323–324.

Comfort, M., Sockloff, A., Loverro, J., & Kaltenbach, K. (2003). Multiple predictors of substance abuse, women's treatments and outcomes: A prospective longitudinal study. *Addiction Behavior, 28*(2), 199–224.

Cooley, M. E., Yeomans, A. C., & Cobb, S. C. (1986). Sexual and reproductive issues for women with Hodgkin's disease. II. Application of PLISSIT model. *Cancer Nursing, 9,* 248–255.

Cutcliffe, J. R. (2004). The inspiration of hope in bereavement counseling. *Issues in Mental Health Nursing, 25*(2), 165–190.

DeFabio, D. C. (2000). Fluid and nutrient maintenance before, during, and after exercise. *Journal of Sports Chiropractic and Rehabilitation, 14*(2), 21–24, 42–43.

Denison, B. (2004). Touch the pain away. *Holistic Nursing Practice, 18*(3), 142–151

Dennis, K. (2004). Weight management in women. *Nursing Clinics of North America, 39*(14), 231–41.

Dochterman, J. M. & Bulechek, G. M. (2008). *Nursing interventions classification (NIC)* (6th ed.). St. Louis: Mosby.

Eakes, G. (1995). Chronic sorrow: The lived experience of parents of chronically mentally ill individuals. *Archives of Psychiatric Nursing, 9*(2), 77–84.

Eckert, R. M. (2001). Understanding anticipatory nausea. *Continuing Education, 28*(10), 1553–1560.

Edgerly, E. S., & Donovick, P. J. (1998). Neuropsychological correlates of wandering in persons with Alzheimer's disease. *American Journal of Alzheimer's Disease, 13*(6), 317–329.

Essen, J., & Blegen, M. (1991). Social isolation. In M. Maas, K. Backwater, & N. Hardy (Eds.), *Nursing diagnoses and interventions for the elderly.* Redwood City, CA: Addison-Wesley Nursing.

Evans, L. K., Strumpf, N. E., & Williams, C. C. (1992). Limiting use of physical restraints: A prerequisite for independent functioning. In E. Calkins, A. Ford, & P. Katz (Eds.),

The practice of geriatrics (2nd ed.). Philadelphia: W. B. Saunders.

Feinstein, N., Torgerson, K.L., & Atterbury, J. (Eds.). (2003). *Fetal heart monitoring principles & practices* (3rd ed.). Dubuque, IA: Kendall-Hunt.

Fetterman, L. G., & Lemburg, L. (2004). A silent killer—Often preventable. *American Journal of Critical Care, 13*(5), 431–436.

Flandermyer, A. A. (1993). The drug exposed neonate. In C. Kenner, A. Brueggemeyer, & L. Gunderson (Eds.), *Comprehensive neonatal nursing.* Philadelphia: W. B. Saunders.

Fleitas, J. (2000). When Jack fell down. . . . Jill came tumbling after. Siblings in the web of illness and disability. *MCN: American Journal of Maternal-Child Nursing, 25*(5), 267–273.

Fuhrman, M. P. (1999), Diarrhea and tube feeding. *Nutritional Clinical Practice, 14*(2), 83–84.

Gardner, D. L., & Campbell, B. (1991). Assessing postpartum fatigue. *Maternal-Child Nursing Journal, 16*(5), 264–266.

Geisman, L. K. (1989). Advances in weaning from mechanical ventilation. *Critical Care Nursing Clinics of North America, 1*(4), 697–705.

Giger, J., & Davidhizar, R. (2009). *Transcultural nursing.* St. Louis: Mosby–Year Book.

Gilbert, E.S. (2007). *Manual of high risk pregnancy and delivery* (4th ed.). St. Louis: Mosby.

Gordon, M. (1994). *Nursing diagnosis: Process and application.* St. Louis: Mosby-Year Book.

Gray, J. (1995). *Mars and Venus in the bedroom: A guide to lasting romance and passion.* New York: Harper Collins.

Hall, G. R. (1991). Altered thought processes: Dementia. In M. Maas, K. Buckwalter, & M. Hardy (Eds.), *Nursing diagnoses and interventions for the elderly.* Menlo Park, CA: Addison-Wesley Nursing.

Hall, G. R. (1994). Caring for people with Alzheimer's disease using the conceptual model of progressively lowered stress threshold in the clinical setting. *Nursing Clinics of North America, 29,* 129–141.

Hall, G. R., & Buckwalter, K. C. (1987). Progressively lowered stress threshold: A conceptual model for care of adults with Alzheimer's disease. *Archives of Psychiatric Nursing, 1,* 399–406.

Harkulich, J., & Brugler, C. (1988). Nursing diagnosis—translocation syndrome: Expert validation study. Partial funding granted by the Peg Schiltz Fund, Delta Xi Chapter, Sigma Theta Tau International. Indianapolis, IN: Sigma Theta Tau International.

Hatton, C. L., & McBride, S. (1984). *Suicide: Assessment and intervention.* Norwalk, CT: Appleton-Century-Crofts.

Heinrich, L. (1987). Care of the female rape victim. *Nurse Practitioner, 12*(11), 9.

Herman-Staab, B. (1994). Screening, management and appropriate referral for pediatric behavior problems. *Nurse Practitioner, 19*(7), 40–49.

Hickey, J. (2006). *The clinical practice of neurological and neurosurgical nursing* (5th ed.). Philadelphia: Lippincott Williams & Wilkins.

Hiltunen, E. (1987). Diagnostic content validity of the nursing diagnosis: Decisional conflict. In A. M. McLane (Ed.), *Classification of nursing diagnoses: Proceedings of the seventh conference.* St. Louis: Mosby.

Hockenberry, M. J. & Wilson, D. (2008) *Wong's essentials of pediatric nursing* (6th ed.). St. Louis: Mosby.

Holmstrom, L., & Burgess, A. W. (1975). Development of diagnostic categories: Sexual traumas. *American Journal of Nursing, 75,* 1288–1291.

Janssen, J., & Giberson, D. (1988). Remotivation therapy. *Journal of Gerontological Nursing, 14*(6), 31–34.

Jenny, J. (1987). Knowledge deficit: Not a nursing diagnosis. *Image: Journal of Nursing Scholarship, 19*(4), 184–185.

Jenny, J., & Logan, J. (1991). Interventions for the nursing diagnosis Dysfunctional Ventilatory Weaning Response: A qualitative study. In R. M. Carroll-Johnson (Ed.), *Classification of nursing diagnoses.* Philadelphia: J. B. Lippincott.

Johnson-Crowley, N. (1993). Systematic assessment and home follow-up. In C. Kenner, A. Brueggemeyer, & L. Gunderson (Eds.), *Comprehensive neonatal nursing.* Philadelphia: W. B. Saunders.

Kavchak-Keyes, M. A. (2000). Autonomic hyperreflexia. *Rehabilitation Nursing, 25*(1), 31–35.

Keegan, L. (2000). Protocols for practice: Applying research at the bedside. Alternative and complementary modalities for managing stress and anxiety. *Critical Care Nurse, 20*(3), 93–96.

Kovalesky, A. (2004). Women with substance abuse concerns. *Nursing Clinics of North America, 39*(1), 205–17.

Krieger, D. (1979). *The therapeutic touch: How to use your hands to help or to heal.* Englewood Cliffs, NJ: Prentice-Hall.

Landis, C., & Moc, K. (2004). Sleep and menopause. *Nursing Clinics of North America, 39*(1), 97–115.

Larson, C. E. (2000). Evidence-based practice. Safety and efficacy of oral rehydration therapy for treatment of diarrhea and gastroenteritis in pediatrics. *Pediatric Nursing, 26*(2), 177–179.

Levin, R. F., Krainovitch, B. C., Bahrenburg, E., & Mitchell, C. A. (1989). Diagnostic content validity of nursing diagnoses. *Image: Journal of Nursing Scholarship, 21*(1), 40–44.

Lindeman, M., Hokanson, J., & Batek, J. (1994). The alcoholic family. *Nursing Diagnosis, 5*(2), 65–73.

Logan, J., & Jenny, J. (1991). Interventions for the nursing diagnosis Dysfunctional Ventilatory Weaning Response: A qualitative study. In R. M. Carroll-Johnson (Ed.), *Classification of nursing diagnoses: Proceedings*

of the ninth conference (pp. 141–147). Philadelphia: J. B. Lippincott.

Lugina, H. I., Christenson, R., et al. (2001). Change in maternal concerns during 6 weeks postpartum period. *Journal of Midwifery and Women's Health, 46*(4), 248–257.

Lyons, B. A. (2002). Cognitive self-care skills: A model for managing stressful lifestyles. *Nursing Clinics of North America, 37*(2), 285–94.

Macauley, M., Pettersen, L., Fader, M., Brooks, R., & Cottenden, R. (2004). A multicenter evaluation of absorbent products for children with incontinence and disabilities. *Journal of WOCN, 31*(4), 235–244.

Magnan, M. A. (1987). *Activity intolerance: Toward a nursing theory of activity.* Paper presented at the Fifth Annual Symposium of the Michigan Nursing Diagnosis Association, Detroit.

Maier-Lorentz, M. M. (2000) Effective nursing interventions for the management of Alzheimer disease. *Journal of Neuroscience Nursing, 32*(2), 117–125.

Maresca, T. (1986). Assessment and management of acute diarrheal illness in adults. *Nurse Practitioner, 11*(11), 15–16.

May, J. (1996). Fathers: The forgotten parent. *Pediatric Nursing, 22*(3), 243–71.

May, K. A., & Mahlmeister, L. R. (1998). *Maternal and neonatal nursing family-centered care* (2nd ed.). Philadelphia: Lippincott-Raven.

May, R. (1987). *The meaning of anxiety.* New York: W. W. Norton.

Maynard, C. K. (2004). Assess and manage somatization. *Holistic Nursing Practice, 18*(2), 54–60.

McFarland, G., & Wasli, E. (2000). Manipulation in nursing diagnosis and process. In B. S. Johnson (Ed.), *Psychiatric-mental health nursing* (5th ed.) (p. 147). Philadelphia: J. B. Lippincott.

McLane, A., & McShane, R. (1986). Empirical validation of defining characteristics of constipation: A study of bowel elimination practices of healthy adults. In M. E. Hurley (Ed.), *Classification of nursing diagnoses: Proceedings of the sixth conference* (pp. 448–455). St. Louis: Mosby.

McMillan, J., DeAngelis, C., Feigin, R., & Warshaw, J. (1999). *Oski's pediatrics: Principles and practice.* Philadelphia: Lippincott Williams & Wilkins.

Meehan, T. G. (1991). Therapeutic touch. In G. Bulechek & J. McCloskey (Eds.), *Nursing interventions: Essential nursing treatments.* Philadelphia: W. B. Saunders.

Merenstein, G. B., & Gardner, S. L. (1998). *Handbook of neonatal intensive care* (4th ed.). St. Louis: Mosby-Year Book.

Miller, C. (2009). *Nursing care of the older adult* (5th ed.). Philadelphia: Lippincott Williams & Wilkins.

Mina, C. (1985). A program for helping grieving parents. *Maternal-Child Nursing Journal, 10,* 118–121.

Moorhead, S., Johnson, M. & Maas, M. L. (2008). *Nursing outcomes classification (NOC).* St. Louis: Mosby.

Morton, P., Fontaine, D., Hudak, C., & Gallo, B. (2005). *Critical care nursing* (8th ed.). Philadelphia: Lippincott Williams & Wilkins.

Murray, J. S. (2000). A concept analysis of social support as experienced by siblings of children with cancer. *Journal of Pediatric Nursing, 15*(5), 313–322.

Murray, R. B., Zentner, J. P., & Yakimo, R. (2009). *Health promotion strategies through the life span* (8th ed.). Upper Saddle River, NJ: Pear-Prentice Hall.

National Safety Council. (2000). *Injury facts.* Itaska, IL: National Safety Council.

Norris, J., & Kunes-Connell, M. (1987). Self-esteem disturbance: A clinical validation study. In A. McLane (Ed.), *Classification of nursing diagnoses: Proceedings of the seventh NANDA national conference.* St. Louis: Mosby.

North American Nursing Diagnosis Association International. (2007). *NANDA nursing diagnosis: Definitions and classifications.* Philadelphia: Author.

Pillitteri, A. (2007). *Maternal and child health nursing* (5th ed.). Philadelphia: Lippincott Williams & Wilkins.

Polomeno, V. (1999). Sex and babies: Couples' postnatal sexual concerns. *Journal of Perinatal Education, 8*(4), 9–18.

Porth, C. (2007). *Pathophysiology* (7th ed.). Philadelphia: Lippincott Williams & Wilkins.

Puterbough, C. (1991). Hypothermia related to exposure and surgical interventions. *Today's OR Nurse, 13*(7), 32–33.

Quinn, C. (1994). The four A's of restraint reduction: Attention, assessment, anticipation, avoidance. *Orthopaedic Nursing, 13*(2), 11–19.

Rateau, M. R. (2000). Confusion and aggression in restrained elderly persons undergoing hip repair surgery. *Applied Nursing Research, 13*(1), 50–54.

Reeder, S., Martin, L., & Koniak-Griffin, D. (1997). *Maternity nursing* (18th ed.). Philadelphia: Lippincott-Raven.

Rhoten, D. (1982). Fatigue and the post surgical patient. In C. Norris (Ed.), *Concept clarification in nursing.* Rockville, MD: Aspen Systems.

Schoenfelder, D. P. (2000). A fall prevention program for elderly individuals. *Journal of Gerontological Nursing, 26*(3), 43–45.

Shields, C. (1992). Family interaction and caregivers of Alzheimer's disease patients: Correlates of depression. *Family Process, 31*(3), 19–32.

Shrago, L., & Bocar, D. (1990). The infant's contribution to breastfeeding. *Journal of Obstetric, Gynecologic, and Neonatal Nursing, 19*(3), 209–211.

Simpson, K. R., & Creehan, P. A. (2007). *AWHONN's perinatal nursing* (3rd ed.). Philadelphia: Lippincott Williams & Wilkins.

Smeltzer, S., Bare, B., Hinkle, J., & Cheever, K. (2008). *Brunner & Suddarth's textbook of medical-surgical nursing* (11th ed.). Philadelphia: Lippincott Williams & Wilkins.

Stanley, M., & Beare, P. G. (2000). *Gerontological nursing*. Philadelphia: F. A. Davis.

Taylor, E. J. (2000). Spiritual and ethical end-of-life concerns. In C. H. Yarbro, M. H. Frogge, M. Goodman & S. L. Groenwald. *Cancer nursing: Principles and practice* (5th ed.). Boston: Jones and Bartlett.

Taylor, S. E., Klein, L. C., Lewis, B., & Petal, C. (2000). Biobehavioral responses to stress in females: Tend and befriend, not fight-or-flight. *Psychology Review, 107*(3), 411–29.

Teel, C. S. (1991). Chronic sorrow: Analysis of the concept. *Journal of Advanced Nursing, 16*(11), 311–319.

Thomas, K. A. (1989). How the NICU environment sounds to a preterm infant. *MCN: American Journal of Maternal Child Nursing, 14*(4), 249–251.

Thomas, S. P. (1998). Assessing and intervening with anger disorders. *Nursing Clinics of North America, 33*(1), 121–134.

Townsend, M. C. (1994). *Nursing diagnosis in psychiatric nursing* (3rd ed.). Philadelphia: F. A. Davis.

Tusaie, K., & Dyer, J. (2004). Resilience: A historical review of the construct. *Holistic Nursing Practice, 18*(1), 3–8.

Vandenberg, K. (1990). The management of oral nippling in the sick neonate, the disorganized feeder. *Neonatal Network, 9*(1), 9–16.

Vanezis, M., & McGee, A. (1999). Mediating factors in the grieving process of the suddenly bereaved. *British Journal of Nursing, 8*(14), 932–937.

Varcarolis, E. (2007). *Foundations of psychiatric mental health nursing* (5th ed.). Philadelphia: W. B. Saunders.

Vickers, J. L., & McGee, A. (2000). Choices and control: Parental experiences in pediatric terminal home care. *Journal of Pediatric Oncology Nursing, 17*(1), 12–21.

Vincent, K. G. (1985). The validation of a nursing diagnosis. *Nursing Clinics of North America, 20*(4), 631–639.

Voith, A. M., Frank, A. M., & Pigg, J. S. (1987). Validations of fatigue as a nursing diagnosis. In A. McLane (Ed.), *Classification of nursing diagnoses: Proceedings of the seventh national conference* (p. 280). St. Louis: Mosby.

Walsh, K. & Kowanko, I. (2002). Nurses' and patients' perceptions of dignity. *International Journal of Nursing Practice, 8*(3), 143–151.

Wilkinson, J., & Van Leuven, K. (2007). *Fundamentals of nursing: Theory, concepts & applications*. Philadelphia: F. A. Davis.

Willis, D. & Porche, D. (2004). Male battering of intimate partners: Theoretical underpinnings, intervention approaches and implications. *Nursing Clinics of North America, 39*(1), 271–282.

Winslow, B., & Carter, P. (1999). Patterns of burden in wives who care for husbands with dementia. *Nursing Clinics of North America, 34*(2), 275–287.

Worden, W. (2002). *Grief counseling and grief therapy* (3rd ed.). New York: Springer.

Yarbro, C. H., Frogge, M. H., Goodman, M., & Groenwald, S. L. (2006). *Cancer nursing: Principles and practice* (6th ed.). Boston: Jones and Bartlett.

Zerwich, J. (1992). Laying the groundwork for family self-help: Locating families, building trust and building strength. *Public Health Nursing, 9*(1), 15–21.

INDEX

Page numbers followed by *t* or *b* indicate tables and boxes, respectively. Nursing diagnoses are in **bold**.